NANOMEDICINE

Edited by:
Dr. Vandana Dahiya, Dr. Archana Gupta, Dr. Manoj Kumar Yadav and Dr. Rakhi Srivastava

ALLIED HEALTH PRESS

Nanomedicine

Editors: **Dr. Vandana Dahiya, Dr. Archana Gupta, Dr. Manoj Kumar Yadav and Dr. Rakhi Srivastava**

Allied Health Press
4164 Lakeshore Road
Burlington ON L7L 1A4
Canada
www.alliedhealthpress.com
Email: orders@arclereducation.com

ISBN: 978-1-77956-767-3

ABOUT THE EDITORS

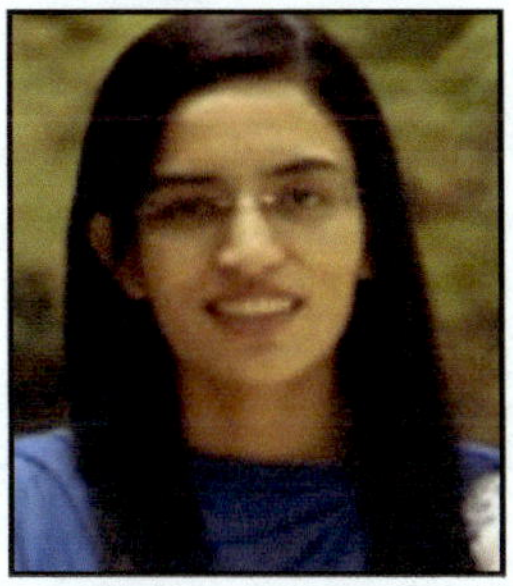

Dr. Vandana Dahiya is an is an Assistant Professor-SG at Amity University Haryana. Dr. Vandana is a DST INSPIRE Fellow (2014), gold medallist and an MHRD research fellow (2014-2020). Her fields of research and interest include biochemistry, spectroscopy, and nanobiotechnology. Dr. Vandana has published several papers in peer-reviewed journals and book chapters with reputed publishers. She has more than five years of teaching and research experience in biomedical engineering.

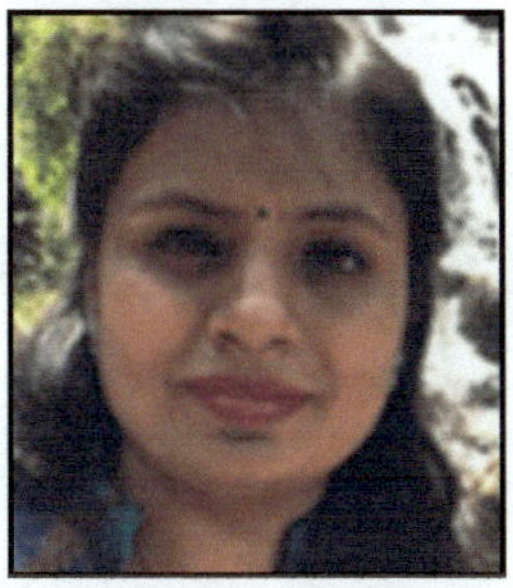

Dr. Archana Gupta is an Associate Professor at SRM University, Delhi-NCR Sonipat. Dr. Gupta is a gold medallist and received a fellowship from the Défense Research and Development Organization (DRDO). Her field of research and interest includes biotechnology and nanobiotechnology. Dr. Gupta has published papers in peer-reviewed journals. She has more than eight years of teaching experience in the field. She has published more than seven book chapters.

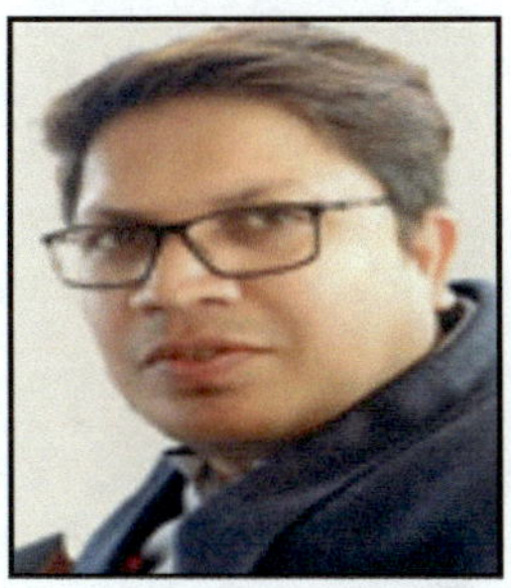

Dr. Manoj Kumar Yadav is an Associate Professor at SRM University, Delhi-NCR, Sonipat. Dr. Yadav is an honorary fellow of the Society of Life Sciences and has more than 10 years of teaching and research experience. Dr. Yadav has published one book and eight book chapters with reputed publishers. He has published more than 28 research papers in esteemed international journals. He has completed several government-funded projects. His research interest includes infectious diseases, cancer biology, COVID-19, and the application of artificial intelligence in healthcare.

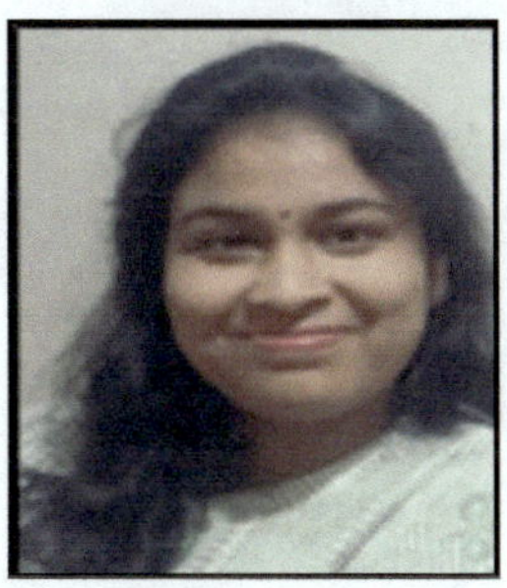

Dr. Rakhi Srivastava is an Assistant Professor at SRM University, Delhi-NCR Sonipat. Her research interests involve the field of medicinal plants, natural products, and the isolation of active principle/s from various plants for anticancer properties. Her research work also includes the establishment of effective combination therapy regimes for the different cancer targets against various cancer types. Dr. Rakhi has published papers in peer-reviewed journals. She has more than nine years of teaching and research experience in the field.

Brief Table of Contents

Detailed Table of Contents

LIST OF FIGURES

LIST OF TABLES

LIST OF CONTRIBUTORS

Amrendra K. Ajay

Department of Medicine, Brigham and Women's Hospital; Harvard Medical School, Boston, MA, USA

Sakshi Bhagat

Department of Chemistry, Indian Institute of Technology, Karwar, Jodhpur, Rajasthan, India

Khushboo Bhutani

Department of Biotechnology, SRM University Delhi-NCR, Sonepat, Haryana, India

Chanchal

Department of Biotechnology, Faculty of Science and Humanities, SRM University Delhi-NCR, Sonepat, Haryana, India

Chung-Ming Chang

Graduate Institute of Biomedical Sciences; Department of Biotechnology Industry, Chang Gung University, Guishan, Taoyuan, Taiwan, Republic of China

Vandana Dahiya

Department of Biomedical Engineering, SRM University Delhi-NCR, Sonipat, Haryana, India; Department of Biomedical Engineering, Amity School of Engineering and Technology (ASET), Amity University, Gurugram, Haryana, India

Ruby Dhiman

School of Health Sciences and Technology (SoHST), University of Petroleum and Energy Studies (UPES), Dehradun, Uttarakhand, India

Diksha

Department of Biotechnology and Microbiology, Faculty of Science and Humanities, SRM University Delhi-NCR, Sonepat, Haryana, India

Pratibha Gaur

Center for Drug Design Discovery and Development, SRM University Delhi-NCR, Rajiv Gandhi Education City, Sonepat, Haryana, India; Department of Biotechnology and Microbiology, School of Science and Humanities, SRM University Delhi-NCR, Sonepat, Haryana, India

Archana Gupta

Department of Biotechnology and Microbiology, Faculty of Science and Humanities, SRM University Delhi-NCR, Sonepat, Haryana, India

Harsh Kashyap

Amity Institute of Biotechnology, Amity University, Noida, Uttar Pradesh, India

Manisha Khatri

Department of Biomedical Sciences, Shaheed Rajguru College of Applied Sciences for Women, University of Delhi, Vasundhara Enclave, Delhi, India

Deepak Kumar

Central Ayurveda Research Institute, Central Council for Research in Ayurvedic Sciences (CCRAS), Kolkata, West Bengal, India

Rishav Kumar

Department of Biotechnology, SRM University, Rajiv Gandhi Education City, Sonepat, Haryana, India; Institute of Nuclear Medicine and Allied Sciences (INMAS), Defense Research and Development Organization (DRDO), Brig S.K. Mazumdar Marg, Timarpur, Delhi, India

Umesh Kumar

Department of Paramedical Sciences, Subharti Medical College, Swami Vivekanand Subharti University, Meerut, Uttar Pradesh, India

Sneh Kumari

Department of Community Medicine, Maharaja Agrasen Medical College, Agroha, Hisar, Haryana, India

Vanshika Makol

Department of Biomedical Sciences, Shaheed Rajguru College of Applied Sciences for Women, University of Delhi, Vasundhara Enclave, Delhi, India

Nikita Malik

Department of Biotechnology and Microbiology, School of Science and Humanities, SRM University Delhi-NCR, Sonepat, Haryana, India

Meenakshi Mishra

Department of Paramedical Sciences, Subharti Medical College, Swami Vivekanand Subharti University, Meerut, Uttar Pradesh, India

Pankaj Kishor Mishra

Department of Paramedical Sciences, Subharti Medical College, Swami Vivekanand Subharti University, Meerut, Uttar Pradesh, India

Ramendra Pati Pandey

School of Health Sciences and Technology (SoHST), University of Petroleum and Energy Studies (UPES), Dehradun, Uttarakhand, India

V. Samuel Raj

Center for Drug Design Discovery and Development, SRM University Delhi-NCR, Rajiv Gandhi Education City, Sonepat, Haryana, India; Department of Biotechnology and Microbiology, School of Science and Humanities, SRM University Delhi-NCR, Sonepat, Haryana, India

Puspendra Kumar Rajput

Department of Paramedical Sciences, Subharti Medical College, Swami Vivekanand Subharti University, Meerut, Uttar Pradesh, India

Kusum Rani

Center for Drug Design Discovery and Development, SRM University Delhi-NCR, Rajiv Gandhi Education City, Sonepat, Haryana, India

Anu Saini

Department of Biomedical Engineering, SRM University Delhi-NCR, Sonipat, Haryana, India

Sakshi

Department of Biotechnology and Microbiology, Faculty of Science and Humanities, SRM University Delhi-NCR, Sonepat, Haryana, India

Sheetal

Department of Biotechnology and Microbiology, Faculty of Science and Humanities, SRM University Delhi-NCR, Sonepat, Haryana, India

Sandeep Kumar Shukla

Institute of Nuclear Medicine and Allied Sciences (INMAS), Defense Research and Development Organization (DRDO), Brig S.K. Mazumdar Marg, Timarpur, Delhi, India

Amisha Singh

Department of Biotechnology, JAIN University, Bangalore, Karnataka, India

Viswanath Pratap Singh

Department of Paramedical Sciences, Subharti Medical College, Swami Vivekanand Subharti University, Meerut, Uttar Pradesh, India

Amrita Soni

School of Paramedical Sciences, NIILM University, Kaithal, Haryana, India

Rakhi Srivastava

Department of Biotechnology, SRM University Delhi-NCR, Sonipat, Haryana, India

Swati

Department of Biotechnology and Microbiology, Faculty of Science and Humanities, SRM University Delhi-NCR, Sonepat, Haryana, India

Shweta Tripathi

Department of Biology, Tuskegee University, Tuskegee, Alabama, USA

Shyam Tripathi

Center for Drug Design Discovery and Development, SRM University Delhi-NCR, Rajiv Gandhi Education City, Sonepat, Haryana, India

Rashmi Tyagi

Department of Pharmacy, GNIT College of Pharmacy, Greater Noida, Uttar Pradesh, India

Arpana Vibhuti

Department of Biotechnology, SRM University, Rajiv Gandhi Education City, Sonepat, Haryana, India

Manoj Kumar Yadav

Department of Biomedical Engineering, SRM University Delhi-NCR, Sonepat, Haryana, India

Priyanka Yadav

Department of Biotechnology, SRM University Delhi-NCR, Sonepat, Haryana, India

LIST OF ABBREVIATIONS

ABC	ATP-Binding Cassette
AD	Alzheimer's Disease
ADME	Absorption, Distribution, Metabolism, and Excretion
AFM	Atomic Force Microscopy
AgNPs	Silver Nanoparticles
AHST	Autologous Hematopoietic Stem Cell Transplantation
AI	Artificial Intelligence
Al_2O_3	Aluminum Oxide
ALS	Amyotrophic Lateral Sclerosis
AMD	Age-Related Macular Degeneration
AMT	Adsorptive-Mediated Transcytosis
AP-1	Atherosclerotic Plaque-Specific Peptide-1
APCs	Antigen-Presenting Cells
APIs	Active Pharmaceutical Ingredients
ASO	Antisense Oligonucleotides
AuNPs/GNPs	Gold Nanoparticles
BBB	Blood–Brain Barrier
BMECs	Brain Microvascular Endothelial Cells
BSI	British Standards Institution
c-CNT	Carboxylated Carbon Nanotubes
CED	Convection-Enhanced Delivery
CH	Chitosan
CH_3HPO_2	Phosphonate
CL	Cardiolipin
CNS	Central Nervous System
CNT	Carbon Nanotubes
COO	Carboxylic Acid

CQDs	Carbon Quantum Dots
cRGD	Cyclic Peptide Ligand (GRGDSPKC)
CT	Computed Tomography
CTLA-4	Cytotoxic T-Lymphocyte-Associated Protein 4
CZP	Certolizumab Pegol
DBT	Department of Biotechnology
DDS	Drug Delivery System
DHA	Docosahexaenoic Acid
DLS	Dynamic Light Scattering
DRDO	Defense Research and Development Organization
EFSA	European Food Safety Authority
EGCG	Epigallocatechin Gallate
EGFR	Epidermal Growth Factor Receptor
EMA	European Medicines Agency
EMU	European Medicines Union
EPA	Eicosapentaenoic Acid
EPR	Enhanced Permeability and Retention
ETPN	European Technology Platform on Nanomedicine
EU	European Union
EU-NCL	European Nanomedicine Characterization Laboratory
EuTe	Europium Telluride
FDA	Food and Drug Administration
FDG	Fluorodeoxyglucose
FEVI	Forced Expiratory Volume
FRET	Fluorescence Resonance Energy Transfer
FSSAI	Food Safety and Standards Authority of India
FVC	Forced Vital Capacity
GBM	Glioblastoma Multiforme
GEEC	Glycosylphosphatidylinositol-Anchored Protein-Enriched
GEMMeD	Global Enterprise for Micronutrient and Medicine Delivery
GHIT	Global Health Innovative Technology
GIST	Gastrointestinal Stromal Tumor
GLP-1	Glucagon-Like Peptide-1
GMP	Good Manufacturing Practice
GQDs	Graphene Quantum Dots

HA	Hyaluronic Acid
HD	Huntington's Disease
HE	High-Efficiency
HPH	High-Pressure Homogenization
HPMC	Hydroxypropyl Methylcellulose
IANC	International Alliance for Nanotechnology in Cancer
ICIs	Immune Checkpoint Inhibitors
ICMR	Institution Indian Council of Medical Research
IL-2	Interleukin-2
IND	Investigational New Drug
irAEs	Immune-Related Adverse Events
ISO	International Standard Organization
LDH	Lactate Dehydrogenase
LFIA	Lateral Flow Immunoassay
LOC	Lab-on-a-Chip
LSH	Liposome-Silica Hybrid
MCC	Microcrystalline Cellulose
miRNAs	microRNAs
ML	Machine Learning
MMPs	Matrix Metalloproteinases
MPS	Mononuclear Phagocyte System
MRI	Magnetic Resonance Imaging
MS	Multiple Sclerosis
MSCs	Mesenchymal Stem Cells
MSNs	Mesoporous Silica Nanoparticles
MTD	Maximum Tolerated Dose
MWNT	Multi-Walled Nanotube
NCI	National Cancer Institute
NH_2	Amine
NIH	National Institutes of Health
NIMS	National Institute for Materials Science
NIOSH	National Institute for Occupational Safety and Health
NIR	Near-Infrared
NLCs	Nanostructured Lipid Carriers
NMs	Nanomaterials

NNI	National Nanotechnology Initiative
NOM	Natural Organic Matter
NPC	Neural Progenitor Cells
NPs	Nanoparticles
NSOM	Near Field Scanning Optical Microscopy
OECD	Organization for Economic Co-operation and Development
OEL	Occupational Limits
OH	Hydroxyl
PA	Phosphatidic Acid
PACA	Poly(Alkyl Cyanoacrylate)
PAMAM	Poly(Amidoamine)
PARP	Poly(ADP-Ribose) Polymerase
PCL	Polycaprolactone
PCR	Polymerase Chain Reaction
PD	Parkinson's Disease
PD-1	Death Protein 1
PDT	Photodynamic Therapy
PEG	Polyethylene Glycol
PEI	Poly(Ethyleneimine)
PEPE	Polyether-Copolyester
PET	Positron Emission Tomography
P-gp	P-Glycoprotein
PLA	Polylactic Acid
PLGA	Poly(Lactic-Co-Glycolic Acid)
PMOXA	Poly(2-Methyl-2-Oxazoline)
POC	Point-of-Care
PPE	Personal Protective Equipment
PSMA	Prostate-Specific Membrane Antigen
PTO	Patent and Trademark Office
PTT	Photothermal Therapy
QC	Quality Control
QD	Quantum Dot
QSAR	Quantitative Structure-Activity Relationship
REL	Recommended Exposure Limit
RES	Reticuloendothelial System
RGD	Arginine-Glycine-Aspartate

ROS	Reactive Oxygen Species
RP	Ropinirole
RPE	Retinal Pigmented Epithelium
SAS-WTS	Supercritical Antisolvent Process – Wurster-Type System
SEM	Scanning Electron Microscopy
SI	International System of Units
SiO_2	Silicon Dioxide
siRNA	Small Interfering RNA
SLNs	Solid Lipid Nanoparticles
SLS	Static Light Scattering
SOPs	Standard Operating Procedures
SPIONs	Superparamagnetic Iron Oxide Nanoparticles
SPR	Surface Plasmon Resonance
STM	Scanning Tunneling Microscopy
SWCNTs	Single-Walled Carbon Nanotubes
SWNTs	Single-Walled Nanotubes
TEM	Transmission Electron Microscopy
TiO_2	Titanium Oxide
tMCAO	Transient Middle Cerebral Artery Occlusion
tPA	Tissue Plasminogen Activator
TWA	Time-Weighted Average
UM	Uveal Melanoma
USA	United States of America
VCAM-1	Vascular Cell Adhesion Molecule-1
VEGFR3	Vascular Endothelial Growth Factor Receptor 3
VTA	Ventral Tegmental Area
WHO	World Health Organization
ZnO	Zinc Oxide
ZVI	Zero-Valent Iron

PREFACE

Nanomedicine is an interdisciplinary branch of science that uses the principles of nanobiotechnology to improve the diagnosis process, treatment, repair, and reproduction of biological systems as well as illness prevention with the help of medicine. Nanomedicine science uses materials and methods of nanoscale and aims to find new effective medical solutions. This field makes it possible to create targeted drug delivery systems (DDS), more effective methods of visual inspection, and new therapeutic approaches—all of which work at the molecular and cellular levels to enable effective and precise medical interventions. Hence the objective of our book "Nanomedicine: Transforming Solutions for Healthcare" is intended to impart a quality knowledge base about Nanomedicines current applications and future perspective.

Many books about nanomedicine are available in the market. While some of them focus on basics, others are more concerned with the application. Very few books cover both portions. This book equally emphasizes fundamentals as well as their applications with recent advancements in the medical sector. The book also highlights the transformational potential of nanoscale interventions highlighting the significance of nanotechnology. This book is written to fulfil the curriculum needs of undergraduate and postgraduate students in the fields of medicine, life sciences, and pharmacy, where they may learn nanomedicine as one of the subjects. This book has been created in a complete manner. The chapters within this book have been drafted by experts in their respective fields, which provide in-depth knowledge and clarity about each topic. This book focuses on the fundamental principles of nanomedicine and its specific applications in many diseases and medical situations.

The first chapter, "Introduction to Nanomedicine," explains the fundamental principles of nanomedicine and their relevance to the healthcare sector. Subsequent chapters explore particular uses such as the use of nanoparticles in drug delivery systems, which offers the potential to improve the targeted treatments with minimal side effects. Its application in Imaging and targeted therapy is the use of nanoparticles to increase the magnitude of imaging methods and promote the delivery of therapeutic agents to disease cells. The next section of the book highlights the significance of nanomedicine in various diseases namely, cancer, neurological disorders, ophthalmology, diabetes, and COVID-19.

Finally, the book ends by examining the obstacles, regulation, ethical considerations and prospects of nanomedicine, providing valuable information on the current research and possible advancements that might further transform healthcare. We hope that this book will play a crucial role in the educational field as well as in guiding researchers towards new areas in healthcare.

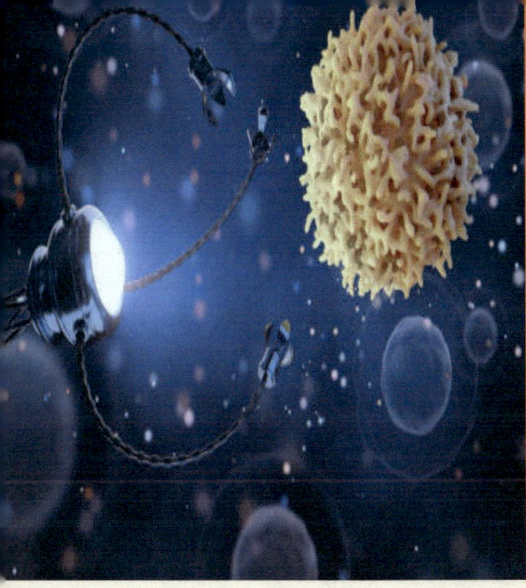

Chapter 1

INTRODUCTION TO NANOMEDICINE: TRANSFORMING HEALTHCARE AT THE NANOSCALE

Contents

Sakshi Bhagat,[1,*] Sneh Kumari,[2] and Deepak Kumar[3,*]

[1]*Department of Chemistry, Indian Institute of Technology, Karwar, Jodhpur, Rajasthan, India*

[2]*Department of Community Medicine, Maharaja Agrasen Medical College, Agroha, Hisar, Haryana, India*

[3]*Central Ayurveda Research Institute, Central Council for Research in Ayurvedic Sciences (CCRAS), Kolkata, West Bengal, India*

**Corresponding author.*

Abstract

Nanomedicines have brought an ingenious revolution in the area of heath cure and medicine by introducing potent drug delivery systems (DDS). It open ups the new possibilities for early disease detection, diagnostic, and therapeutic procedures. Nanomedicines involve the application of medicines in nanoscale, utilizing organic and inorganic nanomaterials (NMs) for drug delivery, imaging, and targeting. The amazing function of natural materials in nanomedicines is further demonstrated by the creation of nanoparticles (NPs) by plants. Most of the complications associated with the traditional DDS including solubility, bioavailability, biocompatibility, toxicity, target-specific, premature degradation, side-effects, stability, and so on, can easily be overcome with the usage of nanomedicine-based drug delivery approaches. Passive and active targeting approaches are used to amplify the drug delivery regulation and to shrink the side effects. This chapter outlines the main influences responsible for the expansion in the development of nanotechnology in medicine and highlighted the various applications of nanotechnology in pharmaceuticals and novel DDS.

1.1. Introduction

Before delving into the origins of nanomedicine within healthcare, it is essential to grasp the essence of medicine and its intersection with nanotechnology, a burgeoning field of recent time (Malik and Waheed, 2023). Medicine, an ancient discipline, encompasses the diagnosis, treatment, and prevention of ailments, with its roots tracing back to the Greek word "medome," signifying to care for (Bârsu, 2017). Conversely, the contemporary term "nanotechnology" derives from the Greek word "nanos," denoting dwarf. In the International System of Units (SI), "nano" serves as a prefix representing 1 billionth of a meter or 10^{-9} m^3. Nanomaterials (NMs) exhibit atom-like behaviors owing to their expansive surface area, fueled by heightened surface energy (Astruc, 2016; Soares et al., 2018). In contrast, bulk materials, irrespective of size, maintain consistent physical properties. However, at the nanoscale, this uniformity does not always hold true (Van Dijken et al., 2000). The inception of nanotechnology traces back to 1959 when Richard Feynman introduced the concept during one of his lectures titled "There's Plenty of Room at the Bottom" at the California Institute of Technology. Around 15 years later, a Japanese scientist Norio Taniguchi became the foremost to employ and state the term "nanotechnology" in the year 1974. He described it as the stratagem and processing of substances at the atomic or molecular level, emphasizing activities such as separation, consolidation, and deformation (Bayda et al., 2020). Nanotechnology finds its application in materials and devices characterized by dimensions ranging from approximately 1 to 100 nanometers. Nanotechnology, being a revolution in the era of emerging technology, spreading its roots deep right from our big industries to our day-to-day routine as well (Bogunia-Kubik and Sugisaka, 2002; Grewal, 2016; Kumar, Mutalik, and Rajanikant, 2010). Over the decades, this technology has taken up various areas of science and application including medicines, bio-imaging, food science, electronics, environmental sciences, transportation, materials, energy, water-air treatment, and so on, and is being applied via holistic approach (Gothandam, 2018). The manipulation of matter on a nanoscale level has yielded remarkable results in the subject of nanotechnology, namely the creation of unique structures, or nanostructures, with physiochemical properties that fall between 1 and 100 nm. Because of changes in their physiochemical, electrical, magnetic, and optical properties, nanostructures behave differently from their bulk counterparts in terms of surface to volume ratio, size distribution, surface energy, particle size, and so on (Chang et al., 2015).

Figure 1.1 depicts the schematic representation of NMs with various biological molecules (Brydson and Hammond, 2005; Kargozar and Mozafari, 2018).

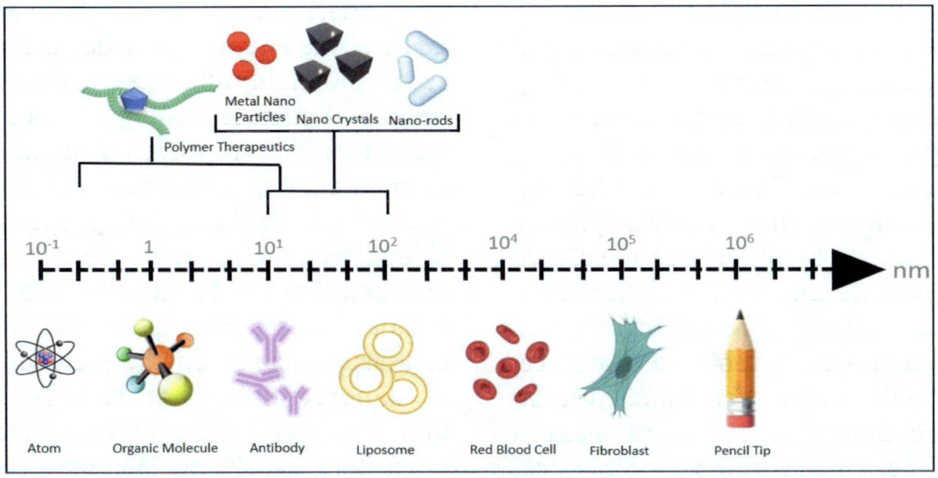

Figure 1.1. Schematic representation of nanomaterials (NMs) with various biological molecules.

The implication of nanotechnology and the use of NMs in medical sciences to full fill demands of various clinical treatment has brought nanomedicine into its existence (Tinkle et al., 2014). Nanomedicine is a sub-branch of nanotechnology which productively trades with different application of medicines in nanoscale. Nanomedicine is a present-day scientific domain that emerged from the blending of medicine and nanotechnology.

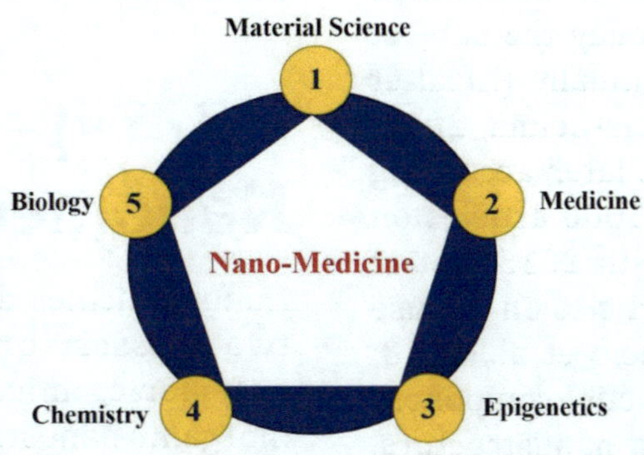

Figure 1.2. Schematic representation of nanomedicine as a multidisciplinary field.

Using the tools and principles of nanotechnology, the field of nanomedicine seeks to enhance human health in every manner. Nanotechnology offers technological platforms and monitoring tools for imaging, bioanalysis, diagnosis, and detection (Verma et al., 2024). One of the most demanding properties of NMs that make them acceptable for clinical applications is their size. Due to its smaller size these particles can easily circulate in human body through blood vessels without any interference (Singh and Singh, 2013). The electronic and optical characteristics of nanoparticles (NPs) which the metal NPs in particular possess are another important characteristic. The surface plasmon resonance (SPR) theory, which describes the oscillation of free electrons within metal NPs, provides the theoretical foundation for these properties. Certain metallic metal oxide NPs (Ghosh and Pal,

2007) have an additional magnetic property that makes them helpful for a range of applications, including targeting, drug administration, imaging, and cell separation (Lin et al., 2010). In general, producing nanomedicines on a small scale is easy and inexpensive; however, scaling up and maintaining stability during large-scale manufacturing has proven to be challenging (Paliwal, Babu, and Palakurthi, 2014). Nanomedicine is an emerging multidisciplinary field which is blended by other area of science and technology including biology, chemistry, physics, genetics, medicine, engineering sciences and develops nano-sized tools to diagnose, treat, and prevent disease (Tahir and Everest, 2016). Nanotechnology is poised to make a significant impact in the domain of medical science, with the overarching target of enhancing quality of life. Figure 1.2 depicts the schematic representation of nanomedicine in various areas of research (Singh and Singh, 2013). The phrase "nanomedicine" did not emerge until the turn of the century, and as of 2005, fewer than 30 papers had contained this term, despite the fact that NPs and biomedicine have been debated since the late 1970s and are today the subject of over 10,000 publications annually (Afzal et al., 2022; Fornaguera and García-Celma, 2017; Nalwa, 2014). Around 10 years later, according to Web of Science, more than 1000 articles on nanomedicine were published in 2015, out of more than 10 times as many articles on the use of NPs in biomedicine (Bonifácio et al., 2013; Mughal et al., 2024). When a bioactive component like drugs is encapsulated in a nanostructure, it is termed as nanomedicine (Psimadas et al., 2012). This innovation in technology is potent enough to provide insight in molecular findings from genomics and proteomics and has brought an ease among patients over the globe (Germain et al., 2020). Surprisingly, there is still debate over the precise definition of nanomedicine despite the fact that many researchers today operate at the nanoscale. The European Science Foundation provides a helpful definition of nanomedicine as "the application of nanoscale tools in disease diagnosis, prevention, and treatment, as well as in the pursuit of a deeper comprehension of the intricate pathophysiology that underlies disease" (Boisseau and Loubaton, 2011). This chapter provides a concise outline about the main influences which is driving the impact of nanotechnology in health care and medicine. The application of nanotechnology in medicine is advancing rapidly, with NMs poised to revolutionize properties such as solubility, polarity, and reactivity at molecular and cellular levels (Brown and Patel, 2015; Yohan and Chithrani, 2014). While this chapter primarily focuses on the medical applications of nanotechnology, it is essential to note that the engineering process often overlooks potential side effects, including environmental concerns related to manufacturing and disposal. Although it significantly complicates decision-making, environmental factors should be taken into account when developing NMs and nanomedicines. In this chapter, we emphasis mainly on nanotechnology being applied to pharmaceuticals and drug development and is considered the "hot growth" area of nanoscience.

1.2. Type of Nanomedicines

Nanomedicines are primarily categorized into two classes: organic nanostructures (like, polymeric, micelles, liposomes, etc.) and inorganic nanostructures (namely, mesoporous silica, gold, iron oxide, zinc oxide (ZnO) and carbon nanotubes [CNTs]) (Astruc, 2016; Brown and Patel, 2015) as shown in Figure 1.3. These NPs have recently found applications in a range of therapeutic and diagnostic scenarios, encompassing treatments for conditions like anemia and hyperthermia, as well as imaging techniques such as lymph node imaging, among others (Astruc, 2016).

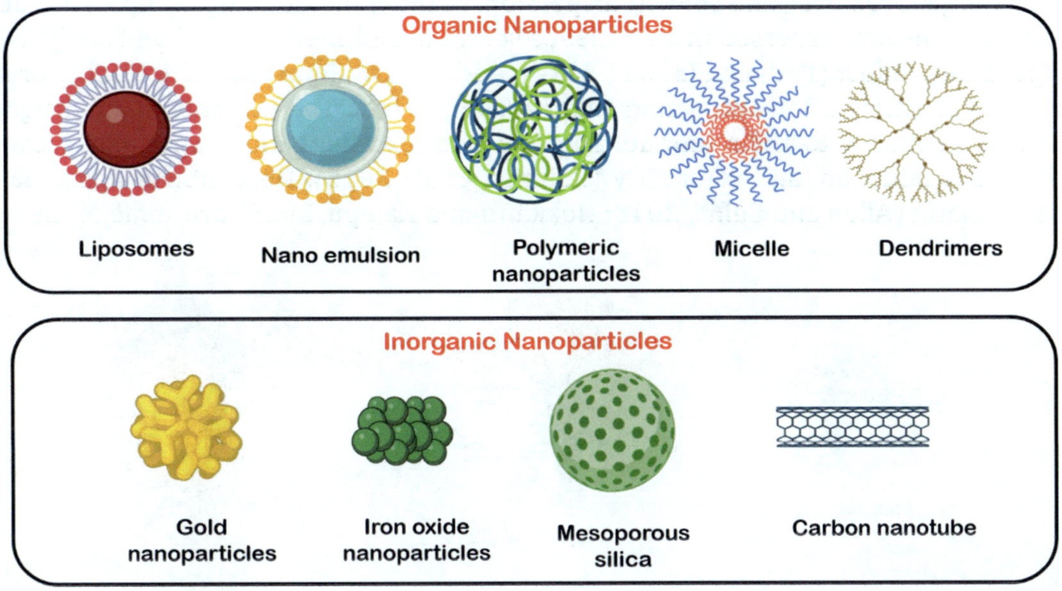

Figure 1.3. Diverse organic and inorganic nanomaterials (NMs) that are widely used in the construction of biomedical applications.

1.2.1. Organic Nanoparticles (NPs)

1.2.1.1. Micelles as Nanomedicine

Micelles are amphiphilic monomers that form nanosized colloidal structures (5–100 nm) with two distinct components: a hydrophilic tail that serves as a shielding layer in the aqueous environment and a tiny hydrophobic head that is absolutely necessary for retaining insoluble substances (Kumar and Balasubramanian, 1980). Because of their multifunctionality and capacity to encapsulate both hydrophobic and hydrophilic molecules, they can be employed in a range of therapeutic applications due to their small size and simplicity of functionalization (Balafouti et al., 2023). Antidotes can be enclosed in micelles and utilized as a means of delivering specific medications to specific tissues. Their nanoscale nature allows them to swiftly traverse capillaries and vascular systems, facilitating rapid targeting (Bose et al., 2021). The release of drugs is primarily influenced by the abundance of micelle moieties, resulting in controlled and precise release dynamics. NK012, Genexol-PM, and NK911 are a few examples of micelles used as nanomedicine (Cagel et al., 2017).

1.2.1.2. Liposomes as Nanomedicine

The discovery of liposomes is credited to Alec D. Bangham in the 1960s at the Babraham Institute, University of Cambridge, marking a significant milestone in the area of lipid-based drug delivery systems (DDS) (Watts, 2010). A liposome refers to a nano-artificial vesicle enclosed within phospholipid bilayer membranes as shown in Figure 1.4. These phospholipid molecules have different polarity due to their hydrophilic head groups and hydrophobic carbon chain tails. These two elements self-organize in a dispersed system so that phospholipid bilayers continuously encapsulate the scattered aqueous media to form vesicles through oscillation (Allen and Cullis, 2013; Nekkanti and Kalepu, 2015). Various methods are employed in liposome preparation, including mechanical dispersion, detergent removal, and solvent dispersion. In these methodologies, lipids are desiccated from the organic solvent, dispersed in an aqueous solution, and then purified and analyzed to yield the final liposome product (Patil and Jadhav, 2014). Additionally, liposomes are gaining prominence in DDS, serving as carriers for optimizing the therapeutic index of anti-rheumatic drugs (Mason, 1964). This is attributed to their unique drug payload, excellent biocompatibility, low toxicity, straightforward production, and versatility (Rahman et al., 2015). Doxorubicin liposomal, Stealth Liposomes, cisplatin (Allen and Cullis, 2013; Nekkanti and Kalepu, 2015) are some of the examples.

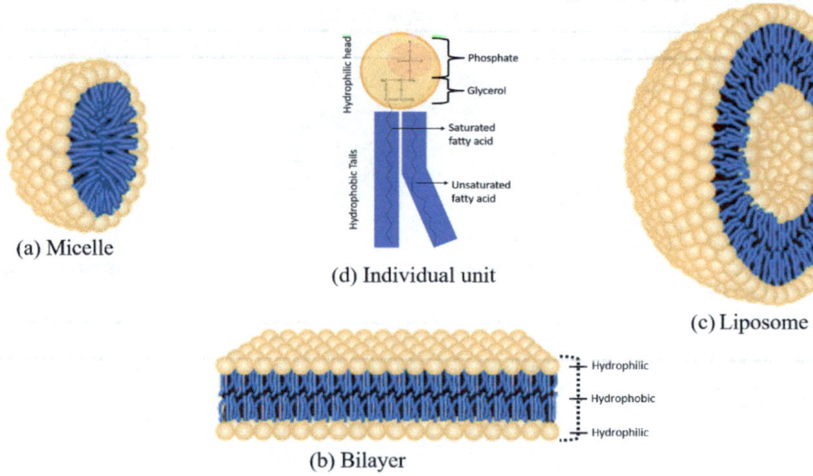

Figure 1.4. Representation of the structure of liposomes: (a) micelle; (b) individual unit; (c) liposome; and (d) lipid bilayer. A micelle is made up of a single lipid layer in which the apolar section is turned inward and the polar heads interact with the environment, whereas liposomes are made up of a lipid bilayer, providing better space for the drug to be loaded.

1.2.1.3. Polymeric Nanoparticle (NP) as Nanomedicine

Polymeric NPs stand as one of the extensively researched organic NPs in the field of nanomedicine. These small solid and colloidal particles (typically 1–1000 nm size) possess versatile structures and morphologies (Venkataraman et al., 2011). They can be layered with active chemicals that are either surface adsorbed onto the polymeric core or trapped and hooked within it (Zielinska et al., 2020). Polymeric NPs are a novel form of material produced from nanotechnology that aids in the development of drug delivery and other healthcare applications. These uses include the conjugation and entrapment of pharmaceuticals, prodrugs, the creation of systems that respond to stimuli, imaging modalities, and therapeutic (Yildiz et al., 2018; Zang et al., 2022). Polymeric NPs are crafted using both natural and synthetic polymers, employing diverse techniques to achieve desired characteristics (Banik, Fattahi, and Brown, 2016). Polysaccharides, polylactides, polyglycolides, and their copolymers are few of the examples of polymeric NPs. One of the most used polymers for protein amalgamation is polyethylene glycol (PEG) (Parveen and Sahoo, 2006).

1.2.1.4. Dendrimers as Nanomedicine

Dendrimers are hugely ordered, repetitively branched nano-molecules that resemble trees. They are sometimes referred to as nano-architectures because of their spherical, branched polymeric molecule shape, high degree of molecular homogeneity, and versatile 3-D morphology. Generation (G) is the name given to each branching (Dias et al., 2020; Nikzamir et al., 2021; Rolland et al., 2009). Dendrimers scale in dimension from 1.5 nm to 8.1 nm, and their molecular weight from 517 to 1,16,493 Daltons (Esfand and Tomalia, 2001). There are three parts to Dendrimer's structure: the outside surface, inner branches, and center core as shown in Figure 1.5. Most of the drugs are targeted into the core of the dendrimer by host-guest chemistry. As shown in Figure 1.5, the surface of dendrimers is susceptible to a variety of ligands, medications, and imaging agents. Anti-cancer medications are delivered by dendrimer-based nanotherapeutics. One major disadvantage of dendrimers is their incapacity to control the rate at which medications are released. Before the drug reaches its target locations, it may leak out quickly into circulation if the contact force between the drug and dendrimer is minimal (Kim, Park, and Na, 2018). Extensively used dendrimer is poly(amidoamine) (PAMAM), popularly known as PAMAM (Esfand and Tomalia, 2001).

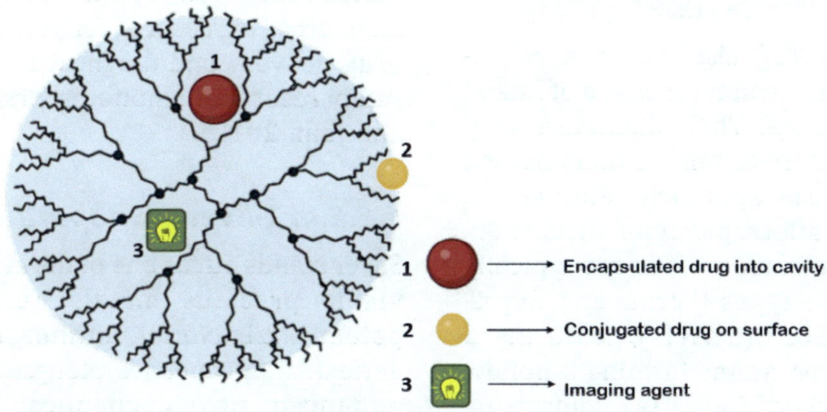

Figure 1.5. Schematic representation of a dendrimer with different agents.

1.2.2. Inorganic Nanoparticles (NPs)

Metal NPs present a viable way to circumvent the drawbacks of conventional methods by administering medication to tumor sites. The size range of metallic nanocarriers is 10–1000 nm. They are stable. They can deliver small to large molecules, stabilize medications, and use both passive and active targeting mechanisms to target tumor cells specifically (Pandey and Dahiya, 2016). Functionalized metal NPs with theragnostic agents and targeting ligands also allow for theragnostic applications like targeted delivery of active agents to tumor specific cells and imaging (Bakunin et al., 2004).

1.2.2.1. Mesoporous Silica

Solid materials with porous inorganic siloxane structures are known as mesoporous silica nanoparticles (MSNs), and they are becoming more and more well-liked as a possible choice for therapeutic uses (Vallet-Regí, 2010). They boast pore sizes ranging from 2 to 50 nm, coupled with a high surface area (exceeding 600 m^2/g) and pore volume (>0.6 cm^3/g). These properties are attributed to the silica network, featuring silanol groups on the outer surface (Rastegari et al., 2021). These meso-structures are more pronounced as drug delivery agents due to their textural properties found in their ordered mesoporosity, inspiring researchers to use them as sensors, catalysts, various kinds of drugs can be selectively loaded and released on demand to the target (Vallet-Regí, 2010). The MSN surface can be functionalized with a range of functional groups, such as phosphonate (CH_3HPO_2), hydroxyl (OH), carboxyl (COOH), amine (NH_2), and PEG (Giret et al., 2015; Lather, Poonia, and Pandita, 2018), due to the flexible and adaptive nature of silica chemical processing. The surface alteration gives MSNs unique charges and influences their behavior and colloidal interactions significantly (Abbasi et al., 2021; Rastegari et al., 2021).

1.2.2.2. Carbon Nano-Tubes (CNT)

Carbon nanotubes (CNTs), also known as "rolled-up" CNTs, are tubular structures made of linked layers of carbon atoms. Their diameters vary from a few nanometers to tens of nanometers, and their lengths can approach centimeters. They are a third allotropic type of carbon, after graphite and diamond. CNTs are typically categorized into two types (Verma and Gupta, 2022): "single-walled" (SWNTs), featuring a single layer of carbon atoms forming a hollow core, and "multi-walled" (MWNTs), comprising concentric hollow cylinders of carbon atoms nested within each other (Harris and Bawa, 2007; Yamashita et al., 2012). Discovered by S. Iijima in 1991, CNTs serve as carbon NMs with potential applications as carriers in DDS. Their notable qualities include a large carrier capacity, excellent chemical stability, and the capacity to efficiently accommodate both hydrophilic and hydrophobic substances (Gupta, Gupta, and Sharma, 2019; Ibrahim, 2013; Revathi, Vuyyuru, and Dhanaraju, 2015).

1.2.2.3. Gold Nanoparticles (AuNPs)

Gold (Au) and other noble metal-based NPs represent some of the most significant types of metal NPs. AuNPs, in particular, have garnered substantial attention due to their ability to interact with light through SPR (Ghosh and Pal, 2007). AuNPs can range in size from 1 to 120 nm and have a gold nucleus that is coated or uncoated. After being initially believed to be inert, AuNPs show excellent stability, low toxicity, and biocompatibility (Li and Lane, 2019; Lopes et al., 2019). They find applications across various fields such as optics, catalysis, materials science, nanotechnology, biology, and nanomedicine. These nanocarriers can efficiently deliver both medication molecules and large biomolecules like proteins, RNA, and DNA (Li and Lane, 2019). The release rate of drugs from gold nanoparticles (AuNPs) is influenced by factors such as the pH of the target site, internal glutathione levels, or external light stimuli. The main areas of research for gold nanocarriers are drug delivery and diagnostics because of their safety record and monodisperse size (Kumawat and Jain, 2012).

1.2.2.4. Silver Nanoparticles (AgNPs)

Silver stands out as one of the most commercially viable precious metals, renowned for its potent antibacterial, antifungal, antiviral, and antioxidant properties, alongside its remarkably enhanced physicochemical characteristics compared to bulk materials (Lee and Jun, 2019). Many drugs face limitations such as toxicity, unpredictable side effects, drug resistance, and lack of specificity. Silver nanoparticles (AgNPs) address these challenges by mitigating side effects and enhancing efficacy (Długosz et al., 2020; Lee and Jun, 2019). They are very appealing for research projects because they are widely used as vehicles for the delivery of controlled drugs. AgNPs have surfaces that can be functionalized with a variety of molecules, such as polymers, peptides, targeting ligands, and imaging probes, and they are easily synthesized in a variety of sizes and shapes (Długosz et al., 2020). A key advantage is their ability to traverse diverse biological barriers, facilitating targeted drug delivery (Pasparakis, 2022).

1.2.2.5. Iron Oxide Nanoparticles (NPs)

Iron oxide NPs, which belong to the ferrimagnetic type of magnetic materials, have a wide range of uses in the bioengineering and biomedical sciences (Vallabani and Singh, 2018). Iron oxide-based NPs come in various forms, such as mixed ferrites (MFe_2O_4, where M = Co, Mn, Ni, or Zn), magnetite (Fe_3O_4), and maghemite (γ-Fe_2O_3), and they stand as the most extensively studied type of magnetic NPs (Boyer et al., 2010). Iron oxide NPs possess several key attributes that make them highly sought-after. These include a wide surface area that is useful for anchoring targeted moieties, stability in colloidal suspension, resistance to *in vivo* degradation, and effective drug administration. Furthermore, they found that MRI scans are useful as diagnostic tools for identifying illnesses or conditions in various body parts (Etemadi et al., 2021; Lin et al., 2010).

1.2.2.6. Zinc Oxide (ZnO) Nanoparticles (NPs)

Compared to other metals like cobalt, iron, and manganese, ZnO has several advantages. It only exists in one chemically stable form, wurtzite structure, and crystallizes primarily in this form at ambient conditions. ZnO NPs are among the most widely used NPs in biosensing, drug delivery, diagnosis, and treatment because of their unique chemical and physical properties (Verma et al., 2023). Additionally, their enormous 3.37 eV band gap and 60 meV exciton binding energy have attracted attention in different areas of food, pharma, electrical industries (Racca et al., 2018; Wang et al., 2017). Because of their unique properties, lower toxicity, and biodegradability, ZnO NPs are naturally more appealing than other NMs (Racca et al., 2018). ZnO NPs have attracted a lot of attention when it comes to anti-cancer drug delivery. ZnO NPs exhibit improved solubility, greater toxicity as compared to individual compounds, and efficient delivery into cancer cells when loaded with a range of medicines, including DNA fragments and doxorubicin, paclitaxel, curcumin, and baicalin (Anjum et al., 2021; Jin and Jin, 2019).

1.3. Plant-Mediated Nanomedicines

Biodiversity has a significant impact on human civilization, and people always rely on plants for their basic needs, including the treatment of illnesses (RC, 2020). The use of plants as medicine has developed alongside human society. Traditionally, Indian and Chinese medicine have employed plants as natural remedies to treat a wide range of physiological disorders since ancient times (Shah, 2021). Since the pores in the lipid layer of the cell membrane are relatively small, the majority of molecules derived from plants are too large to pass through. The best way to address the aforementioned issues and maximize therapeutic activity potential while using a minimal amount of drug molecules and preventing side effects from overdosing on the same is to apply a DDS based on nanotechnology (Yu et al., 2020). Plant based NPs have found diverse application in medicine, that is, nanomedicine. It is interesting to note that plant-based "green" NM synthesis has gained a lot of attention because it is efficient in the treatment process and is low-cost, non-pathogenic, and environmentally friendly. Furthermore, "green" synthesis offers a one-step method that is also easy to scale up for large synthesis needs (Gour and Jain, 2019; Ying et al., 2022).

There have been previous reports in the literature on the "green" synthesis of various metal NPs such as gold (Au), platinum (Pt), silver (Ag), titanium (Ti), nickel (Ni), copper (Cu), zinc (Zn) and selenium (Se), using plant resources. In Ayurveda, these metal NPs exhibit outstanding antidiabetic, anticancer, anti-inflammatory, antimicrobial, immunomodulatory, and antioxidant properties (Gadge et al., 2022). Plant ingredients are combined with minerals or metals and repeatedly crushed and ground during the preparation of Ayurvedic medications (Ying et al., 2022). Plant extracts contain numerous functional groups, including C=N (amide), O=H (phenolic and alcohol), N=H (amine), C=C (alkenyl), and COO (carboxylic acid), among others. These groups are present in significant quantities and possess the capability to bind with metal ions, resulting in the preparation of NPs. Figure 1.6 illustrates the schematic depiction of the synthesis steps required for plant-extracted NPs. The plant-mediated synthesis of NPs progresses through three distinct stages. Firstly, in the activation phase, metal ions are reduced, leading to the formation of nucleated reduced metal atoms.

At this stage, NP formation starts. After then, neighboring tiny NPs spontaneously combine to produce larger particles during the development phase. The NPs' thermodynamic stability is improved by this phase. Ultimately, the ultimate form of the NPs is established at the phase of process termination (El-Shafey, 2020; Ying et al., 2022). In this stage, the NPs obtain the most conformation that is energetically favorable; this process may have been impacted by the plant extract's ability to stabilize metal NPs. All in all, these three steps coordinate the complex process of plant-mediated NP synthesis, highlighting the exceptional contribution of natural materials to nanotechnology. Regardless of the advancements in technology, plants remain the most reliable and sustainable source of therapeutic compounds for all time, making green medicine an essential resource.

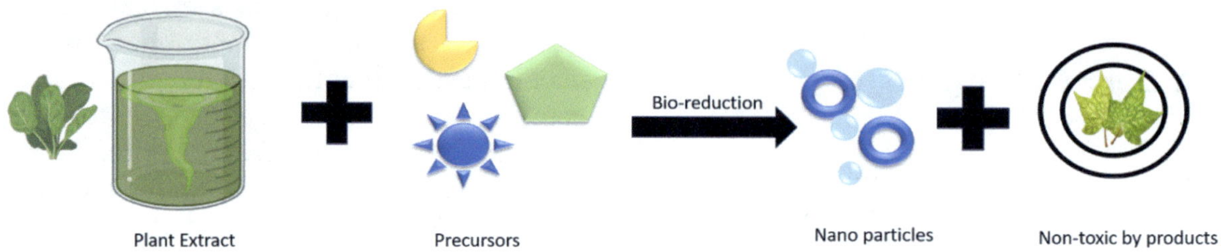

Figure 1.6. Schematic representation of nanoparticle (NP) synthesis using plant extracts.

1.4. Targeting Strategies

Nanoparticle (NP) delivery to its target is categorized into passive, active, and triggered release methods (Villaverde and Baeza, 2019). These methods significantly improve selectivity, allowing for the targeted delivery of therapeutic NPs to diseased tissues while reducing accumulation in healthy cells and organs. Nanomedicine research is actively exploring both passive and active targeting ways to improve drug delivery efficiency and reduce negative effects.

1.4.1. Passive Targeting

It is a strategy which facilitates the delivering of various therapeutic agents like nano-vectors, drugs, macromolecules, and so on, to specific or diseased tissues or cells microenvironment within the body through natural physiological processes, without the need of any external stimulus, intervention, or guidance (Narum et al., 2019). This strategy exploits the properties and characteristics of target tissues and cells and the properties of nanosized drugs as well. A phenomenon known as "Enhanced permeation and retention (EPR) effect" exhibited by tumors which provides the path or direction for the nanomedicine or certain drugs beyond certain size (above 40 kDa) to be accumulated in the infected area of tissues or cells (Narum et al., 2019). This effect is prone in area closed to tumors where blood vessels surrounding the tumors are often leaky and allows the NPs to pass through more easily. Due to lack of lymphatic drainage, nanomedicines tend to be accumulated within the tumor tissues. Passive targeting is quite advantageous as it provides minimum need for complex and potentially invasive procedures (Bazak et al., 2014). However, the type of disease, the stage at which the disease is progressing, and the variability of each patient all have a significant impact on the effectiveness of passive targeting. A schematic illustration of drug targeting techniques for triggered, active, and passive release is presented in Figure 1.7.

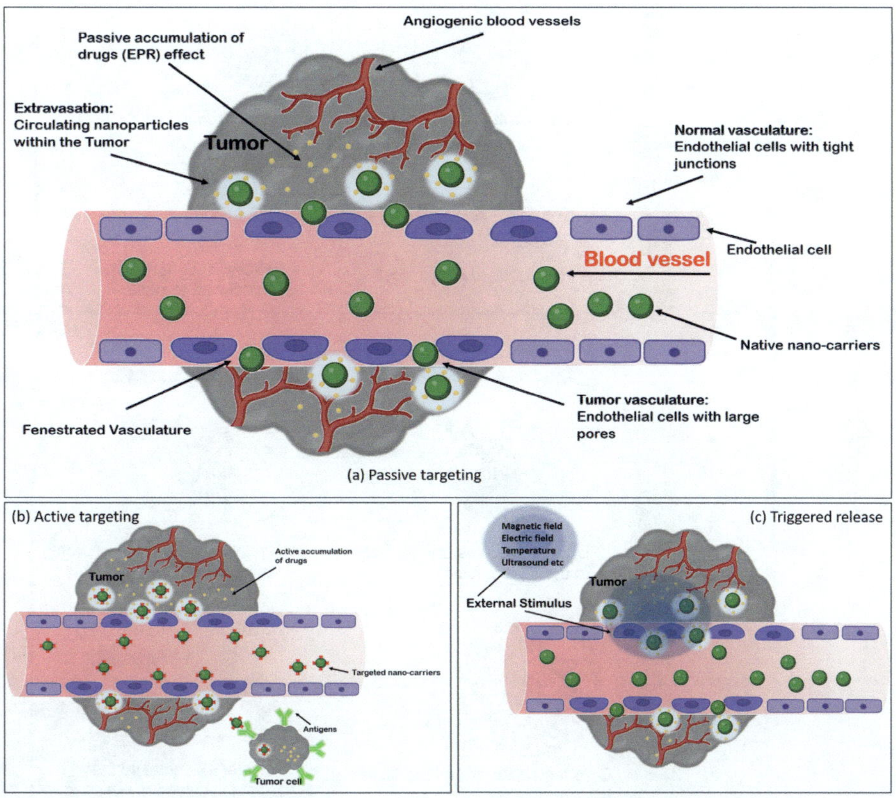

Figure 1.7. Schematic representation of drug-targeting strategies: (a) passive; (b) active targeting; and (c) triggered release.

1.4.2. Active Targeting

Active targeting presents a solution to the limitations inherent in passive targeting. This approach primarily entails modifying nanomedicines with specific ligands and molecules on their surface, which selectively interact with antigens or receptors uniquely expressed on damaged cells compared to normal cells (Pearce and O'Reilly, 2019). Targeting ligands include a wide range of molecules, including larger macromolecules like aptamers, peptides, and antibodies, as well as smaller ones like folic acid and carbohydrates (Wicki et al., 2015). These ligands exhibit a high affinity for specific receptors or biomarkers present on the surface of target cells or tumors (Chen et al., 2017). These ligands or molecules helps in governing nanomedicine to its appropriate location. Selecting a ligand that predominantly binds to target cells while minimizing binding to healthy cells is crucial. Nanocarriers need to maintain adequate stability to prevent premature drug release and degradation in the bloodstream, ensuring effective targeting.

1.4.3. Triggered Release

The previous discussion emphasized the shortcomings of drug nanocarriers in passive targeting, but active targeting is of interest because it has the potential to improve drug capabilities.

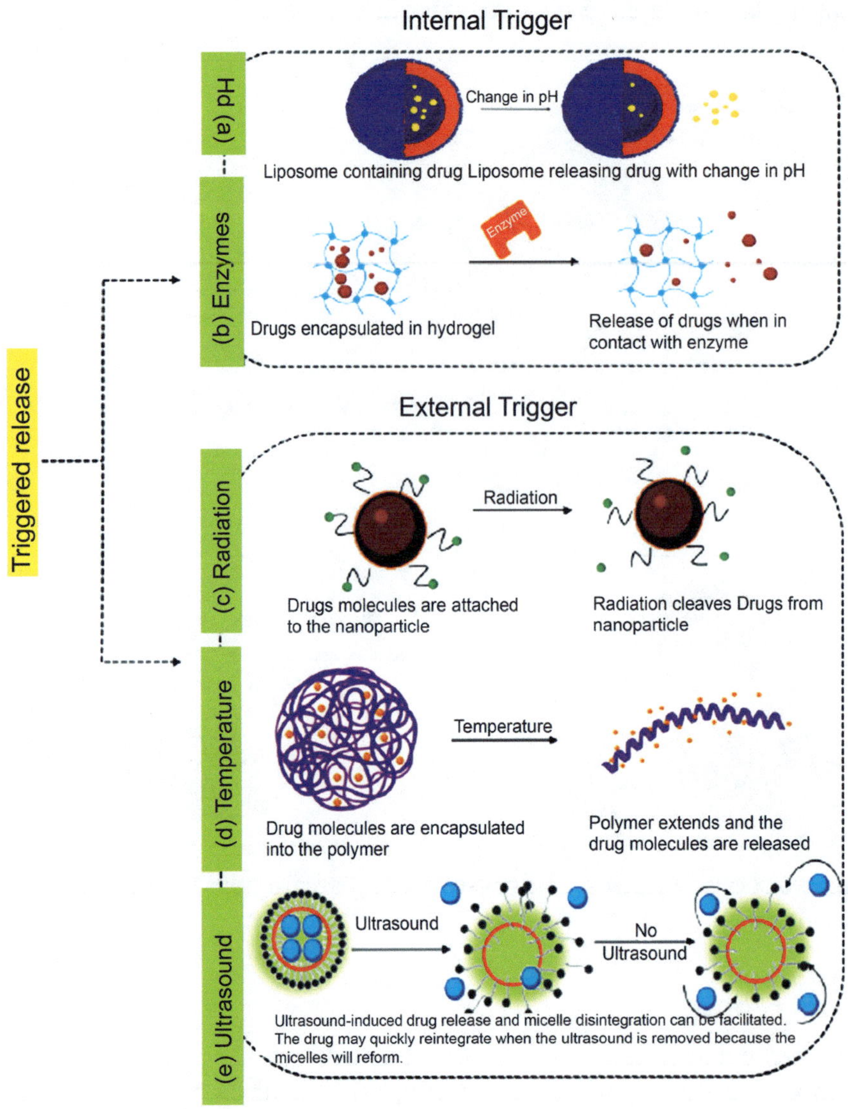

Figure 1.8. Schematic representation of triggered release mechanisms. Internal triggers: (a) pH; (b) enzyme; external triggers: (c) radiation; (d) temperature; and (e) ultrasound.

However, because receptors are also expressed in healthy cells and tissues, active targeting presents difficulties because of the possibility of off-target effects, making these ligands less appropriate (Li, Zhang, and Wang, 2018; Loomis, McNeeley, and Bellamkonda, 2011). Stimulus-triggered targeting systems are being developed to improve disease site selectivity. These systems change the phase, structure, or conformation of the nanocarrier in response to organic, biological, or external stimuli, facilitating the release of the drug (Wang and Kohane, 2017). Among the three targeting strategies, this approach boosts therapeutic efficiency and reduces toxicity by selectively delivering drugs to the appropriate site. Advances in inorganic and organic chemistry have led to the development of smart stimuli carriers sensitive to various stimuli, for example, light, ultrasound, magnetic fields, pH, ionic strength, heat, and enzymes (Wang and Kohane, 2017). Triggered release is further categorized into internal triggers (pH (Bibi et al., 2012; Cajot et al., 2012) and enzymes) and external triggers (radiation, temperature, and ultrasound (Sirsi and Borden, 2014)), as depicted in Figure 1.8.

1.5. Nanotoxicity and Biocompatibility

Even while products based on nanotechnology are becoming more and more common in the market, there is still a dearth of thorough knowledge on the toxicological dangers that are involved. The available literature addressing the toxicological risks related to the utilization of nanotechnology in medical applications is limited. NPs pose a distinct challenge in the field of toxicology, recognized as nanotoxicology, which delves into the interactions between the host organism and nanostructured constructs, with a specific emphasis on the impact of structure, size, and other factors on human health (Oberdörster, Oberdörster, and Oberdörster, 2005). Additionally, the reduction of material sizes to the nano-level results in unique properties, where very small sizes become key indicators of potential drastic or toxic effects. Keck and Muller (2013) introduced a nanotoxicology classification system categorizing NMs into four groups based on properties such as biodegradability and size. This classification is vital, particularly considering the crucial role of size effects, where reduced size enhances solubility, especially evident in poorly soluble NMs (Khare, Saxena, and Gupta, 2015). Another crucial consideration regarding size is the potential for phagocytosis by macrophages. While endocytosis allows any type of cell to internalize NMs smaller than 100 nm, macrophages are the primary internalizers of NMs larger than 100 nm (Mosquera, García, and Liz-Marzán, 2018; Yue et al., 2010). As a result, compared to NMs over 100 nm, those below 100 nm are linked to increased toxicity risks. Creating medication delivery systems requires materials that are biocompatible, or able to be eliminated by the body. Even if they irritate or inflame the body, the immune system returns to normal once they are eliminated. Nonbiodegradable NMs, on the other hand, remain in the body eternally and modify the immune system's normal function (Hussain et al., 2015).

1.6. Challenges and Future Prospects

Nanomedicines have brought tremendous increment in the medical field and have simultaneously increased the use of therapeutics due to the usage of highly efficient drugs delivery systems for the target site with reduced toxicity and less accumulation in the healthy site of the body. It provides convenient solubilization of drugs and also protects the degradation of nanomedicines in the biological environment. With the growing use and application of nanomedicine to treat various diseases, there is an urgent need to introduce or validate certain novel approaches and practices, which will certainly be able to determine potential short-term and long-term health risks (Hua and Wu, 2018). There are certain challenges in the path of implementation of nanomedicines. Firstly, its clinical trials are an expensive and prolonged process and require manpower. Secondly, in comparison to conventional methodology containing free drugs dispersed in a base like tablets, capsules, and injections, the nanoencapsulation process is a far more complex approach. Thirdly, its extensive manufacturing, safety, biocompatibility, compliance with laws, and general cost-effectiveness in relation to continuous therapies (Yamashita et al., 2012). All these factors prove to be a challenging milestone in the road of nanomedicine application in therapeutics (Hua and Wu, 2018). Nanotechnology will be significant to the future of medicine in the years to come. It will open up new possibilities for early disease detection, diagnostics, and therapeutic procedures; better health and physical abilities; and patient-specific, patient-centered therapy (Soares et al., 2018). Nanomedicines can be fervently envisaged as an emergence for the treatment of various kinds of dreadful diseases, including cancer, cardiovascular, respiratory, diabetes, and so on (Abeer, 2012). Nanotechnology will fundamentally change science, technology, and society in response to the increasing demand for its products. It also presents a significant opportunity to improve human health in previously unexplored ways, mainly by enabling accurate and successful patient-specific therapy as well as early disease detection and diagnosis.

KEY TERMS FROM THIS CHAPTER

- drug delivery systems
- drug targeting strategies
- inorganic nanomaterials
- nanomedicine
- nanotoxicity
- organic nanomaterials

References

1. Abbasi, M., Ghoran, S. H., Niakan, M. H., Jamali, K., Moeini, Z., Jangjou, A., Izadpanah, P., & Amani, A. M. (2021). Mesoporous silica nanoparticle: Heralding a brighter future in cancer nanomedicine. *Microporous and Mesoporous Materials, 319*, Article 110967. https://doi.org/10.1016/j.micromeso.2021.110967.

2. Abeer, S. (2012). Future medicine: Nanomedicine. *Journal of the Indian Medical Sciences Academy, 25*(3), 187–192.

3. Afzal, O., Altamimi, A. S. A., Nadeem, M. S., Alzarea, S. I., Almalki, W. H., Tariq, A., Mubeen, B., Murtaza, B. N., Iftikhar, S., Riaz, N., & Kazmi, I. (2022). Nanoparticles in drug delivery: From history to therapeutic applications. *Nanomaterials, 12*(24), 1–27. https://doi.org/10.3390/nano12244494.

4. Allen, T. M. & Cullis, P. R. (2013). Liposomal drug delivery systems: from concept to clinical applications. *Adv Drug Deliv Rev,* 65(1), 36-48. https://doi.org/10.1016/j.addr.2012.09.037.

5. Anjum, S., Hashim, M., Malik, S. A., Khan, M., Lorenzo, J. M., Abbasi, B. H., & Hano, C. (2021). Recent advances in zinc oxide nanoparticles (ZnO NPs) for cancer diagnosis, target drug delivery, and treatment. *Cancers, 13*(18), 4570. https://doi.org/10.3390/cancers13184570.

6. Astruc, D. (2016). Introduction to nanomedicine. *Molecules, 21*(1), Article 4. https://doi.org/10.3390/molecules21010004.

7. Bakunin, V. N., Suslov, A. Y., Kuzmina, G. N., & Parenago, O. P. (2004). Synthesis and application of inorganic nanoparticles as lubricant components—A review. *Journal of Nanoparticle Research, 6*(2), 273–284. https://doi.org/10.1023/B:NANO.0000034720.79452.e3.

8. Balafouti, M., Gerardos, A. M., Balafouti, A., & Pispas, S. (2023). Mixed copolymer micelles for nanomedicine. *Nanomanufacturing, 3*(2), 233–247. https://doi.org/10.3390/nanomanufacturing3020015.

9. Banik, B. L., Fattahi, P., & Brown, J. L. (2016). Polymeric nanoparticles: The future of nanomedicine. *Wiley Interdisciplinary Reviews: Nanomedicine and Nanobiotechnology, 8*(2), 271–299. https://doi.org/10.1002/wnan.1364.

10. Bârsu, C. (2017). History of Medicine between tradition and modernity" *Clujul medical (1957),* 90(2), 243-245. https://doi.org/10.15386/cjmed-794.

11. Bayda, S., Adeel, M., Tuccinardi, T., Cordani, M., & Rizzolio, F. (2020). The history of nanoscience and nanotechnology: From chemical-physical applications to nanomedicine. *Molecules, 25*(1), Article 112. https://doi.org/10.3390/molecules25010112.

12. Bazak, R., Houri, M., Achy, S. El, Hussein, W., & Refaat, T. (2014). Passive targeting of nanoparticles to cancer: A comprehensive review of the literature. *Molecular and Clinical Oncology, 2*(6), 904–908. https://doi.org/10.3892/mco.2014.356.

13. Bibi, S., Lattmann, E., Mohammed, A. R., & Perrie, Y. (2012). Trigger release liposome systems: Local and remote-controlled delivery? *Journal of Microencapsulation, 29*(3), 262–276. https://doi.org/10.3109/02652048.2011.646330.

14. Bogunia-Kubik, K., & Sugisaka, M. (2002). From molecular biology to nanotechnology and nanomedicine. *BioSystems, 65*(2, 3), 123–138. https://doi.org/10.1016/S0303-2647(02)00010-2.

15. Boisseau, P., & Loubaton, B. (2011). Nanomedicine, nanotechnology in medicine. *Comptes Rendus Physique, 12*(7), 620–636. https://doi.org/10.1016/j.crhy.2011.06.001.

16. Bonifácio, B. V., da Silva, P. B., dos Santos Ramos, M. A., Negri, K. M. S., Bauab, T. M., & Chorilli, M. (2013). Nanotechnology-based drug delivery systems and herbal medicines: A review. *International Journal of Nanomedicine, 9*(1), 1–15. https://doi.org/10.2147/IJN.S52634.

17. Bose, A., Burman, D. R., Sikdar, B., & Patra, P. (2021). Nanomicelles: Types, properties and applications in drug delivery. *IET Nanobiotechnology, 15*(1), 19–26. https://doi.org/10.1049/nbt2.12018.

18. Boyer, C., Whittaker, M. R., Bulmus, V., Liu, J., & Davis, T. P. (2010). The design and utility of polymer-stabilized iron-oxide nanoparticles for nanomedicine applications. *NPG Asia Materials, 2*(1), 23–30. https://doi.org/10.1038/asiamat.2010.6.

19. Brown, P. D., & Patel, P. R. (2015). Nanomedicine: A pharma perspective. *Wiley Interdisciplinary Reviews: Nanomedicine and Nanobiotechnology, 7*(2), 125–130. https://doi.org/10.1002/wnan.1288.

20. Brydson, R. M., & Hammond, C. (2005). *Generic Methodologies for Nanotechnology: Classification and Fabrication*. https://doi.org/10.1002/0470020873.ch1.

21. Cagel, M., Tesan, F. C., Bernabeu, E., Salgueiro, M. J., Zubillaga, M. B., Moretton, M. A., & Chiappetta, D. A. (2017). Polymeric mixed micelles as nanomedicines: Achievements and perspectives. *European Journal of Pharmaceutics and Biopharmaceutics : Official Journal of Arbeitsgemeinschaft fur Pharmazeutische Verfahrenstechnik e.V*, 113, 211–228. https://doi.org/10.1016/j.ejpb.2016.12.019.

22. Cajot, S., Van Butsele, K., Paillard, A., Passirani, C., Garcion, E., Benoit, J. P., Varshney, S. K., & Jérôme, C. (2012). Smart nanocarriers for pH-triggered targeting and release of hydrophobic drugs. *Acta Biomaterial*, *8*(12), 4215–4223. https://doi.org/10.1016/j.actbio.2012.08.049.

23. Chang, E. H., Harford, J. B., Eaton, M. A. W., Boisseau, P. M., Dube, A., Hayeshi, R., Swai, H., & Lee, D. S. (2015). Nanomedicine: Past, present and future–A global perspective. *Biochemical and Biophysical Research Communications, 468*(3), 511–517. https://doi.org/10.1016/j.bbrc.2015.10.136.

24. Chen, M., Daddy, K. A., Xiao, Y., Ping, Q., & Zong, L. (2017). Advanced nanomedicine for rheumatoid arthritis treatment: Focus on active targeting. *Expert Opinion on Drug Delivery, 14*(10), 1141–1144. https://doi.org/10.1080/17425247.2017.1372746.

25. Dias, A. P., da Silva Santos, S., da Silva, J. V., Parise-Filho, R., Igne Ferreira, E., Seoud, O. E., & Giarolla, J. (2020). Dendrimers in the context of nanomedicine. *International Journal of Pharmaceutics*, 573, 118814. https://doi.org/10.1016/j.ijpharm.2019.118814.

26. Długosz, O., Szostak, K., Staroń, A., Pulit-Prociak, J., & Banach, M. (2020). Methods for reducing the toxicity of metal and metal oxide NPs as biomedicine. *Materials, 13*(2), 279. https://doi.org/10.3390/ma13020279.

27. El-Shafey, A. M. (2020). Green synthesis of metal and metal oxide nanoparticles from plant leaf extracts and their applications: A review. *Green Processing and Synthesis, 9*(1), 304–339. https://doi.org/10.1515/gps-2020-0031.

28. Esfand, R., & Tomalia, D. A. (2001). Poly(amidoamine) (PAMAM) dendrimers: From biomimicry to drug delivery and biomedical applications. *Drug Discovery Today*, *6*(8), 427–436. https://

doi.org/10.1016/S1359-6446(01)01757-3.

29. Etemadi, H., Buchanan, J. K., Kandile, N. G., & Plieger, P. G. (2021). Iron oxide nanoparticles: Physicochemical characteristics and historical developments to commercialization for potential technological applications. *ACS Biomaterials Science & Engineering, 7*(12), 5432–5450. https://doi.org/10.1021/acsbiomaterials.1c00938.

30. Fornaguera, C., & García-Celma, M. J. (2017). Personalized nanomedicine: A revolution at the nanoscale. *Journal of Personalized Medicine, 7*(4), 14–21. https://doi.org/10.3390/jpm7040012.

31. Gadge, S., Mahavidyalaya, M., Arts, S. A., Veronin, M., & Schumaker, R. (2022). *Current Aspects in Pharmaceutical Research and Development* (Vol. 8). https://doi.org/10.9734/bpi/caprd/v8.

32. Germain, M., Caputo, F., Metcalfe, S., Tosi, G., Spring, K., Åslund, A. K. O., Pottier, A., Schiffelers, R., Ceccaldi, A., & Schmid, R. (2020). Delivering the power of nanomedicine to patients today. *Journal of Controlled Release, 326*, 164–171. https://doi.org/10.1016/j.jconrel.2020.07.007.

33. Ghosh, S. K., & Pal, T. (2007). Interparticle coupling effect on the surface plasmon resonance of gold nanoparticles: From theory to applications. *Chemical Reviews, 107*(11), 4797–4862. https://doi.org/10.1021/cr0680282.

34. Giret, S., Wong Chi Man, M., & Carcel, C. (2015). Mesoporous-silica-functionalized nanoparticles for drug delivery. *Chemistry–A European Journal, 21*(40), 13850–13865. https://doi.org/10.1002/chem.201500578.

35. Gothandam, K. M. (2018). *Food Security and Water Treatment.*

36. Gour, A., & Jain, N. K. (2019). Advances in green synthesis of nanoparticles. *Artificial Cells, Nanomedicine, and Biotechnology, 47*(1), 844–851. https://doi.org/10.1080/21691401.2019.1577878.

37. Grewal, D. S. (2016). Nanotechnologies for the future. *International Journal of Nanotechnology & Nanomedicine, 1*(1), 1–7. https://doi.org/10.33140/ijnn/01/01/00002.

38. Gupta, N., Gupta, S. M., & Sharma, S. K. (2019). Carbon nanotubes: Synthesis, properties and engineering applications. *Carbon Letters, 29*(5), 419–447. https://doi.org/10.1007/s42823-019-00068-2.

39. Harris, D. L., & Bawa, R. (2007). The carbon nanotube patent landscape in nanomedicine: An expert opinion. *Expert Opinion on Therapeutic Patents, 17*(9), 1165–1174. https://doi.org/10.1517/13543776.17.9.1165.

40. Hua, S., & Wu, S. Y. (2018). Editorial: Advances and challenges in nanomedicine. *Frontiers in Pharmacology, 9*, Article 1397. https://doi.org/10.3389/fphar.2018.01397.

41. Hua, S., de Matos, M. B. C., Metselaar, J. M., & Storm, G. (2018). Current trends and challenges in the clinical translation of nanoparticulate nanomedicines: Pathways for translational development and commercialization. *Frontiers in Pharmacology, 9*, Article 790. https://doi.org/10.3389/fphar.2018.00790.

42. Hussain, S. M., Warheit, D. B., Ng, S. P., Comfort, K. K., Grabinski, C. M., & Braydich-Stolle, L. K. (2015). At the crossroads of nanotoxicology *in vitro*: Past achievements and current challenges. *Toxicological Sciences, 147*(1), 5–16. https://doi.org/10.1093/toxsci/kfv106.

43. Ibrahim, K. S. (2013). Carbon nanotubes—Properties and applications: A review. *Carbon Letters, 14*(3), 131–144. https://doi.org/10.5714/cl.2013.14.3.131

44. Jin, S. E., & Jin, H. E. (2019). Synthesis, characterization, and three-dimensional structure generation of zinc oxide-based nanomedicine for biomedical applications. *Pharmaceutics, 11*(11), 575. https://doi.org/10.3390/pharmaceutics11110575.

45. Kargozar, S., & Mozafari, M. (2018). Nanotechnology and nanomedicine: Start small, think big. *Materials Today: Proceedings, 5*(7), 15492–15500. https://doi.org/10.1016/j.matpr.2018.04.155.

46. Keck, C. M., & Müller, R. H. (2013). Nanotoxicological classification system (NCS)–A guide for the risk-benefit assessment of nanoparticulate drug delivery systems. *European Journal of Pharmaceutics and Biopharmaceutics, 84*(3), 445–448. https://doi.org/10.1016/j.ejpb.2013.01.001.

47. Khare, V., Saxena, A. K., & Gupta, P. N. (2015). Toxicology considerations in nanomedicine. In *Nanomedicine in Drug Delivery* (pp. 377–399). Elsevier. https://doi.org/10.1016/B978-0-323-32889-0.00015-7.

48. Kim, Y., Park, E. J., & Na, D. H. (2018). Recent progress in dendrimer-based nanomedicine development. *Archives of Pharmacal Research, 41*(6), 571–582. https://doi.org/10.1007/s12272-018-1008-4.

49. Kumar Teli, M., Mutalik, S., & Rajanikant, G. K. (2010). Nanotechnology and nanomedicine: Going small means aiming big. *Current Pharmaceutical Design, 16*(16), 1882–1892. https://doi.org/10.2174/138161210791208992.

50. Kumar, C., & Balasubramanian, D. (1980). Structural features of water-in-oil microemulsions. *Journal of Physical Chemistry, 84*, 1895–1899.

51. Kumawat, L., & Jain, A. (2012). Review on gold nano particle for novel drug delivery system. *International Journal of Pharmaceutical Sciences, 3*(1), 53–58.

52. Lather, V., Poonia, N., & Pandita, D. (2018). Mesoporous silica nanoparticles. In *Nanopharmaceuticals: Principles and Applications* (pp. 192–246). IGI Global. https://doi.org/10.4018/978-1-5225-4781-5.ch008.

53. Lee, S. H., & Jun, B. H. (2019). Silver nanoparticles: Synthesis and application for nanomedicine. *International Journal of Molecular Sciences, 20*(4), 865. https://doi.org/10.3390/ijms20040865.

54. Li, B., & Lane, L. A. (2019). Probing the biological obstacles of nanomedicine with gold nanoparticles. *Wiley Interdisciplinary Reviews: Nanomedicine and Nanobiotechnology, 11*(3), e1542. https://doi.org/10.1002/wnan.1542.

55. Li, Y., Zhang, Y., & Wang, W. (2018). Photo triggered targeting of nanocarriers for drug delivery. *Nano Research, 11*(10), 5424–5438. https://doi.org/10.1007/s12274-018-2132-7.

56. Lin, M. M., Kim, H. H., Kim, H., Muhammed, M., & Kim, D. K. (2010). Iron oxide-based nanomagnets in nanomedicine: Fabrication and applications. *Nano Reviews, 1*(1), 4883. https://doi.org/10.3402/nano.v1i0.4883.

57. Loomis, K., McNeeley, K., & Bellamkonda, R. V. (2011). Nanoparticles with targeting, triggered release, and imaging functionality for cancer applications. *Soft Matter, 7*(3), 839–856. https://doi.org/10.1039/c0sm00534g.

58. Lopes, T. S., Alves, G. G., Pereira, M. R., Granjeiro, J. M., & Leite, P. E. C. (2019). Advances and potential application of gold nanoparticles in nanomedicine. *Journal of Cellular Biochemistry, 120*(10), 16370–16378. https://doi.org/10.1002/jcb.29044.

59. Malik, S., & Waheed, Y. (2023). Emerging applications of nanotechnology in dentistry. *Dentistry Journal, 11*(11), 1–30. https://doi.org/10.3390/dj11110266.

60. Mason, R. M. (1964). Use of drugs in the treatment of rheumatoid arthritis. *Physiotherapy, 50*, 86–88.

61. Mosquera, J., García, I., & Liz-Marzán, L. M. (2018). Cellular uptake of nanoparticles versus small molecules: A matter of size. *Accounts of Chemical Research, 51*(9), 2305–2313. https://doi.org/10.1021/acs.accounts.8b00292.

62. Mughal, T. A., Ali, S., Hassan, A., Kazmi, S. A. R., Saleem, M. Z., Shakir, H. A., Nazer, S., Farooq, M. A., Awan, M. Z., Khan, M. A., Andleeb, S., Mumtaz, S., Mumtaz, S., Tahir, H. M., & Gulzar, N. (2024). Phytochemical screening, antimicrobial activity, *in vitro* and *in vivo* antioxidant activity of *Berberis lycium* Royle root bark extract. *Brazilian Journal of Biology, 84*, 1–10. https://doi.org/10.1590/1519-6984.249742.

63. Nalwa, H. S. (2014). A special issue on reviews in nanomedicine, drug delivery and vaccine development. *Journal of Biomedical Nanotechnology, 10*(9), 1635–1640. https://doi.org/10.1166/jbn.2014.2033.

64. Narum, S. M., Le, T., Le, D. P., Lee, J. C., Donahue, N. D., Yang, W., & Wilhelm, S. (2019). Passive targeting in nanomedicine: Fundamental concepts, body interactions, and clinical potential. In *Characterization of Nanoparticles* (pp. 69–94). Elsevier. https://doi.org/10.1016/B978-0-12-816662-8.00004-7.

65. Nekkanti, V., & Kalepu, S. (2015). Recent advances in liposomal drug delivery: A review. *Pharmaceutical Nanotechnology, 3*(1), 35–55. https://doi.org/10.2174/2211738503666150709173905.

66. Nikzamir, M., Hanifehpour, Y., Akbarzadeh, A., & Panahi, Y. (2021). Applications of dendrimers in nanomedicine and drug delivery: A review. *Journal of Inorganic and Organometallic Polymers and Materials, 31*(6), 2246–2261. https://doi.org/10.1007/s10904-021-01925-2.

67. Oberdörster, G., Oberdörster, E., & Oberdörster, J. (2005). Nanotoxicology: An emerging discipline evolving from studies of ultrafine particles. *Environmental Health Perspectives, 113*(7), 823–839. https://doi.org/10.1289/ehp.7339.

68. Paliwal, R., Babu, R. J., & Palakurthi, S. (2014). Nanomedicine scale-up technologies: Feasibilities and challenges. *AAPS PharmSciTech, 15*(6), 1527–1534. https://doi.org/10.1208/s12249-014-0177-9.

69. Pandey, P., & Dahiya, M. (2016). A brief review on inorganic nanoparticles. *Journal of Critical Reviews, 3*(3), 18–26.

70. Parveen, S., & Sahoo, S. K. (2006). Nanomedicine: Clinical applications of polyethylene glycol conjugated proteins and drugs. *Clinical Pharmacokinetics, 45*(10), 965–988. https://doi.org/10.2165/00003088-200645100-00002.

71. Pasparakis, G. (2022). Recent developments in the use of gold and silver nanoparticles in biomedicine. *Wiley Interdisciplinary Reviews: Nanomedicine and Nanobiotechnology, 14*(5), e1817. https://doi.org/10.1002/wnan.1817.

72. Patil, Y. P., & Jadhav, S. (2014). Novel methods for liposome preparation. *Chemistry and Physics of Lipids, 177*, 8–18. https://doi.org/10.1016/j.chemphyslip.2013.10.011.

73. Pearce, A. K., & O'Reilly, R. K. (2019). Insights into active targeting of nanoparticles in drug

delivery: Advances in clinical studies and design considerations for cancer nanomedicine. *Bioconjugate Chemistry, 30*(9), 2300–2311. https://doi.org/10.1021/acs.bioconjchem.9b00456.

74. Psimadas, D., Georgoulias, P., Valotassiou, V., & Loudos, G. (2012). Molecular nanomedicine towards cancer. *Journal of Pharmaceutical Sciences, 101*(7), 2271–2280. https://doi.org/10.1002/jps.

75. Racca, L., Canta, M., Dumontel, B., Ancona, A., Limongi, T., Garino, N., Laurenti, M., Canavese, G., & Cauda, V. (2018). Zinc oxide nanostructures in biomedicine. In *Nanostructures for the Engineering of Cells, Tissues and Organs* (pp. 249–274). Elsevier Inc. https://doi.org/10.1016/B978-0-12-814156-4.00012-4.

76. Rahman, M., Beg, S., Sharma, G., Anwar, F., & Kumar, V. (2015). Emergence of lipid-based vesicular carriers as nanoscale pharmacotherapy in rheumatoid arthritis. *Recent Patents on Nanomedicine, 5*(2), 111–121. https://doi.org/10.2174/1877912305666150616215800.

77. Rastegari, E., Hsiao, Y. J., Lai, W. Y., Lai, Y. H., Yang, T. C., Chen, S. J., Huang, P. I., Chiou, S. H., Mou, C. Y., & Chien, Y. (2021). An update on mesoporous silica nanoparticle applications in nanomedicine. *Pharmaceutics, 13*(7), Article 1067. https://doi.org/10.3390/pharmaceutics13071067.

78. RC, J. (2020). Plant extracts-based nanoparticles, a good perspective in the development of drugs in nanomedicine. *Modern Approaches in Drug Designing, 3*(2), 1–8. https://doi.org/10.31031/madd.2020.03.000556.

79. Revathi, S., Vuyyuru, M., & Dhanaraju, M. D. (2015). Carbon nanotube: A flexible approach for nanomedicine and drug delivery. *Asian Journal of Pharmaceutical and Clinical Research, 8*(1), 25–31.

80. Rolland, O., Turrin, C. O., Caminade, A. M., & Majoral, J. P. (2009). Dendrimers and nanomedicine: Multivalency in action. *New Journal of Chemistry, 33*(9), 1809–1824. https://doi.org/10.1039/b901054h.

81. Shah, S. M. A. (2021). Nano biomedicine: A new approach of medicinal plants and their therapeutic modalities. *Journal of Materials and Environmental Science, 12*(1), 1–14.

82. Singh, S., & Singh, A. (2013). Current status of nanomedicine and nano surgery. *Anesthesia: Essays and Researches, 7*(2), 237–242. https://doi.org/10.4103/0259-1162.118976.

83. Sirsi, S. R., & Borden, M. A. (2014). State-of-the-art materials for ultrasound-triggered drug delivery. *Advanced Drug Delivery Reviews, 72*, 3–14. https://doi.org/10.1016/j.addr.2013.12.010.

84. Soares, S., Sousa, J., Pais, A., & Vitorino, C. (2018). Nanomedicine: Principles, properties, and regulatory issues. *Frontiers in Chemistry, 6*, Article 360. https://doi.org/10.3389/fchem.2018.00360.

85. Tahir, E., & Everest, E. (2016). *Nanomedicine* (pp. 579–587). https://doi.org/10.1007/978-3-319-25340-4.

86. Tinkle, S., McNeil, S. E., Mühlebach, S., Bawa, R., Borchard, G., Barenholz, Y. C., Tamarkin, L., & Desai, N. (2014). Nanomedicines: Addressing the scientific and regulatory gap. *Annals of the New York Academy of Sciences, 1313*(1), 35–56. https://doi.org/10.1111/nyas.12403.

87. Vallabani, N. V. S., & Singh, S. (2018). Recent advances and future prospects of iron oxide nanoparticles in biomedicine and diagnostics. *3 Biotech, 8*(6), 279. https://doi.org/10.1007/s13205-018-1286-z.

88. Vallet-Regí, M. (2010). Nanostructured mesoporous silica matrices in nanomedicine. *Journal of Internal Medicine, 267*(1), 22–43. https://doi.org/10.1111/j.1365-2796.2009.02190.x.

89. Van Dijken, A., Meulenkamp, E. A., Vanmaekelbergh, D., & Meijerink, A. (2000). Identification of the transition responsible for the visible emission in ZnO using quantum size effects. *Journal of Luminescence, 90*(3), 123–128. https://doi.org/10.1016/S0022-2313(99)00599-2.

90. Venkataraman, S., Hedrick, J. L., Ong, Z. Y., Yang, C., Ee, P. L. R., Hammond, P. T., & Yang, Y. Y. (2011). The effects of polymeric nanostructure shape on drug delivery. *Advanced Drug Delivery Reviews, 63*(14, 15), 1228–1246. https://doi.org/10.1016/j.addr.2011.06.016.

91. Verma, G., & Gupta, A. (2022). Recent development in carbon nanotubes-based gas sensors. *Journal of Materials Nanoscience, 9*(1), 3–12.

92. Verma, G., Mondal, K., Islam, M., & Gupta, A. (2024). Recent advances in advanced micro and nanomanufacturing for wastewater purification. *ACS Applied Engineering Materials, 2,* 262–285. https://doi.org/10.1021/acsaenm.3c00711.

93. Verma, G., Singhal, S., Kumar Rai, P., & Gupta, A. (2023). A simple approach to develop a paper-based biosensor for real-time uric acid detection. *Analytical Methods, 15*(24), 2955–2963. https://doi.org/10.1039/D3AY00613A.

94. Villaverde, G., & Baeza, A. (2019). Targeting strategies for improving the efficacy of nanomedicine in oncology. *Beilstein Journal of Nanotechnology, 10,* 168–181. https://doi.org/10.3762/bjnano.10.16.

95. Wang, J., Lee, J. S., Kim, D., & Zhu, L. (2017). Exploration of zinc oxide nanoparticles as a multitarget and multifunctional anticancer nanomedicine. *ACS Applied Materials & Interfaces, 9*(46), 39971–39984. https://doi.org/10.1021/acsami.7b11219.

96. Wang, Y., & Kohane, D. S. (2017). External triggering and triggered targeting strategies for drug delivery. *Nature Reviews Materials, 2,* 17020. https://doi.org/10.1038/natrevmats.2017.20.

97. Warner, J. H. (1985). *Science in Medicine* (Vol. 1). https://doi.org/10.1086/368637.

98. Watts, G. (2010). Alec Douglas Bangham. *The Lancet, 375*(9731), 2070. https://doi.org/10.1016/S0140-6736(10)60950-6.

99. Wicki, A., Witzigmann, D., Balasubramanian, V., & Huwyler, J. (2015). Nanomedicine in cancer therapy: Challenges, opportunities, and clinical applications. *Journal of Controlled Release, 200,* 138–157. https://doi.org/10.1016/j.jconrel.2014.12.030.

100. Yamashita, T., Yamashita, K., Nabeshi, H., Yoshikawa, T., Yoshioka, Y., Tsunoda, S., & Tsutsumi, Y. (2012). Carbon nanomaterials: Efficacy and safety for nanomedicine. *Materials, 5*(2), 350–363. https://doi.org/10.3390/ma5020350.

101. Yildiz, T., Gu, R., Zauscher, S., & Betancourt, T. (2018). Doxorubicin-loaded protease-activated near-infrared fluorescent polymeric nanoparticles for imaging and therapy of cancer. *International Journal of Nanomedicine, 13,* 6961–6986. https://doi.org/10.2147/IJN.S174068.

102. Ying, S., Guan, Z., Ofoegbu, P. C., Clubb, P., Rico, C., He, F., & Hong, J. (2022). Green synthesis of nanoparticles: Current developments and limitations. *Environmental Technology & Innovation, 26,* 102336. https://doi.org/10.1016/j.eti.2022.102336.

103. Yohan, D., & Chithrani, B. D. (2014). Applications of nanoparticles in nanomedicine. *Journal of Biomedical Nanotechnology, 10*(9), 2371–2392. https://doi.org/10.1166/jbn.2014.2015.

104. Yu, L., Deng, Z., Liu, L., Zhang, W., & Wang, C. (2020). Plant-derived nanovesicles: A novel form of nanomedicine. *Frontiers in Bioengineering and Biotechnology*, *8*, 584391. https://doi.org/10.3389/fbioe.2020.584391.

105. Yue, H., Wei, W., Yue, Z., Lv, P., Wang, L., Ma, G., & Su, Z. (2010). Particle size affects the cellular response in macrophages. *European Journal of Pharmaceutical Sciences*, *41*(5), 650–657. https://doi.org/10.1016/j.ejps.2010.09.006.

106. Zang, X., Song, J., Yi, X., & Piyu, J. (2022). Polymeric indoximod based prodrug nanoparticles with doxorubicin entrapment for inducing immunogenic cell death and improving the immunotherapy of breast cancer. *Journal of Materials Chemistry B*, *10*(12), 2019–2027. https://doi.org/10.1039/d2tb00197g.

107. Zielinska, A., Carreiró, F., Oliveira, A. M., Neves, A., Pires, B., Nagasamy Venkatesh, D., Durazzo, A., Lucarini, M., Eder, P., Silva, A. M., Santini, A., & Souto, E. B. (2020). Polymeric nanoparticles: Production, characterization, toxicology and ecotoxicology. *Molecules*, *25*(16), Article 3731. https://doi.org/10.3390/molecules25163731.

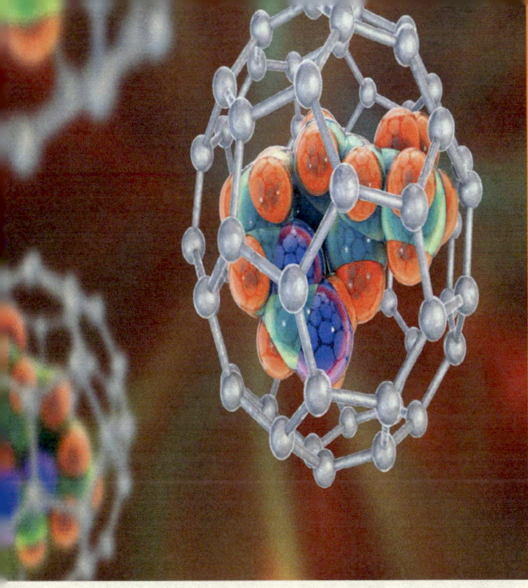

Chapter 2

NANOPARTICLES IN DRUG DELIVERY SYSTEMS

Contents

Ruby Dhiman,[1] Chung-Ming Chang,[2,3] Amrendra K. Ajay,[4,5] and Ramendra Pati Pandey[1,*]

[1]*School of Health Sciences and Technology (SoHST), University of Petroleum and Energy Studies (UPES), Dehradun, Uttarakhand, India*

[2]*Graduate Institute of Biomedical Sciences, Chang Gung University, Guishan, Taoyuan, Taiwan, Republic of China*

[3]*Department of Biotechnology Industry, Chang Gung University, Guishan, Taoyuan, Taiwan, Republic of China*

[4]*Department of Medicine, Brigham and Women's Hospital, Boston, MA, USA*

[5]*Department of Medicine, Harvard Medical School, Boston, MA, USA*

Corresponding author.

Abstract

The objective of this chapter is to better understand the essential role that nanoparticles play in improving medication delivery. It aims to accomplish several goals that together highlight the tremendous importance of nanoparticles in this field. We begin by exploring the complex realm of nanoparticle kinds and their categorization, identifying the several types and their essential features. We next discuss the various methods used in the synthesis of nanoparticles, distinguishing between top-down and bottom-up strategies and looking at chemical, physical, mechanical, and biological synthesis methods. The crucial element of drug loading and encapsulation is then emphasized in the chapter. We additionally look into drug loading strategies that are effective as well as encapsulation techniques that are critical to maximizing drug delivery. As we advance, we uncover the processes underlying targeted drug release, such as active and passive targeting techniques along with the novel field of stimuli-responsive nanoparticles that provide precise drug release patterns. Additionally, we discuss the crucial aspects of safety and biocompatibility in the design of nanoparticles, such as regulatory concerns and toxicity evaluation.

The last section of the chapter highlights a variety of uses for nanoparticle-based drug delivery in the treatment of diseases including cancer treatments, infectious diseases, neurological disorders, and inflammatory disorders. All of these applications demonstrate the revolutionary potential of this approach. Furthermore, we consider the challenges that this area is encountering, novel developments that are emerging and opportunities that lie in the future giving a thorough rundown of the ground-breaking discoveries and possible directions. As a whole, the goals of this chapter highlight the critical role that nanoparticles play in improving drug delivery and paving the way for a new age in therapeutics that will be marked by improved efficiency, efficiency, and improved outcomes for patients.

2.1. Introduction

In recent years, research in the fields of biomedicine and pharmacology is paying more attention to the use of nanomaterials (NMs). Nanoparticles (NPs) smaller than 100 nm have the potential to improve biodistribution, improve patient compliance, and deliver drugs to particular sites (Patil et al., 2019). In the pharmaceutical and biomedical sectors, a number of sophisticated NMs are used. Biological, carbon nanostructures, metal and metal-oxide NMs, magnetic nanoparticles, and silica-based NMs are a few examples of these functional NMs (Bitar et al., 2012; Reddy et al., 2012). NPs can be used in drug delivery systems (DDS) that deliver drugs at suitable, therapeutic concentrations through controlled or sustained release. The usage of nano-size carriers may have an impact on improving pharmacokinetic profiles and bioavailability, as well as increasing the half-life of medications and reducing the frequency of administration (Jurak et al., 2021; Kim et al., 2019). With the advent of solid lipid nanoparticles (SLNs), magnetic nanoparticles, micelles, dendrimers, polymeric nanoparticles, and quantum dots (QDs) all of which have significant physical and chemical characteristics in addition to having nanoscale effects nanotechnology has grown into an extensive field with applications in biomedicine (Stevanović, and Uskoković, 2009). The administration and effectiveness of pharmaceutical molecules, such as antibodies, peptides, vaccines, medicines, and enzymes, are enhanced by DDS. Injections and tablets taken orally are now the most often used medication delivery methods. Most small molecule medications are administered as tablets. Every year, tens of billions of tablets are taken throughout the world only for aspirin. The most common way to give proteins and peptides is still via injection. Worldwide, more than 10 billion injections are administered annually (Kermode, 2004). The DDS that has been investigated the most are nanoparticles (NPs). Using NPs for targeted medication delivery has been the subject of more than 25,000 papers over the past 10 years (Web of Science keyword: targeted nanoparticles, Jan. 2014). Even when it comes to NP-based DDS, cancer is still the most researched application. There are definite benefits to using NPs to administer chemotherapy medications. NPs target wounded tissue, prevent drug breakdown *in vivo*, and regulate drug release at the target location. They also profit from synthesis techniques that enable large-scale manufacture of almost identical batches with similar characteristics (Barenholz, 2012). Nanoparticles (NPs) has the capability to enhance the stability and solubility of cargos that are encapsulated, facilitate transportation across membranes, and extend circulation times to augment safety and effectiveness. These factors have led to the extensive use of NP research, which has produced encouraging *in vitro* and small animal model outcomes. Nevertheless, the quantity of nanomedicines accessible to patients is far less than anticipated for the sector, in part due to a translational gap between animal and human studies, even with this substantial research funded by the NNI (Kou et al., 2018; Mitragotri et al., 2017). Many factors including their physical and chemical characteristics, drug loading capacity, drug release, and most importantly low or non-toxicity of the carrier itself, determine their therapeutic application (Puri et al., 2009).

Studies have indicated that NPs may be hazardous even when they have the potential for therapeutic use. These investigations have shown that NPs may build up in cells and cause toxicity that is unique to certain organs. These findings highlight the critical necessity for the creation of safe nanoparticles and the establishment of stringent rules for their development in terms of toxicity assessment, given the rising levels of human exposure (Missaoui, Arnold, and Cummings, 2018).

This chapter will go into the intriguing field of nanoparticles in DDS. As the demand for efficient and targeted medication delivery grows, nanocarriers have emerged as potential vehicles for delivering therapeutic chemicals to particular areas of the body. Nanocarriers such as core-shell structures, polymers, liposomes, dendrimers, and metallic NP-based nanocarriers have been widely explored. Approximately, 250 nanocarrier-based DDS are now in various phases of preclinical and clinical research.

2.2. Nanoparticle Types and Characterization

Nanoparticles are vulnerable to aggregation and protein opsonization (protein binding to the surface of the nanoparticle as a tag for identification by the immune system) as soon as they are incorporated into the circulation. The opsonized nanoparticles may be removed from circulation by filtration in the kidney, spleen, or liver, or by phagocytosis. The immune system's quick and indiscriminate clearance causes a shorter retention period, which reduces bioavailability. Retention duration can be changed by coating the surface of the nanoparticle with polyethylene glycol (PEG), carbohydrates, acetyl groups, or protein moieties (albumin, arginine-glycine-aspartate (RGD) peptide) (Shreffler et al., 2019). One of the most important factors in assuring the security and effectiveness of pharmaceutical medicines is stability. Physical and chemical stability are two types of stability. Physical stability problems are often associated with sedimentation, agglomeration, crystal growth, and recrystallisation. On the other hand, problems with chemical stability arise from the breakdown of functional groups, such as the oxidative breakdown of amino groups and the hydrolytic breakdown of amides and esters. Chemical stabilities are drug-specific in contrast to physical stability problems, which are often seen. The development of bigger particles (>5 μm) in response to intravenously delivered nanosuspensions is one instance of agglomeration or crystal growth that can cause embolism and capillary obstruction (Patravale, Date, and Kulkarni, 2004). Lipid-based nanoparticles have a variety of component configurations, but they are generally spherical platforms with at least one lipid bilayer encircling at least one interior aqueous compartment. Lipid-based nanoparticles (NPs) have several benefits as a delivery vehicle, such as easy formulation, self-assembly, biocompatibility, high bioavailability, capacity to transport large payloads, and a variety of physicochemical properties that may be adjusted to modify their biological features (Fonseca-Santos, Gremião, and Chorilli, 2015; Sercombe et al., 2015). Natural or synthetic materials, monomers, or preformed polymers can all be used to create polymeric nanoparticles (NPs), opening up a vast range of potential shapes and properties (Brown et al., 2019). Nanostructured materials for diverse medication delivery and imaging purposes have been synthesized using inorganic materials including gold, iron, and silica. These carefully designed inorganic NPs may be made to have a broad range of sizes, topologies, and geometries. The most thoroughly researched NPs, gold (AuNPs), are employed in a variety of configurations, including nanospheres, nanorods, nanostars, nanoshells, and nanocages. Additionally, because to the characteristics of the base material itself, inorganic nanoparticles have special physical, electrical, magnetic, and optical capabilities (Wang et al., 2020; Yang et al., 2019).

2.2.1. Size, Shape, and Surface Properties

Particle size distribution in polymeric NPs) produced by various processes can have mean diameters ranging from 100 to 300 nm. The size distribution should be unimodal and the polydispersity as low as feasible ideally, almost nil. It is also possible to obtain particles with sizes as small as 50 nm or as small as 60 to 70 nm. The most widely used methods for measuring the size of nanoparticles are dynamic (DLS) and static light scattering (SLS), but TEM, SEM, and AFM are also often employed (Brar and Verma, 2011; Hickey et al., 2015). According to some research, there is a direct relationship between the amount of ROS produced in the kidneys and the size and dispersion of NPs (Elsaesser and Howard, 2012). There has also been evidence of this size-dependent toxicity in the liver. When compared to bigger NPs (40 and 100 nm), silver nanoparticles (AgNPs) with a 10 nm size showed greater tissue dispersion and more severe toxic effects in the liver (Wu and Tang, 2014). Another study suggests that therapeutic nanoparticles smaller than 100 nm in size take longer to circulate through the bloodstream. Numerous investigations revealed that because therapeutic nanoparticles in the 20–200 nm size range are not recognized by the RES and cannot be removed by the kidney, they exhibit a greater incidence of accumulation in tumors (Bhatia, 2016). In addition, compared to normal tissues, the quantity and volume of blood vessels are greater in tumor sites. Because of this, nanoparticles of the right size can enter the tumor relatively quickly and stay there for a longer period of time; this phenomenon is called the enhanced permeability and retention (EPR) effect (Fang, Nakamura, and Maeda, 2011; Nakamura et al., 2016).

2.3. Nanoparticle Synthesis

Various particle-engineering methods have been employed by the pharmaceutical sector to regulate the micro- and nano-sized crystals' size/distribution, porosity, crystallinity, and purity. Three main categories can be used to broadly classify the preparation techniques for API nanocrystals or nanosuspensions: top-down techniques, which involve reduction of particle size through mechanical attrition. Bottom-up techniques, which involve controlled precipitation or crystallization (Keck and Müller, 2006), are chosen based on the physicochemical characteristics of the medications, such as solubility and material hardness.

2.3.1. Top-Down Approach

The NP synthesis from bulk materials into tiny ones is described by the top-down method. The top-down approach is primarily classified as a physical technique of NP synthesis since it uses a large tube furnace to break large materials into tiny pieces (Ramanathan et al., 2021). High-energy methods are used in top-down (Figure 2.1) techniques to get pharmaceutical medication particles down to the nanoscale. There are two primary categories of top-down approaches: media milling and high-pressure homogenization (HPH). In order to reduce the particle size, both of these methods rely on collisions, stress, attrition, and shearing forces (Chin et al., 2014). Both dry and wet media milling are types of media milling, which is sometimes referred to as a mechanochemical process (Rasenack and Müller, 2004). Top-down methods are more environmentally friendly since they primarily employ water as a non-solvent to spread poorly soluble medications. Most of the commercial and experimental nanosuspension-based pharmaceutical formulations have been made using top-down approaches due to their more efficient process flow, regulated particle size, and non-solvent nature (Hanafy et al., 2007).

2.3.2. Bottom-Up Approach

Bottom-up approaches are advantageous when a great degree of control and modifications are required.

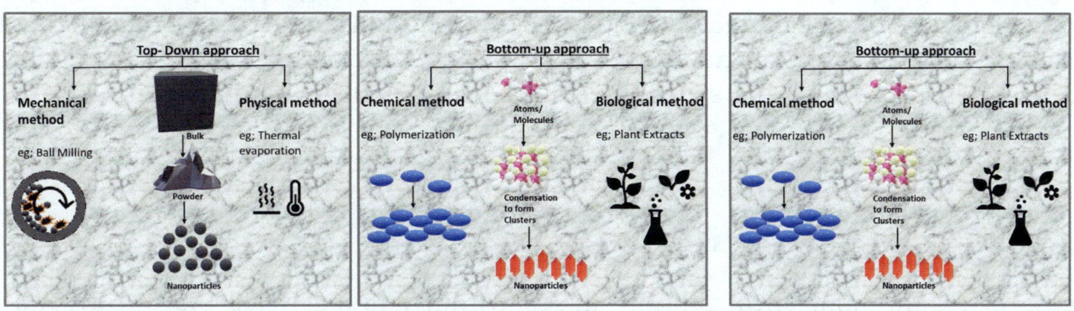

Figure 2.1. Diagrammatic illustration of top-down and bottom-up methods for making nanomaterials (NMs).

Chemical approaches are commonly used in the bottom-up strategy to create nanoparticles. These approaches include sol-gel, co-precipitation, and hydrothermal synthesis. Co-precipitation is often utilized in the development of magnetic nanoparticles for applications drug delivery (Laurent et al., 2008). Biological processes, such as the utilization of microbes or plant extracts, are eco-friendly bottom-up approaches that generate nanoparticles with inbuilt biocompatibility (Mittal, Chisti, and Banerjee, 2013). A diagram of top-down and bottom-up methods for making NMs is depicted in Figure 2.1, different methods for nanoparticles synthesis have been shown in it. The selection between top-down and bottom-up techniques is dependent upon several criteria including the intended particle properties, production scale, and particular drug delivery requirements. The performance and modification of nanoparticles can be further improved by combining these strategies into hybrid systems (Jokerst et al., 2011).

2.3.3. Physical and Mechanical Methods

Another technique, Evaporation-Condensation technique provides excellent control over particle size and uniformity used for the synthesis of metallic nanoparticles, QDs, and carbon-based nanoparticles for drug delivery and imaging (Hessel et al., 2011; Sun et al., 2005). Then we have Spray drying method is valuable for producing inhalable nanoparticles for pulmonary drug delivery. The fine particle size and high surface area of the resulting nanoparticles enhance drug dispersion and absorption in the lungs (Liversidge and Cundy, 1995). Mechanical methods are advantageous for producing drug carriers with controlled particle size and a high surface area. They have been used in the production of nanocrystals which improve the solubility and bioavailability of poorly water-soluble drugs (Merisko-Liversidge, Liversidge, and Cooper, 2003). Also, sonication and HPH often employed in the preparation of liposomal and polymeric nanoparticles for drug delivery.

2.3.4. Biological Synthesis

2.3.4.1. Plant-Mediated Synthesis

Biological synthesis methods are environmentally sustainable as they reduce the need for hazardous chemicals and high-temperature conditions. Many biological agents like plant extracts provide natural capping and stabilizing agents which helps in preventing agglomeration and enhancing colloidal stability. By using different biological agents or modifying the synthesis conditions researchers can modify the surface properties of nanoparticles for specific drug delivery needs. Despite these advantages, biological synthesis methods may have limitations related to scalability, batch-to-batch variability, and control over nanoparticle properties. Researchers must carefully select the biological agents and optimize the synthesis conditions to ensure reproducibility and consistent particle characteristics (Kalimuthu et al., 2008; Sathishkumar et al., 2009).

2.4. Drug Loading and Encapsulation

The process of loading and encapsulating drugs within nanoparticles plays a pivotal role in determining the efficiency, release kinetics, and specificity of DDS.

1. **Selection of Drug:** The choice of drug is very important in drug loading. Different drugs have distinct physicochemical properties, solubility, and compatibility with nanoparticles. Hydrophobic drugs such as paclitaxel, curcumin can be incorporated into hydrophobic nanoparticles. Whereas hydrophilic drugs like doxorubicin, insulin require hydrophilic or amphiphilic nanoparticles for effective encapsulation (Attia et al., 2011; Blanco, Shen, and Ferrari, 2015).
2. **Loading Techniques:** Several methods are employed for drug loading and encapsulation in nanoparticles.

2.4.1. Drug Selection and Compatibility

Selecting the appropriate drug for nanoparticle-based DDS is a critical step that determines the success of the therapy. The compatibility between the drug and the nanoparticle carrier plays a pivotal role in achieving the desired therapeutic outcome while maintaining stability and efficacy.

1. **Drug Properties:** The choice of a drug for nanoparticle encapsulation should consider its physicochemical properties including solubility, hydrophobicity, and molecular weight. Drugs with poor water solubility often benefit from encapsulation in nanoparticles which can enhance their solubility and bioavailability (Liu et al., 2016). For example, paclitaxel, a hydrophobic chemotherapeutic drug can be effectively delivered using various nanoparticles (Li and Guo, 2015). Some drugs are pH-sensitive and may degrade in the harsh acidic environment of the stomach. Nanoparticles can be designed to protect these drugs enabling them to reach the target site intact, where they can release the drug payload in response to local pH changes.
2. **Drug Loading Methods:** Following drugs selection, drug loading is another crucial component. One of the most used methods of encapsulating drugs is co-precipitation encapsulation. For instance, this technique is frequently used to load medications into superparamagnetic iron oxide nanoparticles (SPIONs), resulting in a multipurpose DDS (Wang, 2001). Another factor is adsorption onto nanoparticle surfaces, which involves physically binding of drug molecules to the surface of nanoparticles. This method is simple and allows for high drug loading, making it suitable for both hydrophobic and hydrophilic drugs (Maeda et al., 2000). Emulsion and Solvent Evaporation technique involves dissolving the drug and the polymer used to make the nanoparticles in a common solvent. The resulting emulsion is then subjected to solvent evaporation leading to drug encapsulation.

2.4.2. Encapsulation Techniques

One extremely promising method for the development of nanomedicine is the encapsulation of medicinal substances or therapeutic agents in various NCs. Nanotechnology is often utilized to solve some of the limits of medication delivery, particularly in cancer, and to increase the efficacy of drug administration. The only available treatments for malignancies are surgery, radiation, chemotherapy, and immunotherapy due to their diverse qualities (Kievit and Zhang, 2011). Since they can be included into a variety of food products and drinks and contain lipids, which the bioactive may dissolve in, nanoemulsions are a great choice for encapsulating lipid-soluble bioactives. They are also rather clear. Additionally, the nanoemulsions can be freeze- or spray-dried to create various solid formulations (Öztürk, 2017). In the pharmaceutical industry, freeze drying nanosuspensions to produce dry nanoparticles is a well-recognized technique. Matrix forming is frequently added to the nanosuspension in order to preserve the major goals of the nanoparticulate system, which include quick dissolution, the breakdown of solid forms, and redispersion of individual nanoparticles (Abdelwahed et al., 2006). Drug nanoparticles are also encapsulated utilizing supercritical CO_2 methods. Many supercritical CO_2 procedures have been employed in the past to isolate nanoparticles by coating or encapsulating techniques. A supercritical fluid approach was developed in 2000 by Benoit et al. to facilitate the encapsulation of API microparticles with lipids or polymers (Verma et al., 2021). The encapsulation strategy to encapsulate caffeine-loaded microcrystalline cellulose (MCC, 1–1.4 mm) beads with ethyl cellulose was described by Niu et al. The supercritical antisolvent process integrated with a Wurster-type coater (SAS-WTS) was used in this process (Niu et al., 2012).

2.5. Biocompatibility and Safety

2.5.1. Toxicity Assessment

1. ***In Vivo* Studies:** Animal studies are conducted to evaluate nanoparticle toxicity in living organisms. These studies help determine how nanoparticles interact with biological systems and their impact on various organs and tissues. Toxicological endpoints, such as histopathology and biochemistry, are assessed to gauge the safety profile (Fadeel and Garcia-Bennett, 2010).
2. **Nanoparticle Characterization:** Detailed characterization of nanoparticles, including size, shape, surface charge, and stability, is essential to understand their potential toxicity. Poorly characterized nanoparticles may pose unexpected risks (Clogston and Patri, 2011). Dose-Response Assessments; Evaluating the relationship between nanoparticle dose and biological responses is vital for determining safe dosage levels in drug formulations. Establishing the maximum tolerated dose (MTD) and therapeutic index is crucial for clinical translation (Monopoli, Åberg, Salvati, and Dawson, 2012). Long-term and Chronic Toxicity; Nanoparticle safety assessment should consider long-term and chronic exposure scenarios, as well as potential accumulation and persistence in the body over time (Colombo et al., 2012).

2.5.2. Biocompatible Nanoparticle Design

2.5.2.1. Surface Functionalization

Modifying nanoparticle surfaces with biocompatible polymers, such as PEG, can improve their stability, reduce immune recognition, and prolong circulation time in the body (Owens and Peppas, 2006).

1. **Natural Materials:** Using biodegradable and biocompatible materials, such as chitosan (CH), hyaluronic acid (HA), or lipids, for nanoparticle synthesis can enhance their biocompatibility and reduce the risk of toxicity (Silva et al., 2017).
2. **Incorporating Targeting Ligands:** Nanoparticles have the potential to revolutionize drug delivery by improving drug pharmacokinetics, reducing side effects, and enhancing therapeutic efficacy. However, for these benefits to be fully realized, nanoparticles must efficiently and selectively reach their target sites. Incorporating targeting ligands into nanoparticles is a strategy that addresses this challenge by enhancing their specificity for specific cells, tissues, or disease sites. The surface of nanoparticles is engineered to display targeting ligands called surface modification.

2.6. Applications in Disease Treatment

2.6.1. Cancer Therapy

Multifunctional nanoparticles can carry multiple therapeutic agents including chemotherapy drugs, genes, and imaging agents, facilitating combination therapy for enhanced cancer treatment (Liu and Lu, 2007). Globally, cancer continues to be the second most common cause of death. Because cancer is so diverse, it can be extremely difficult to create effective treatments for the disease. However, tailored chemotherapy has been created to treat patients who exhibit certain biomarkers, and precision medicine has emerged as a viable strategy. Patients with chronic myeloid leukemia who express the BCR-ABL fusion protein from the Philadelphia chromosome are treated with imatinib, the first medication of this kind (American Cancer Society, 2019; Dalby et al., 2019). By directly targeting the cancer cell, administering the agent at a regulated pace, and maximizing the therapeutic drug efficacy, recent advancements in nano-delivery systems have circumvented these restrictions (Mishra, Patel, and Tiwari, 2010). Two main techniques are employed to deliver anti-cancer drugs to the tumor site: passive targeting and active targeting. A variety of nanoparticles have been produced for this purpose. The basis for passive targeting is the build-up of therapeutic agents in tumors because of their unique characteristics in contrast to normal tissues. The EPR effect, which is the transport and retention of therapeutic nanoparticles, is frequently observed in tumors due to their leaky vasculature and defectively lymphatic drainage (Danhier, Feron, and Preat, 2010; Maeda, Bharate, and Daruwalla, 2009).

2.6.2. Infectious Diseases

Nanoparticles are used in the fight against infectious diseases with applications in drug delivery and diagnostics. Antibacterial Nanoparticles like AgNPs and other antimicrobial NMs have demonstrated efficacy in combating bacterial infections (Raghunath and Perumal, 2017). Nanoparticles can serve as vaccine carriers providing controlled release and enhanced immune responses, which is critical for addressing infectious diseases (Karch and Burkhard, 2016). Also, functionalized nanoparticles enable the sensitive and rapid detection of pathogens aiding in early diagnosis and monitoring of infectious diseases. An illustration of various applications of Nanoparticles in healthcare sector has been shown in Figure 2.2 (Patra et al., 2018). Polymer-based and non-polymeric nanoparticles, as well as liposomes that enhance the anti-microbial action of medications, are examples of nano-delivery applications for the treatment of infectious disorders (Zazo, Colino, and Lanao, 2016). Antiviral medications can also be made with nanoparticles. Viral adjuvants such toll-like receptors, viral glycoproteins, or protein fractions are carried by virosome vaccines. Such vaccinations such as Epaxal for influenza and Inflexal V for hepatitis-A, are already utilized in clinics for therapeutic purposes (Ghaffar et al., 2014). AgNPs in central venous catheters are examples of anti-microbial nano-drugs that are used to adorn medical equipment to prevent biofilm development. Additionally, certain nanoparticles, such as *Verigene*, *Silverline*, *Acticoat*, or *Endorem* SPIONs, are employed as medical devices or in diagnostics (Bozzuto and Molinari, 2015; Wang, Hu, and Shao, 2017; Wu et al., 2015).

2.6.3. Neurological Disorders

Nanoparticles hold promise in treating neurological disorders by overcoming the blood–brain barrier (BBB) and enhancing drug delivery. Liposomes and polymeric nanoparticles can transport drugs across the BBB, enabling targeted therapy for conditions like Alzheimer's and Parkinson's disease (PD) (Liu and Lu, 2007).

Nanoparticles can encapsulate neuroprotective drugs and facilitate their controlled release, potentially reducing neuronal damage and promoting recovery (Nance et al., 2012). Due to a progressive loss of neurons, patients with neurological disorders, such as those with Alzheimer's, PD, and multiple sclerosis (MS), experience symptoms pertaining to movement, memory, and dementia. To preserve the homeostasis of the central nervous system (CNS), the BBB is a highly selective semipermeable membrane that divides the brain from the circulation and blocks the passage of most molecules in the blood (Pardridge, 2012). Consequently, large dosages are needed, which might have negative systemic consequences. Targeted delivery and sustained local release of therapeutic drugs into the afflicted area of the brain once they pass the BBB are the key goals of nanoparticle-based treatment methods in neurological disorders (Wohlfart, Gelperina, and Kreuter, 2012). Only a small number of methods have been described for other neurodegenerative illnesses, such as MS and amyotrophic lateral sclerosis (ALS), despite the fact that several research publications on the creation of innovative therapeutic nanoparticles for AD and PD have been published. The progressive neurodegenerative illness known as ALS affects the motor neurons in the brain and spinal cord that regulate voluntary muscular movements, such as chewing, walking, and speaking. Clinically, respiratory failure leading to increasing muscular weakening is fatal. Riluzole is currently the sole medication authorized for the treatment of ALS. Riluzole is more likely to reach the CNS when loaded into SLNs. This also results in pH-based regulated release with less random biodistribution in organs such the liver, spleen, heart, kidneys, and lung (Bondi et al., 2010; Mazibuko et al., 2015).

2.6.4. Inflammatory Conditions

Nanoparticles are utilized in managing inflammatory conditions by delivering anti-inflammatory drugs or modulating the immune response. Nanoparticles can be administered directly to the site of inflammation, enabling sustained drug release and reducing systemic side effects (Butoescu et al., 2012).

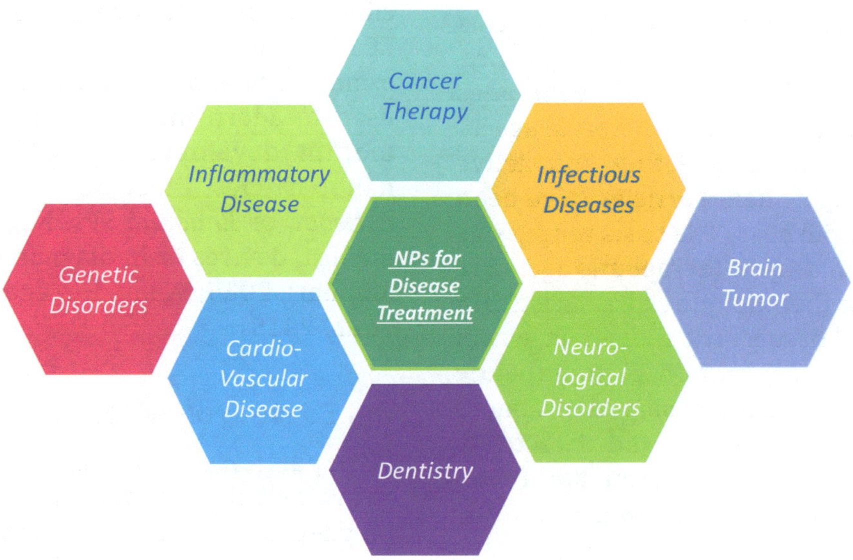

Figure 2.2. Schematic representation of how different nanoparticles are used in healthcare and medicine.

Immunomodulation, some nanoparticles can modulate immune responses offering potential in treating autoimmune and inflammatory disorders (Loutfy et al., 2017). Systems of nanoparticles provide promise for the delivery of therapeutic drugs, especially to target inflammatory tissue (synovial membrane), limiting unwanted and systemic effects. Certolizumab pegol (CZP) is a commonly used inhibitor of TNF-α. When CZP is nano-formulated with PEG, its half-life is increased to around 14 days, and clinical studies have produced encouraging outcomes for RA patients' long-term treatment. Using non-drug loaded, stand-alone C_{60} fullerenes to target inflammatory tissues shown encouraging outcomes in RA therapy by lowering synovitis and decreasing bone resorption and degradation (Horton, Walsh, and Emery, 2012; Lim et al., 2018; Yudoh et al., 2009).

2.7. Challenges and Future Directions

Nanoparticle-based DDS have witnessed significant progress, yet they face several challenges that are driving innovation and shaping future prospects. Ensuring the biocompatibility of nanoparticles is a key challenge, as some materials may induce immune responses or toxicity (Butoescu et al., 2012). Bridging the gap between promising preclinical results and clinical translation poses significant challenges (Loutfy et al., 2017). Scaling up nanoparticle production while maintaining quality and consistency is a complex issue (Nel et al., 2006). Regulatory approvals and safety assessments for nanoparticle-based DDS require clear guidelines and standards (Soppimath et al., 2001).

Tailoring drug-loaded nanoparticles to individual patient profiles for precision medicine is an emerging trend (Puri et al., 2009). Designing nanoparticles with responsiveness to environmental cues, such as pH or temperature, for controlled drug release (Etheridge et al., 2013). Developing nanoparticles that can deliver multiple therapeutic agents simultaneously, enhancing treatment efficacy (Ventola, 2013). Integrating nanoparticles into immunotherapy strategies for enhanced immune system response against diseases like cancer (Soppimath et al., 2001). Exploring nanoparticles for delivering gene-editing tools and RNA-based therapies (Wang et al., 2012).

Utilizing novel biomaterials with improved biocompatibility, safety, and functionality (Batrakova and Kabanov, 2008). Customizing DDS based on genetic and physiological factors for optimized treatment (Yin and Kanasty, 2014). Advancing minimally invasive methods for precise and targeted nanoparticle delivery (Hossen et al., 2018). Implementing artificial intelligence (AI) and data analytics for better DDS design (Guo et al., 2021).

Encouraging international collaboration to address regulatory and safety concerns and promote global acceptance of nanoparticle-based drug delivery (Vahrmeijer et al., 2013). In summary, the challenges in nanoparticle drug delivery are driving innovation and fostering promising future directions. With advancements in personalized medicine, smart nanoparticles, and regulatory harmonization, the field holds tremendous potential to revolutionize healthcare. A table summarizing nanoparticle usage and their limitations has been added in Table 2.1 (Alkilani et al., 2015; Kirtane et al., 2021; Orrantia-Borunda et al., 2022; Smith and Edelman, 2023; Sun, 2022).

Table 2.1. Summary of Nanoparticle Usage in Various Diseases along with Their Limitations

SL. No.	Medical Condition	Nanomaterial Type	Usage in Disease	Limitations	References
1.	Breast cancer	Carbon nanostructures	May be useful in the early phases of breast cancer diagnosis and therapy, even if there are only a few cancerous cells present.	May cause toxicity	Orrantia-Borunda et al. (2022)
2.	Infectious diseases (e.g., HIV, HSV)	PEGylated PLGA nanoparticles	Maximum tissue absorption has been attained using PEG-coated nanoparticles; however, tissue uptake was restricted to the lower reproductive tract. The increased diffusivity of PEGylated nanoparticles across the mucous layer may account for their improved tissue absorption.	Low nanoparticle absorption in the upper reproductive canal, bringing the coverage offered by these systems into doubt. Medication concentrations in mouse models become undetectable roughly 24 hours after administration, indicating that continuous delivery may be achievable for only a short period.	Kirtane et al. (2021)
3.	Neurological diseases	Gold nanoparticles (CNM-Au8 [Clene Nanomedicine Inc.])	Intended to assist brain cells in enhancing their energy stores and stress resistance. Potentially broad-reaching neurotherapeutic that can restore neurodegenerative disease–impaired cellular bioenergetics. Studied for neurodegenerative conditions such as MS and ALS.	Clinical trial results are expected in late 2024	Sun (2022)
4.	Cardiovascular disease	Single-walled carbon nanotubes (SWNTs)	Abolished all adverse effects, including anemia, reticulocytosis, and splenomegaly.	Toxicity and safety issues depending on material and size. Long-term biocompatibility, circulation half-life, repeatability, and serum stability.	Smith and Edelman (2023)

2.8. Conclusion

In summary, although there have been great achievements in the field of nanoparticle-based DDS, there are still substantial obstacles that will likely spur further research and development as well as determine future paths. Assuring biocompatibility and safety, negotiating the complexity of clinical translation, resolving scalability and manufacturing concerns, and setting clear regulatory requirements are only a few of the essential parts of the current challenges. And overcoming the obstacles related to choosing the right emulsifiers to stabilize nanoemulsions and optimizing encapsulation settings. The kind of emulsifier, core materials, and manufacturing parameters all affect the chemical and physical stability of nanoemulsions, hence it is important to research and optimize these factors. Although there are several benefits to using nanoparticles in the biomedical area, there is currently little study on the safety of different NPs for this usage. Our ability to control cell fate will probably increase with new approaches to direct nano-bio-interactions at subcellular compartments, such as mitochondrial or epigenetic targeting.

Additionally, new approaches to sub-cellular analysis, such as super-resolution microscopy, cryo-electron microscopy, high content analytics, and imaging cytometry, will likely yield new insights into how disease can be modulated or reversed using nanoscale technologies. The creation of nanoparticles that can successively navigate these barriers will be made possible by advancements in materials science and a deeper comprehension of the biological mechanisms regulating these barriers and how they change in different disease conditions. Lastly, until a thorough understanding of the toxicological status of current NPs is achieved, it is critical to recognize the challenge of establishing practical techniques to generate safer NPs.

KEY TERMS FROM THIS CHAPTER

- disease treatment
- drug delivery systems
- drug loading
- immune responses
- multiple therapeutic agents
- nanoparticles
- safety assessment

References

1. Abdelwahed, W., Degobert, G., Stainmesse, S., & Fessi, H. (2006). Freeze-drying of nanoparticles: Formulation, process, and storage considerations. *Advanced Drug Delivery Reviews, 58*(15), 1688–1713.

2. Alkilani, A. Z., McCrudden, M. T., Donnelly, R. F., & Mills, A. (2015). Laser-engineered dissolving microneedle arrays for protein delivery: Potential for enhanced intradermal vaccination. *Journal of Pharmacy and Pharmacology, 67*(3), 409–425.

3. American Cancer Society. (2019). *Cancer Facts & Figures 2019*. American Cancer Society.

4. Attia, A. B. E., Ong, Z. Y., Hedrick, J. L., & Lee, P. P. (2011). Drug delivery to solid tumors. *Chemical Society Reviews, 41*(19), 6641–6655.

5. Barenholz, Y. (2012). Doxil®—The first FDA-approved nano-drug: Lessons learned. *Journal of Controlled Release, 160*(2), 117–134.

6. Batrakova, E. V., & Kabanov, A. V. (2008). Pluronic block copolymers: Evolution of drug delivery concept from inert nanocarriers to biological response modifiers. *Journal of Controlled Release, 130*(2), 98–106.

7. Bhatia, S. (2016). Nanoparticles types, classification, characterization, fabrication methods, and drug delivery applications. In *Natural Polymer Drug Delivery Systems: Nanoparticles, Plants, and Algae* (pp. 33–93). Springer International Publishing.

8. Bitar, A., Ahmad, N. M., Fessi, H., & Elaissari, A. (2012). Silica-based nanoparticles for biomedical applications. *Drug Discovery Today, 17*(21, 22), 1147–1154.

9. Blanco, E., Shen, H., & Ferrari, M. (2015). Principles of nanoparticle design for overcoming biological barriers to drug delivery. *Nature Biotechnology, 33*(9), 941–951.

10. Bondi, M. L., Craparo, E. F., Giammona, G., & Drago, F. (2010). Brain-targeted solid lipid nanoparticles containing riluzole: Preparation, characterization, and biodistribution. *Nanomedicine: Nanotechnology, Biology and Medicine, 5*, 25–32.

11. Bozzuto, G., & Molinari, A. (2015). Liposomes as nanomedical devices. *International Journal of Nanomedicine, 10*, 975–999.

12. Brar, S. K., & Verma, M. (2011). Measurement of nanoparticles by light-scattering techniques. *Trends in Analytical Chemistry, 30*(1), 4–17.

13. Brown, S. B., Wang, L., Jungels, R. R., & Sharma, B. (2019). Effects of cartilage-targeting moieties on nanoparticle biodistribution in healthy and osteoarthritic joints. *Acta Biomaterial, 101*, 469–483.

14. Butoescu, N., Jordan, O., Burdet, P., Stadelmann, P., Petri-Fink, A., & Hofmann, H. (2012). Dexamethasone-containing biodegradable superparamagnetic microparticles for local drug delivery to the inner ear. *Advanced Functional Materials, 22*(4), 718–728.

15. Chin, W., Lim, W., Wei, W., Parmentier, J., Widzinski, M., Tan, E. H., & Gokhale, R. (2014). A brief literature and patent review of nanosuspensions to a final drug product. *Journal of Pharmaceutical Sciences, 103*(9), 2980–2999.

16. Clogston, J. D., & Patri, A. K. (2011). Characterization of nanoparticles intended for drug delivery. In *Methods in Enzymology* (Vol. 464, pp. 163–194). Academic Press.

17. Colombo, M., Carregal-Romero, S., Casula, M. F., Gutiérrez, L., Morales, M. P., Böhm, I. B., & Parak, W. J. (2012). Biological applications of magnetic nanoparticles. *Chemical Society Reviews, 41*(11), 4306–4334.

18. Dalby, M., Cree, I. A., Challoner, B. R., Ghosh, S., & Thurston, D. E. (2019). The precision medicine approach to cancer therapy: Part 1 solid tumors. *Pharmaceutical Journal*. https://doi.org/10.1211/PJ.2019.20207119.

19. Danhier, F., Feron, O., & Preat, V. (2010). To exploit the tumor microenvironment: Passive and active tumor targeting of nanocarriers for anti-cancer drug delivery. *Journal of Controlled Release, 148*, 135–146.

20. Elsaesser, A., & Howard, C. V. (2012). Toxicology of nanoparticles. *Advanced Drug Delivery Reviews, 64*(2), 129–137.

21. Etheridge, M. L., Campbell, S. A., Erdman, A. G., Haynes, C. L., Wolf, S. M., & McCullough, J. (2013). The big picture on nanomedicine: The state of investigational and approved nanomedicine products. *Nanomedicine: Nanotechnology, Biology and Medicine, 9*(1), 1–14.

22. Fadeel, B., & Garcia-Bennett, A. E. (2010). Better safe than sorry: Understanding the toxicological properties of inorganic nanoparticles manufactured for biomedical applications. *Advanced Drug Delivery Reviews, 62*(3), 362–374.

23. Fang, J., Nakamura, H., & Maeda, H. (2011). The EPR effect: Unique features of tumor blood vessels for drug delivery, factors involved, and limitations and augmentation of the effect. *Advanced Drug Delivery Reviews, 63*(3), 136–151.

24. Fonseca-Santos, B., Gremião, M. P. D., & Chorilli, M. (2015). Nanotechnology-based drug delivery systems for the treatment of Alzheimer's disease. *International Journal of Nanomedicine, 10*, 4981–5003.

25. Ghaffar, K. A., Giddam, A. K., Zaman, M., Skwarczynski, M., & Toth, I. (2014). Liposomes as nano vaccine delivery systems. *Current Topics in Medicinal Chemistry, 14*, 1194–1208.

26. Guo, C., Shi, F., Sun, J., Feng, R., & Shi, W. (2021). Biomimetic drug delivery systems for precision cancer therapy. *Molecules, 26*(12), 3694.

27. Hanafy, A., Spahn-Langguth, H., Vergnault, G., Grenier, P., Tubic Grozdanis, M., Lenhardt, T., & Langguth, P. (2007). Pharmacokinetic evaluation of oral fenofibrate nanosuspensions and SLN in comparison to conventional suspensions of micronized drug. *Advanced Drug Delivery Reviews, 59*(5), 419–426.

28. Hessel, C. M., Pattani, V. P., Rasch, M., Panthani, M. G., Koo, B., Tunnell, J. W., & Korgel, B. A. (2011). Copper selenide nanocrystals for photothermal therapy. *Nano Letters, 11*(6), 2560–2566.

29. Hickey, J. W., Santos, J. L., Williford, J. M., & Mao, H. Q. (2015). Control of polymeric nanoparticle size to improve therapeutic delivery. *Journal of Controlled Release, 219*, 536–547.

30. Horton, S., Walsh, C., & Emery, P. (2012). Certolizumab pegol for the treatment of rheumatoid arthritis. *Expert Opinion on Biological Therapy, 12*, 235–249.

31. Hossen, S., Hossain, M. K., Basher, M. K., & Mia, M. N. H. (2018). A concise review of analytical methods for quantification of paclitaxel in biological matrices. *Journal of Applied Pharmaceutical Science, 8*(7), 154–159.

32. Jokerst, J. V., Lobovkina, T., Zare, R. N., & Gambhir, S. S. (2011). Nanoparticle PEGylation for imaging and therapy. *Nanomedicine*, *6*(4), 715–728.

33. Jurak, M., Wiącek, A. E., Ładniak, A., Przykaza, K., & Szafran, K. (2021). What affects the biocompatibility of polymers? *Advances in Colloid and Interface Science*, *294*, 102451.

34. Kalimuthu, K., Suresh Babu, R., Venkataraman, D., Bilal, M., & Gurunathan, S. (2008). Biosynthesis of silver nanocrystals by *Bacillus licheniformis*. *Colloids and Surfaces B: Bio Interfaces*, *65*(1), 150–153.

35. Karch, C. P., & Burkhard, P. (2016). Vaccine technologies: From whole organisms to rationally designed protein assemblies. *Biochemical Pharmacology*, *120*, 1–14.

36. Keck, C. M., & Müller, R. H. (2006). Drug nanocrystals of poorly soluble drugs produced by high pressure homogenization. *European Journal of Pharmaceutical Sciences*, *62*(1), 3–16.

37. Kermode, M. (2004). Unsafe injections in low-income country health settings: Need for injection safety promotion to prevent the spread of blood-borne viruses. *Health Promotion International*, *19*(1), 95–103.

38. Kievit, F. M., & Zhang, M. (2011). Surface engineering of iron oxide nanoparticles for targeted cancer therapy. *Accounts of Chemical Research*, *44*(10), 853–862. https://doi.org/10.1021/ar2000277.

39. Kim, H. S., Sun, X., Lee, J. H., Kim, H. W., Fu, X., & Leong, K. W. (2019). Advanced drug delivery systems and artificial skin grafts for skin wound healing. *Advanced Drug Delivery Reviews*, *146*, 209–239.

40. Kirtane, A. R., Verma, M., Karandikar, P., et al. (2021). Nanotechnology approaches for global infectious diseases. *Nature Nanotechnology*, *16*, 369–384.

41. Kou, L., et al. (2018). Transporter-guided delivery of nanoparticles to improve drug permeation across cellular barriers and drug exposure to selective cell types. *Frontiers in Pharmacology*, *9*, Article 790.

42. Laurent, S., Forge, D., Port, M., Roch, A., Robic, C., Vander Elst, L., & Müller, R. N. (2008). Magnetic iron oxide nanoparticles: Synthesis, stabilization, vectorization, physicochemical characterizations, and biological applications. *Chemical Reviews*, *108*(6), 2064–2110.

43. Li, J., & Guo, Y. (2015). Liposomal paclitaxel formulations: A comprehensive study on different formulations and their pharmacokinetics. *Expert Opinion on Drug Delivery*, *12*(1), 129–142.

44. Lim, H., Lee, S. H., Lee, H. T., Lee, J. U., Son, J. Y., Shin, W., & Heo, Y. S. (2018). Structural biology of the TNF-alpha antagonists used in the treatment of rheumatoid arthritis. *International Journal of Molecular Sciences*, *19*(7), 1–18.

45. Liu, D., Yang, F., Xiong, F., & Gu, N. (2016). The smart drug delivery system and its clinical potential. *Theragnostic*, *6*(9), 1306–1323.

46. Liu, Y., & Lu, W. (2007). Recent advances in brain tumor-targeted nano-drug delivery systems. *Expert Opinion on Drug Delivery*, *4*(2), 149–164.

47. Liversidge, G. G., & Cundy, K. C. (1995). Particle size reduction for improvement of oral bioavailability of hydrophobic drugs: I. Absolute oral bioavailability of nanocrystalline danazol in beagle dogs. *International Journal of Pharmaceutics*, *125*(1), 91–97.

48. Loutfy, S. A., El-Sherbiny, I. M., Abdel-Monem, R. A., Mohamed, M. B., & Mohamed, A. A. (2017). Surface modification of PLGA nanoparticles for the delivery of dexamethasone sodium phosphate: Cellular uptake, intracellular localization, and *in vitro* anti-inflammatory activities. *Journal of Pharmaceutical Sciences, 106*(2), 272–281.

49. Maeda, H., Bharate, G. Y., & Daruwalla, J. (2009). Polymeric drugs for efficient tumor-targeted drug delivery based on EPR effect. *European Journal of Pharmaceutical Sciences, 71*, 409–419.

50. Maeda, H., Wu, J., Sawa, T., Matsumura, Y., & Hori, K. (2000). Tumor vascular permeability and the EPR effect in macromolecular therapeutics: A review. *Journal of Controlled Release, 65*(1, 2), 271–284.

51. Mazibuko, Z., Choonara, Y. E., Kumar, P., Du Toit, L. C., Modi, G., Naidoo, D., & Pillay, V. (2015). A review of the potential role of nano-enabled drug delivery technologies in amyotrophic lateral sclerosis: Lessons learned from other neurodegenerative disorders. *Journal of Pharmaceutical Sciences, 104*, 1213–1229.

52. Merisko-Liversidge, E., Liversidge, G. G., & Cooper, E. R. (2003). Nanosizing: A formulation approach for poorly-water-soluble compounds. *European Journal of Pharmaceutical Sciences, 18*(2), 113–120.

53. Mishra, B., Patel, B. B., & Tiwari, S. (2010). Colloidal nanocarriers: A review on formulation technology, types, and applications toward targeted drug delivery. *Nanomedicine: Nanotechnology, Biology and Medicine, 6*, 9–24.

54. Missaoui, W. N., Arnold, R. D., & Cummings, B. S. (2018). Toxicological status of nanoparticles: What we know and what we don't know. *Chemical-Biological Interactions, 295*, 1–12.

55. Mitragotri, S., et al. (2017). Drug delivery research for the future: Expanding the nano horizons and beyond. *Journal of Controlled Release, 246*, 183–184.

56. Mittal, A. K., Chisti, Y., & Banerjee, U. C. (2013). Synthesis of metallic nanoparticles using plant extracts. *Biotechnology Advances, 31*(2), 346–356.

57. Monopoli, M. P., Åberg, C., Salvati, A., & Dawson, K. A. (2012). Biomolecular coronas provide the biological identity of nanosized materials. *Nature Nanotechnology, 7*(12), 779–786.

58. Nakamura, Y., Mochida, A., Choyke, P. L., & Kobayashi, H. (2016). Nanodrug delivery: Is the enhanced permeability and retention effect sufficient for curing cancer? *Bioconjugate Chemistry, 27*(11), 2225–2238.

59. Nance, E. A., Woodworth, G. F., Sailor, K. A., Shih, T. Y., Xu, Q., Swaminathan, G., & Hanes, J. (2012). A dense poly (ethylene glycol) coating improves penetration of large polymeric nanoparticles within brain tissue. *Science Translational Medicine, 4*(149), 149ra119.

60. Nel, A., Xia, T., Mädler, L., & Li, N. (2006). Toxic potential of materials at the nano level. *Science, 311*(5761), 622–627.

61. Niu, F., Haslam, J., Rajewski, R., & Subramaniam, B. (2012). A fluidized-bed coating technology using near-critical carbon dioxide as fluidizing and drying medium. *Journal of Pharmaceutical Sciences, 66*(3), 315–320.

62. Orrantia-Borunda, E., Acuña-Aguilar, L. E., & Ramírez-Valdespino, C. A. (2022). Nanomaterials for breast cancer. In H. N. Mayrovitz (Ed.), *Breast Cancer*. Exon Publications. Online first. https://doi.org/10.1093/.

63. Owens, D. E., & Peppas, N. A. (2006). Opsonization, biodistribution, and pharmacokinetics of polymeric nanoparticles. *International Journal of Pharmaceutics, 307*(1), 93–102.

64. Öztürk, B. (2017). Nano emulsions for food fortification with lipophilic vitamins: Production challenges, stability, and bioavailability. *European Journal of Lipid Science and Technology, 119*(12), 1500539.

65. Pardridge, W. M. (2012). Drug transport across the blood-brain barrier. *Journal of Cerebral Blood Flow and Metabolism, 32*, 1959–1972.

66. Patil, A., Mishra, V., Thakur, S., Riyaz, B., Kaur, A., Khursheed, R., Patil, K., & Sathe, B. (2019). Nanotechnology derived nanotools in biomedical perspectives: An update. *Current Nanoscience, 15*(2), 137–146.

67. Patra, J. K., Das, G., Fraceto, L. F., Campos, E. V. R., Rodriguez-Torres, M. D. P., Acosta-Torres, L. S., & Parveen, A. (2018). Nano-based drug delivery systems: Recent developments and future prospects. *Journal of Nanobiotechnology, 16*(1), 71.

68. Patravale, V. B., Date, A. A., & Kulkarni, R. M. (2004). Nanosuspensions: A promising drug delivery strategy. *Journal of Pharmacy and Pharmacology, 56*(7), 827–840.

69. Puri, A., Loomis, K., Smith, B., Lee, J. H., & Yavlovich, A. (2009). Scale-up and scale-down methodologies for the rapid evaluation of critical material attributes of PLGA nanoparticles for drug delivery. *AAPS Pharm SciTech, 10*(2), 728–738.

70. Puri, A., Loomis, K., Smith, B., Lee, J. H., Yavlovich, A., Heldman, E., & Blumenthal, R. (2009). Lipid-based nanoparticles as pharmaceutical drug carriers: From concepts to clinic. *Critical Reviews in Therapeutic Drug Carrier Systems, 26*(6), 523–580.

71. Raghunath, A., & Perumal, E. (2017). Metal oxide nanoparticles as antimicrobial agents: A promise for the future. *International Journal of Antimicrobial Agents, 49*(2), 137–152.

72. Ramanathan, S., et al. (2021). Nanoparticle synthetic methods: Strength and limitations. *Nanotechnology, 32*(3), 1320–1334.

73. Rasenack, N., & Müller, B. W. (2004). Micron-size drug particles: Common and novel micronization techniques. *Pharmaceutical Development and Technology, 9*(1), 1–13.

74. Reddy, L. H., Arias, J. L., Nicolas, J., & Couvreur, P. (2012). Magnetic nanoparticles: Design and characterization, toxicity and biocompatibility, pharmaceutical and biomedical applications. *Chemical Reviews, 112*(11), 5818–5878.

75. Sathishkumar, M., Sneha, K., Won, S. W., Cho, C. W., Kim, S., & Yun, Y. S. (2009). Cinnamon zeylanicum bark extract and powder mediated green synthesis of nano-crystalline silver particles and its bactericidal activity. *Colloids and Surfaces B: Bio Interfaces, 73*(2), 332–338.

76. Sercombe, L., et al. (2015). Advances and challenges of liposome assisted drug delivery. *Frontiers in Pharmacology, 6*, Article 286.

77. Shreffler, J. W., Pullan, J. E., Dailey, K. M., Mallik, S., & Brooks, A. E. (2019). Overcoming hurdles in nanoparticle clinical translation: The influence of experimental design and surface modification. *International Journal of Molecular Sciences, 20*(24), 6056.

78. Silva, A. C., Santos, D., Ferreira, L., Lino, M. M., & Pereira, M. C. (2017). Lipid-based nanoparticles in pharmaceutical development: What is new? *Current Medicinal Chemistry, 24*(20), 2179–2201.

79. Smith, B. R., & Edelman, E. R. (2023). Nanomedicines for cardiovascular disease. *Nature Cardiovascular Research*, *2*, 351–367.

80. Soppimath, K. S., Aminabhavi, T. M., Kulkarni, A. R., & Rudzinski, W. E. (2001). Biodegradable polymeric nanoparticles as drug delivery devices. *Journal of Controlled Release*, *70*(1, 2), 1–20.

81. Stevanović, M., & Uskoković, D. (2009). Poly(lactide-co-glycolide)-based micro and nanoparticles for the controlled drug delivery of vitamins. *Current Nanoscience*, *5*(1), 1–14.

82. Sun, J. S. (2022). Use of nanoparticles to combat neurodegenerative disease. *Neurology Live*, *5*(5).

83. Sun, Y. P., Atorngitjawat, P., Meziani, M. J., Tang, L., Kelly, K. F., & Carroll, D. L. (2005). Preparation of gold nanoparticles via vaporization of a gold foil and their size-dependent catalytic activity. *Nano Letters*, *5*(4), 685–693.

84. Vahrmeijer, A. L., Hutteman, M., van der Vorst, J. R., van de Velde, C. J., Frangioni, J. V., & Swijnenburg, R. J. (2013). Image-guided cancer surgery using near-infrared fluorescence. *Nature Reviews Clinical Oncology*, *10*(9), 507–518.

85. Ventola, C. L. (2013). Progress in personalized medicine. *Pharmacy and Therapeutics*, *38*(4), 225–240.

86. Verma, V., et al. (2021). Production and isolation of pharmaceutical drug nanoparticles. *International Journal of Pharmaceutics*, *603*, 120708. https://doi.org/10.1016/j.ijpharm.2021.120708.

87. Wang, A. Z., Langer, R., & Farokhzad, O. C. (2012). Nanoparticle delivery of cancer drugs. *Annual Review of Medicine*, *63*, 185–198.

88. Wang, J., Potocny, A. M., Rosenthal, J., & Day, E. S. (2020). Gold nano shell–linear tetrapyrrole conjugates for near infrared–activated dual photodynamic and photothermal therapies. *ACS Omega*, *5*(2), 926–940.

89. Wang, L., Hu, C., & Shao, L. (2017). The antimicrobial activity of nanoparticles: Present situation and prospects for the future. *International Journal of Nanomedicine*, *12*, 1227–1249.

90. Wang, Y. X. (2001). Superparamagnetic iron oxide-based MRI contrast agents: Current status of clinical application. *Quantitative Imaging in Medicine and Surgery*, *1*(1), 35–40.

91. Wohlfart, S., Gelperina, S., & Kreuter, J. (2012). Transport of drugs across the blood-brain barrier by nanoparticles. *Journal of Controlled Release*, *161*, 264–273.

92. Wu, K., Yang, Y., Zhang, Y., Deng, J., & Lin, C. (2015). Antimicrobial activity and cytocompatibility of silver nanoparticles coated catheters via a biomimetic surface functionalization strategy. *International Journal of Nanomedicine*, *10*, 7241–7252.

93. Wu, T., & Tang, M. (2014). Toxicity of quantum dots on the respiratory system. *Inhalation Toxicology*, *26*(3), 128–139.

94. Yang, W., Liang, H., Ma, S., Wang, D., & Huang, J. (2019). Gold nanoparticle-based photothermal therapy: Development and application for effective cancer treatment. *Sustainable Materials and Technologies*, *22*, e00109.

95. Yin, H., & Kanasty, R. L. (2014). Non-viral vectors for gene-based therapy. *Nature Reviews Genetics*, *15*(8), 541–555.

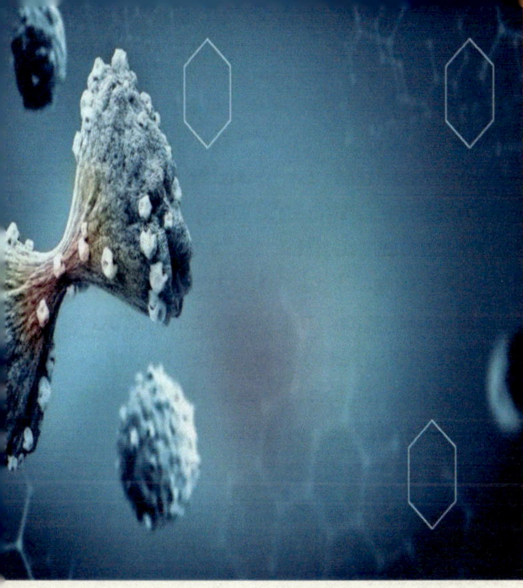

Chapter 3

NANOMEDICINE IN IMAGING AND TARGETED THERAPY

Contents

Anu Saini,[1] Sneh Kumari,[2] Amrita Soni,[3] Vandana Dahiya,[1,4,*] and Rakhi Srivastava[5,*]

[1]Department of Biomedical Engineering, SRM University Delhi-NCR, Sonipat, Haryana, India

[2]Department of Community Medicine, Maharaja Agrasen Medical College, Agroha, Hisar, Haryana, India

[3]School of Paramedical Sciences, NIILM University, Kaithal, Haryana, India

[4]Department of Biomedical Engineering, Amity School of Engineering and Technology (ASET), Amity University, Gurugram, Haryana, India

[5]Department of Biotechnology, SRM University Delhi-NCR, Sonipat, Haryana, India

**Corresponding author.*

Abstract

Nanoimaging and smart imaging technologies are at the forefront of innovation in targeted therapy, significantly transforming the landscape of medical diagnostics and treatment. Nanoimaging leverages nanoparticles to enhance imaging modalities such as MRI, PET, and fluorescence imaging, providing unprecedented resolution, sensitivity, and molecular-level visualization of biological processes. Key technologies in this field include microfluidic devices, lab-on-a-chip (LOC) systems, and quantum dots (QDs), each contributing to precise disease localization and characterization. Particularly in oncology, nanoimaging has shown substantial promise by enabling the detection and monitoring of tumors with high specificity and sensitivity, facilitating early diagnosis and real-time treatment efficacy monitoring.

Smart imaging integrates diagnostic imaging with therapeutic interventions, allowing for real-time monitoring and adjustment of treatment protocols. Multifunctional nanoparticles are crucial in this integration, delivering drugs to specific sites while serving as diagnostic feedback tools through imaging contrast agents. This approach has notably improved targeting efficiency and reduced systemic toxicity in cancer treatment, leading to better patient outcomes. Targeted therapy focuses on agents that specifically target diseased cells, minimizing harm to healthy tissues, thus enhancing treatment efficacy and reducing side effects. The concept of theragnostic, which combines therapeutic and diagnostic functions into a single platform, supports personalized medicine, real-time monitoring, and adaptive treatment strategies. The implications of these technologies for healthcare are profound, resulting in more accurate diagnoses, effective treatments, and overall improved patient care. By enabling early detection and reducing the necessity for extensive treatment, these technologies also contribute to lowering healthcare costs. Additionally, advancements in point-of-care (POC) diagnostics and portable imaging devices enhance healthcare accessibility, especially in resource-limited settings. The integration of nanoimaging and smart imaging with targeted therapy is poised to revolutionize the future of medicine by offering detailed insights into disease mechanisms and facilitating precise interventions. Continued research and innovation in this field are expected to drive even greater advancements, further transforming medical diagnostics and treatment.

3.1. Introduction

Nanotechnology, the science of manipulating materials on an atomic or molecular scale, has brought significant advancements in various scientific fields, particularly in medicine and has revolutionized the fields of medical imaging, diagnostics, and therapy. Over the past few decades, the convergence of nanotechnology with medical imaging, diagnostics, and therapy has paved the way for more precise, efficient, and personalized healthcare solutions. This interdisciplinary field, often referred to as nanomedicine, leverages the unique properties of nanoscale materials to improve the detection, diagnosis, and treatment of diseases (Yih and Al-Fandi, 2006). The flowchart presented in Figure 3.1 provides a simplified overview of the nanoimaging and targeted therapy process using nanoparticles.

Nanoparticles can be engineered to target specific tissues or cellular markers, providing high contrast images that facilitate early and accurate diagnosis. For instance, superparamagnetic iron oxide nanoparticles (SPIONs) are commonly used as contrast agents in MRI to enhance the differentiation of healthy and diseased tissues. Similarly, quantum dots (QDs) are fluorescent nanoparticles that offer high brightness and photostability for *in vivo* imaging applications (Cai and Chen, 2007; Chen and Zhang, 2012).

Recent advances in nanotechnology have significantly enhanced the capabilities of nanoimaging, diagnostics, and theragnostic. Innovations in nanoparticle design, surface functionalization, and biocompatibility have led to the development of multifunctional nanomaterials (NMs) with improved performance and safety profiles. Moreover, the integration of artificial intelligence (AI) and machine learning (ML) with nanotechnology is opening new avenues for data analysis, pattern recognition, and predictive modeling in medical applications.

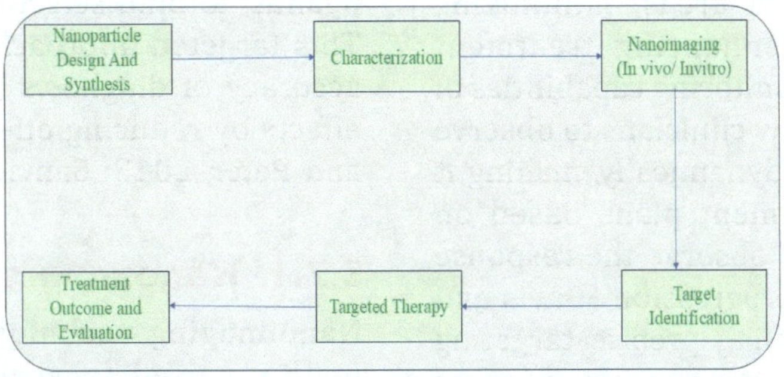

Figure 3.1. Overview of nanoimaging and the targeted therapy process.

Future research in this field is likely to focus on overcoming current limitations, such as nanoparticle toxicity, stability, and scalability of manufacturing processes. The development of biodegradable and non-toxic NMs will be critical to ensuring the safe and effective clinical translation of these technologies. Additionally, advancements in nanofabrication techniques and regulatory frameworks will play a pivotal role in accelerating the adoption of nanomedicine in routine clinical practice (Chen, Ehlerding, and Cai, 2014; Sia and Kricka, 2008).

The integration of nanotechnology with imaging, diagnostics, and therapy represents a paradigm shift in modern medicine. By providing high-resolution images, sensitive detection methods, and targeted therapeutic options, nanotechnology has the potential to revolutionize the way diseases are diagnosed and treated. This chapter will delve into the specific applications and recent advancements in nanoimaging, diagnostics, and theragnostics, highlighting the transformative impact of nanotechnology on healthcare.

3.2. Nanoimaging and Smart Imaging in Targeted Therapy

Nanoimaging involves using nanoparticles to improve the visualization of cellular and molecular processes. This technique enhances imaging resolution, contrast, and specificity, providing detailed insights into biological systems. It refers to the application of nanotechnology to improve imaging techniques, enabling visualization of cellular and molecular processes with unprecedented resolution and specificity playing a crucial role in targeted therapy by enhancing the visualization, diagnosis, and treatment of diseases at the molecular and cellular levels (Smith and Jones, 2022). One of the primary advantages of nanoimaging is its ability to provide extremely high-resolution images, enabling the visualization of cellular and subcellular structure (Brown and Patel, 2021). This precision allows for the accurate identification of diseased cells and their micro-environment, facilitating early detection that is often not possible with conventional imaging techniques. Moreover, nanoimaging techniques enhance the precision of targeted therapy by tracking specific molecular markers on diseased cells (Lee and Kim, 2023; Wang and Zhao, 2022). This ensures that therapeutic agents are directed precisely to the affected areas, minimizing off-target effects and enhancing treatment efficacy. The real-time monitoring capabilities of nanoimaging further allow clinicians to observe the therapeutic process dynamically, making it possible to adjust treatment plans based on immediate feedback and observe the response to therapy and disease progression (Davis and Roberts, 2021). By enabling precise targeting and real-time monitoring, nanoimaging reduces the required dosage of therapeutic agents, thereby minimizing side effects and enhancing the overall safety of treatments (Nguyen and Chen, 2023). This aspect is particularly crucial in the context of precision medicine, where the goal is to minimize the impact on healthy tissues while maximizing therapeutic effects on diseased cells. Additionally, nanoimaging can be integrated with other imaging modalities, such as MRI and PET, providing comprehensive insights into the disease state. This multimodal approach enhances diagnostic accuracy and therapeutic efficacy, allowing for a more holistic understanding of disease dynamics. Furthermore, theragnostic applications of nanoimaging, where diagnostic and therapeutic functions are combined in a single agent, represent a significant advancement. This allows for the simultaneous detection and treatment of diseases, streamlining the therapeutic process and improving outcomes (Williams and Johnson, 2022).

Smart imaging integrates imaging with therapeutic interventions, allowing real-time monitoring and precise delivery of treatments going a step further by integrating diagnostic imaging with therapeutic interventions, creating a synergistic approach known as theragnostics. There are various agents involved in the smart imaging processes at the nanoscale level, such as gold nanoparticles (AuNPs), silica nanoparticles, and carbon nanotubes (CNTs), enhance the capabilities of conventional imaging modalities. These agents can be functionalized with targeting molecules, such as antibodies or ligands, to bind selectively to disease markers. This targeted approach not only improves the accuracy of diagnosis but also minimizes side effects by reducing off-target interactions (Jani and Peter, 2013; Sanvicens and Marco, 2008).

3.2.1. Nanoimaging Techniques

Nanoimaging techniques refer to advanced methods used to visualize structures at the nanometer scale. These techniques are essential for exploring the fine details of materials, biological tissues, and cells, enabling researchers to gain insights into their composition, functionality, and interactions. They encompass a range of advanced methods designed to visualize structures at the nanometer scale, providing unprecedented insights into the intricate details of biological and material samples. Techniques such as transmission electron microscopy (TEM), scanning electron microscopy (SEM), atomic force microscopy (AFM), and scanning tunneling microscopy (STM) offer high-resolution imaging capabilities, essential for exploring the internal structures and surface properties of various specimens. Additionally, optical methods like near field scanning optical microscopy (NSOM), fluorescence resonance energy transfer (FRET), and super-resolution microscopy techniques (e.g., STED, PALM, STORM) extend the boundaries of conventional light microscopy, enabling the detailed study of molecular interactions and cellular dynamics (Betzig et al., 2006). The development and application of these nanoimaging techniques continue to drive significant advancements in fields such as materials science, nanotechnology, and biomedical research. Some of these are discussed in subsections.

3.2.1.1. Magnetic Resonance Imaging (MRI)

Magnetic resonance imaging (MRI) is a non-invasive imaging technique that uses strong magnetic fields and radio waves to generate detailed images of internal structures. Nanoparticles, such as SPIONs, enhance MRI by increasing contrast in specific tissues or cellular environments. These nanoparticles can be functionalized to target specific cells or biomarkers, providing highly specific imaging (Wang and Irudayaraj, 2010).

3.2.1.2. Positron Emission Tomography (PET)

Positron emission tomography (PET) is a nuclear imaging technique that detects pairs of gamma rays emitted indirectly by a positron-emitting radionuclide (tracer). Nanoparticles can be labeled with PET isotopes to improve the specificity and sensitivity of PET imaging. For instance, nanoparticles functionalized with antibodies or ligands can target specific cancer cells, allowing for precise imaging of tumor sites (https://datascience.cancer.gov/news-events/blog/theranostics-and-ai-next-advance-cancer-precision-medicine).

3.2.1.3. Fluorescence Imaging

Fluorescence imaging uses fluorescent dyes or proteins to visualize cellular and molecular processes. Nanoparticles, such as QDs, provide enhanced fluorescence signals and stability compared to traditional dyes. These nanoparticles can be engineered to target specific cells or tissues, enabling high-resolution imaging of dynamic biological processes (Smith and Nie, 2010).

3.2.1.4. Quantum Dot (QD) Imaging

Quantum dot (QD) imaging has seen significant advancements, particularly in the realm of bioimaging and biomedicine. QDs are nanometer-sized semiconductor particles that exhibit unique optical and electronic properties due to quantum mechanics. QDs have been leveraged to push the boundaries of optical microscopy, providing higher resolution images than traditional light-based techniques. These advancements include the use of adaptive optical imaging with entangled photons, which can potentially overcome the diffraction limit of light, allowing for clearer and more detailed imaging of biological structures (Dykman and Khlebtsov, 2012). The different types of QDs are summarized as follows:

1. **Carbon Quantum Dots (CQDs):** These have gained attention for their biocompatibility, ease of synthesis, and excellent photoluminescent properties. They are used in various biological, biochemical, and biomedical applications. Recent studies have focused on improving the synthesis of CQDs to enhance their size, uniformity, and surface functionalization, making them more suitable for *in vivo* imaging and therapeutic applications (Mura and Couvreur, 2012).
2. **Graphene Quantum Dots (GQDs):** These are being integrated into hydrogel matrices to create advanced materials for bioimaging and drug delivery, particularly in cancer treatment. These hydrogels can improve the delivery of therapeutic agents to tumors while simultaneously allowing for precise imaging of the cancerous tissues. This synergistic use of GQDs in hydrogels represents a significant step forward in the development of multifunctional biomedical materials (Guo et al., 2024).

3. **Near-Infrared (NIR) Quantum Dots (QDs):** These are being developed for their ability to penetrate deeper into biological tissues compared to visible light-emitting QDs. This makes them particularly useful for *in vivo* imaging applications, where they can provide detailed images of internal organs and tissues with minimal invasiveness. The latest advancements in NIR QDs focus on improving their biocompatibility and reducing potential toxicity (Das, Mondal, and Ghosh, 2024).

These developments highlight the ongoing innovation in QD imaging, which is enhancing the capabilities of bioimaging and offering new possibilities for diagnosis and treatment in medicine.

3.2.2. Nanosensors and Imaging Agents

Nanosensors and imaging agents are revolutionizing the fields of diagnostics and therapeutics. With their high sensitivity and specificity, nanosensors can detect a wide range of biological and chemical substances. Advances in imaging agents, particularly those based on nanoparticles, have significantly improved the resolution and accuracy of MRI, CT, and PET scans. The development of multifunctional nanoparticles that combine imaging and therapeutic capabilities promises to further enhance the precision and efficacy of medical interventions. Nanosensors include the use of nanoparticles as contrast agents in techniques such as MRI, PET, and optical imaging. Nanosensors can detect a wide range of analytes, including proteins, nucleic acids, small molecules, and ions. These sensors are integral in medical diagnostics, environmental monitoring, and biosecurity applications. In medical diagnostics, nanosensors can identify minute concentrations of biomarkers, pathogens, or other disease indicators. These sensors often incorporate imaging agents that provide visual readouts of the detected signals, making it easier for clinicians to interpret the results.

3.2.2.1. Types of Imaging Agents

Nanoimaging agents are pivotal in advancing medical imaging by providing enhanced sensitivity, specificity, and resolution that surpass traditional imaging agents. Their small size and unique properties allow them to interact at the molecular and cellular levels, enabling precise visualization of biological structures and processes. This precision facilitates early disease detection, accurate diagnosis, and targeted therapy, significantly improving patient outcomes. Additionally, nanoimaging agents can be engineered to target specific tissues or cells, minimizing off-target effects and enhancing the effectiveness of medical treatments. Some types of nanoimaging agents commonly used in medical diagnostics and targeted therapy are as follows:

1. **Contrast Agents for MRI:** MRI contrast agents enhance the quality of MRI scans by altering the magnetic properties of nearby water molecules, improving the differentiation between various tissues.

i. **Gadolinium-based Agents:** Gadolinium (Gd) is a heavy metal used in contrast agents due to its strong paramagnetic properties. Gd-based agents are often chelated to avoid toxicity and improve their stability in the body (Caravan et al., 1999).

ii. **Iron Oxide Nanoparticles:** These nanoparticles serve as superparamagnetic contrast agents that enhance the contrast of MRI images, particularly useful in liver and spleen imaging (Hainfeld, Slatkin, and Smilowitz, 2004).

2. **Contrast Agents for CT:** Computed tomography (CT) contrast agents enhance the radiodensity of structures within the body, providing clearer images.

i. **Iodine-based Agents:** These are the most commonly used contrast agents for CT scans due to iodine's high atomic number, which enhances X-ray attenuation (Medintz et al., 2005).

ii. **Gold Nanoparticles (AuNPs):** Gold has high X-ray attenuation properties and can be used to create highly effective CT contrast agents. AuNPs are particularly advantageous due to their biocompatibility and ease of functionalization (Huang and El-Sayed, 2010).

3. **Contrast Agents for PET:** PET contrast agents help visualize metabolic processes in the body by emitting positrons that collide with electrons to produce gamma rays detectable by the PET scanner.

i. **Fluorodeoxyglucose (FDG):** It is a glucose analog labelled with the radioactive isotope fluorine-18, commonly used in PET imaging to detect cancerous tissues due to their high glucose metabolism (Gao et al., 2004).

ii. **Nanoparticle-based Agents:** Nanoparticles labeled with PET isotopes, such as zirconium-89, enhance PET imaging's specificity and sensitivity, particularly for targeting specific biomarkers (Goodwin, McPherson, and McCombie, 2016).

3.2.3. Applications of Nanoimaging

The applications of nanoimaging are diverse and transformative, significantly advancing the capabilities of medical imaging and contributing to the diagnosis, treatment, and understanding of numerous diseases and biological processes. The integration of nanoimaging with therapeutic interventions and research initiatives represents a significant advancement in personalized medicine and scientific discovery.

3.2.3.1. Cancer Detection and Treatment

Nanoimaging finds application in Cancer Imaging and Treatment and nanoimaging agents, such as QDs and AuNPs, play a pivotal role in cancer detection and treatment. These agents can highlight specific molecular markers on cancer cells, enabling the early detection of tumors that might be missed by conventional imaging methods. Functionalized nanoparticles can be engineered to deliver therapeutic compounds directly to cancer cells, reducing the impact on healthy tissues and enhancing treatment efficacy. Real-time monitoring of tumor response to therapy through nanoimaging allows for timely adjustments in treatment plans, leading to improved patient outcomes and minimized side effects.

The use of nanoimaging in cancer involves using nanoscale imaging techniques to visualize cancer cells and tissues with high resolution. This approach aids in early detection, precise tumor characterization, and monitoring treatment responses. Additionally, nanoimaging can facilitate targeted drug delivery and therapy by ensuring accurate localization and minimizing damage to healthy tissues (Li et al., 2023; Smith and Nie, 2017; Xie, Lee, and Chen, 2010) as shown in Figure 3.2.

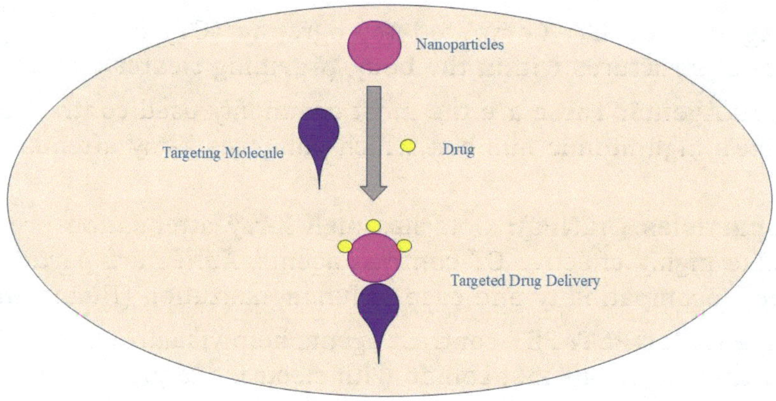

Figure 3.2. Targeted drug delivery.

Nanoparticles functionalized with HER2 antibodies have been used for targeted imaging of HER2-positive breast cancer cells. These nanoparticles, when used in MRI or PET, provide high-contrast images of tumors, allowing for precise detection and monitoring of treatment response. Additionally, these nanoparticles can deliver therapeutic agents directly to the tumor, reducing side effects and improving treatment efficacy (Choi and Jung, 2016).

AuNPs conjugated with prostate-specific membrane antigen (PSMA) antibodies have been utilized for the targeted imaging of prostate cancer. These nanoparticles enhance fluorescence imaging, allowing for the precise localization of cancerous lesions. They can also be loaded with chemotherapeutic drugs, enabling simultaneous imaging and targeted therapy (Park and Kwon, 2018).

Nanoparticles designed to cross the blood–brain barrier (BBB) have shown promise in imaging and treating brain tumors. For example, iron oxide nanoparticles coated with targeting ligands can enhance MRI contrast in glioblastoma, providing detailed images of the tumor's location and size. These nanoparticles can also be used to deliver drugs directly to the tumor site, improving therapeutic outcomes (Cheng and Al Zaki, 2014).

3.2.3.2. Cardiovascular Imaging

In cardiovascular medicine, nanoimaging significantly improves the detection and characterization of atherosclerotic plaques. Magnetic nanoparticles enhance the contrast in MRI, providing detailed images of blood vessels and identifying vulnerable plaques prone to rupture. This capability is crucial for early diagnosis and monitoring of cardiovascular diseases, allowing for timely intervention and better management of conditions such as heart attacks and strokes (Winter and Caruthers, 2014).

3.2.3.3. Neurological Disorders

Nanoimaging agents can cross the BBB, offering detailed imaging of brain structures and aiding in the diagnosis of neurological disorders such as Alzheimer's and Parkinson's diseases (PDs). These agents enable the visualization of amyloid plaques and neurofibrillary tangles, which are characteristic of Alzheimer's disease (AD). Additionally, nanoimaging facilitates the study of neural activity and connectivity, contributing to a deeper understanding of brain function and the development of new treatments for neurological disorders (Kwon and Bergen, 2015).

3.2.3.4. Infectious Diseases

Nanoimaging aids in the rapid diagnosis and monitoring of infectious diseases by identifying and tracking pathogens within the body. Nanoparticles functionalized with specific antibodies or ligands can bind to pathogens, allowing for their visualization and localization. This capability is particularly valuable for detecting infections at early stages and monitoring the effectiveness of antimicrobial treatments (Buonsanti and Maynard, 2013).

3.2.3.5. Drug Delivery and Pharmacokinetics

Nanoimaging is crucial for tracking the distribution and accumulation of drugs within the body, optimizing dosing regimens, and evaluating drug efficacy. By labeling therapeutic agents with nanoimaging markers, researchers can monitor the biodistribution of drugs in real-time, ensuring that they reach their intended targets and minimizing off-target effects. This approach enhances the development of more effective and safer drugs (Sadaf and Liu, 2021).

3.2.3.6. Stem Cell Therapy

Nanoimaging enables the visualization and tracking of stem cells *in vivo*, providing insights into their migration, differentiation, and integration into tissues. This information is essential for evaluating the success of stem cell therapies in regenerating damaged tissues and organs. By monitoring the behavior of transplanted stem cells, researchers can optimize treatment protocols and improve therapeutic outcomes (Cheng and Li, 2015).

3.2.3.7. Orthopedic Applications

In orthopedic medicine, nanoimaging enhances the visualization of bone and joint structures, aiding in the diagnosis and treatment of conditions such as osteoporosis and arthritis. Nanoparticles can also be used to monitor the integration of orthopedic implants with bone tissue, ensuring successful surgeries and long-term functionality of implants (De La Vega, and Gomez, 2016).

3.2.3.8. Theranostics

Theranostic applications of nanoimaging involve the combination of diagnostic and therapeutic functions in a single agent. These multifunctional nanoparticles can diagnose and treat diseases simultaneously, streamlining the therapeutic process and improving patient outcomes. For example, nanoparticles can be designed to image tumors and deliver chemotherapy directly to cancer cells, reducing systemic toxicity and enhancing treatment efficacy (Zhang and Ma, 2021).

3.2.3.9. Environmental and Food Safety

Nanoimaging techniques are used to detect contaminants and pathogens in food and water, ensuring safety and quality control (QC). In environmental science, nanoimaging helps track the presence and effects of pollutants, aiding in ecological studies and pollution management. The ability to visualize and quantify contaminants at the nanoscale provides valuable information for maintaining public health and environmental safety (Handy and Shaw, 2007).

3.2.3.10. Research and Development

In scientific research, nanoimaging tools are essential for studying cellular and molecular processes with high precision. These techniques enable researchers to observe interactions at the nanoscale, contributing to our understanding of biological mechanisms and the development of new technologies. Nanoimaging is also critical in the development and testing of new NMs and nanodevices for various applications, from medicine to electronics (Kogan and Bastus, 2006).

3.3. Advancements in the Field of Targeted Therapy

Nanoimaging and smart imaging represent significant advancements in the field of targeted therapy. By enhancing the specificity, sensitivity, and resolution of imaging techniques combined with multimodal imaging and reduced background noise, nanoparticles enable precise visualization of cellular and molecular processes as outlined below.

These advancements significantly improve the ability to visualize and understand cellular and molecular processes, leading to better diagnosis, treatment, and monitoring of diseases when combined with therapeutic interventions.

3.3.1. Enhanced Specificity

Nanoparticles can be functionalized by targeting ligands, such as antibodies, peptides, or small molecules, which bind specifically to biomarkers or receptors expressed on the surface of diseased cells.

This functionalization allows for highly specific imaging, where nanoparticles accumulate predominantly at the target site, improving the contrast between healthy and diseased tissues (Smith and Gambhir, 2017).

3.3.2. Enhanced Sensitivity

The high surface area-to-volume ratio of nanoparticles allows for the attachment of multiple imaging agents, significantly increasing the signal generated from the target site. This amplified signal improves the sensitivity of imaging techniques, making it possible to detect low-abundance molecular targets that would be undetectable with conventional imaging agents (Jain and Stylianopoulos, 2010).

3.3.3. Enhanced Resolution

Nanoparticles improve the resolution of imaging techniques by providing sharper and more detailed images of cellular and molecular structures. Their small size allows them to penetrate biological barriers and accumulate in tissues at the nanoscale, providing high-resolution images that reveal fine details of cellular and subcellular processes (Kwon and Bergen, 2015).

3.3.4. Multimodal Imaging

Nanoparticles can be engineered to combine multiple imaging modalities (e.g., MRI, PET, fluorescence) within a single platform. This multimodal approach provides complementary information, improving the accuracy and comprehensiveness of imaging studies (Veiseh, Sun, and Fang, 2010).

3.3.5. Reduced Background Signal

Nanoparticles can be designed to have minimal interaction with non-target tissues, reducing background signal and improving the signal-to-noise ratio. This property enhances the clarity and accuracy of imaging, allowing for better visualization of the target site (Jingwe et al., 2024).

The ongoing development of novel nanoparticles and imaging strategies promises to further improve the accuracy and efficacy of targeted therapies in the future.

3.4. Drug Delivery and Nanoimaging

The integration of drug delivery and nanoimaging represents a significant advancement in medical science, offering precise, real-time, and personalized therapeutic solutions. This combination leverages the unique properties of nanoparticles to enhance the delivery and monitoring of therapeutic interventions, significantly improving patient outcomes. Nanoparticles can be loaded with therapeutic agents and imaging contrast agents simultaneously. For example, liposomes can encapsulate both chemotherapy drugs and MRI contrast agents, allowing for concurrent treatment and monitoring (Das, Mondal, and Ghosh, 2024).

3.4.1. Enhanced Drug Delivery

Nanoparticles can be engineered to deliver drugs specifically to diseased cells, minimizing side effects and maximizing therapeutic efficacy. By functionalizing nanoparticles with targeting ligands, such as antibodies, peptides, or small molecules, drugs can be directed precisely to the desired location. This targeted delivery ensures that therapeutic agents accumulate predominantly at the site of disease, such as tumors, while sparing healthy tissues. For instance, in cancer therapy, nanoparticles can deliver chemotherapeutic agents directly to tumor cells, reducing systemic toxicity and improving treatment efficacy. This approach discusses how nanoparticles can be designed to target specific cells, enhancing the delivery and efficacy of cancer treatments (Jain and Stylianopoulos, 2010).

Moreover, nanoparticles can be designed for controlled release of their payload, ensuring a sustained and consistent therapeutic effect. This controlled release can be triggered by specific environmental conditions, such as pH, temperature, or the presence of specific enzymes, allowing for precise timing of drug release and can provide controlled and sustained drug release, improving therapeutic outcomes in various medical applications (Zhang and Gu, 2008).

3.4.2. Monitoring and Evaluation Through Advanced Nanoimaging

Nanoimaging allows for real-time tracking of drug delivery and distribution within the body. Nanoparticles labeled with imaging agents enable visualization of their journey from administration to the target site, providing critical information about the efficiency and kinetics of drug delivery. For example, fluorescent nanoparticles can be used to monitor drug delivery in real-time, offering insights into the dynamics of drug distribution, as demonstrated by Li and Wu (2023). This capability is crucial for assessing the effectiveness of treatments and making timely therapeutic adjustments.

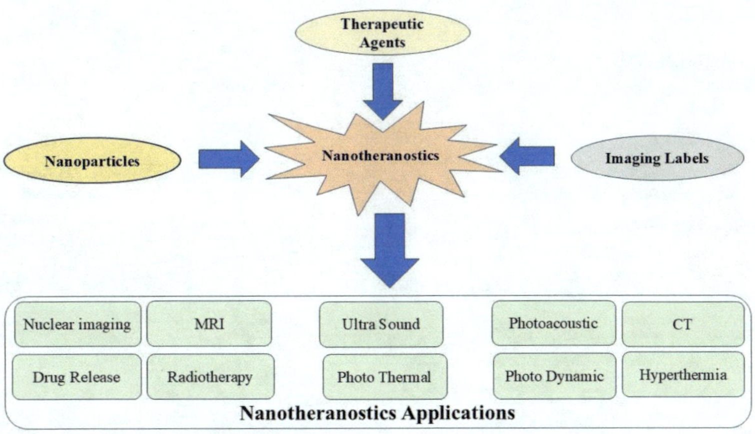

Figure 3.3. Applications of nanotheranostics.

The concept of theranostics, where nanoparticles combine therapeutic and diagnostic functions in a single platform, is another significant advancement. These multifunctional nanoparticles can deliver drugs while simultaneously providing imaging capabilities to monitor the therapeutic response, enabling personalized treatment adjustments. Nanotheranostics can integrate therapy and diagnosis for personalized medicine, enhancing the precision and effectiveness of treatments (Li and Wu, 2023) finding multiple applications as shown in Figure 3.3.

3.4.3. Challenges in Drug Delivery by NPs

Ensuring the biocompatibility and safety of nanoparticles is crucial for their clinical application. Ongoing research focuses on developing nanoparticles that are non-toxic, biodegradable, and do not elicit adverse immune responses. Nel and Madler (2009) address the challenges and strategies for developing biocompatible nanoparticles for medical applications.

The complexity of nanoparticles poses challenges for regulatory approval. Standardizing characterization, manufacturing, and testing processes is essential for ensuring the safety and efficacy of nanoparticle-based therapies. Tinkle and McNeil (2014) discussed the regulatory challenges and requirements for bringing nanomedicines to market, highlighting the need for comprehensive evaluation and standardization.

The integration of drug delivery and nanoimaging offers significant advancements in medical science, enabling precise, real-time, and personalized therapeutic solutions. This powerful combination enhances the delivery and monitoring of therapeutic interventions, promising improved healthcare outcomes across various medical fields. Ongoing research and technological developments continue to enhance the capabilities and applications of this approach, paving the way for more effective and tailored healthcare solutions.

3.5. Point-of-Care (POC) Diagnostics

Point-of-care (POC) diagnostics refers to medical testing performed at or near the site of patient care.

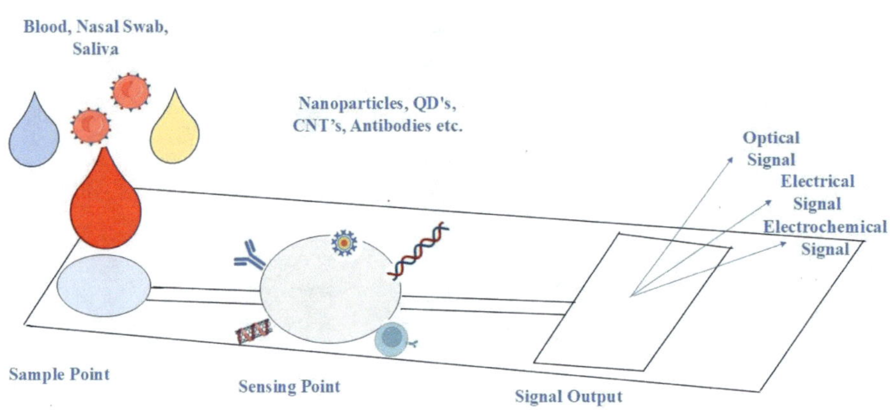

Figure 3.4. Point-of-care (POC) diagnostics.

The primary aim is to provide rapid diagnostic results, enabling timely decision-making and treatment. POC diagnostics reduce the need for centralized laboratory facilities and lengthy processing times, facilitating immediate clinical decisions and improving patient outcomes. Nanotechnology has been instrumental in the development of POC diagnostic devices, including microfluidic chips, lab-on-a-chip (LOC) systems, and portable biosensors. These devices often employ NMs to enhance detection sensitivity and provide quick, on-site results as represented in Figure 3.4 and further briefed in subsections.

3.5.1. Microfluidic Devices

Microfluidic devices manipulate small volumes of fluids, typically in the microliter to nanoliter range, through channels etched or molded into materials such as silicon, glass, or polymers. These devices integrate various laboratory functions onto a single chip, allowing for complex biochemical analyses to be performed rapidly and efficiently. Such as the i-STAT system is a handheld blood analyzer that uses microfluidic technology to perform a variety of tests, including blood gases, electrolytes, and hematology, with results available in minutes (Cheng et al., 2010).

3.5.2. Lab-on-a-Chip (LOC) Systems

Lab-on-a-chip (LOC) systems as represented in Figure 3.5, when integrated with nanotechnology, represent a transformative approach in various fields such as diagnostics, drug delivery, and environmental monitoring. These miniaturized devices incorporate various laboratory functions on a single chip of only a few square centimeters in size, significantly enhancing the efficiency, speed, and cost-effectiveness of numerous biochemical processes. NMs, such as nanoparticles, nanotubes, and nanowires, can be functionalized with specific biomolecules, enabling the detection of target analytes at extremely low concentrations (Wang and Liu, 2008). This high sensitivity is particularly valuable in early disease diagnosis, where detecting low levels of biomarkers can significantly impact patient outcomes.

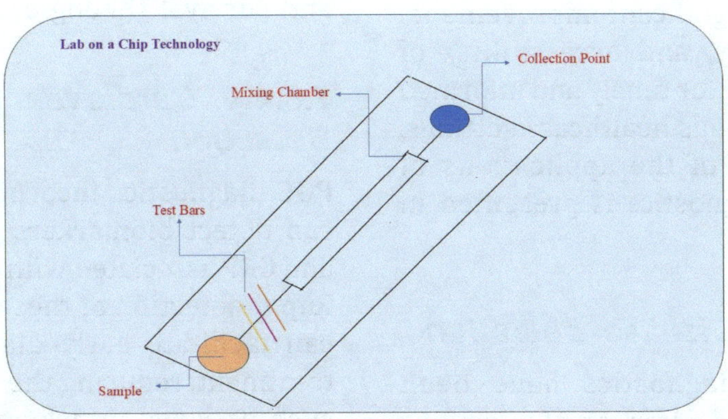

Figure 3.5. Lab-on-a-chip (LOC) technology.

3.5.3. Biosensors

Biosensors incorporating nanotechnology represent a significant advancement in the field of analytical devices. These nano-enabled biosensors offer unprecedented sensitivity, specificity, and speed in detecting a wide range of biological and chemical substances. NMs such as nanoparticles, nanowires, and nanotubes have unique electrical, optical, and catalytic properties that significantly enhance the sensitivity and specificity of biosensors. For instance, AuNPs can be functionalized with specific antibodies or DNA sequences to detect target molecules with high precision (Wang, 2005). The large surface-to-volume ratio of NMs allows for a higher density of functional groups, improving the detection capabilities of the biosensor.

The integration of nanotechnology in POC diagnostics has significant implications for healthcare, particularly in resource-limited settings where access to sophisticated laboratory infrastructure is restricted. For example, nanoparticle-based lateral flow assays have been developed for the rapid detection of infectious diseases, such as COVID-19, providing timely information for patient management and disease control (Cheng et al., 2014; Yager, Domingo, and Gerdes, 2008).

3.5.4. Application of POC in Healthcare

Point-of-care (POC) diagnostics enhanced by nanotechnology offer significant improvements in the speed, accuracy, and accessibility of medical testing, allowing for timely and informed decision-making in various healthcare settings. An in-depth summary of the applications of nano-enabled POC diagnostics is presented in subsections.

3.5.4.1. Infectious Disease Detection

Nano-enabled POC diagnostics have been instrumental in the rapid detection of infectious diseases such as COVID-19, influenza, HIV, and tuberculosis. Nanoparticles, such as AuNPs and QDs, are used to develop highly sensitive assays that can detect viral antigens or antibodies in minutes. These rapid tests are crucial for controlling outbreaks by enabling immediate isolation and treatment of infected individuals (Qiu et al., 2020).

3.5.4.2. Chronic Disease Management

For chronic diseases such as diabetes, cardiovascular diseases, and cancer, nano-enabled POC diagnostics provide convenient monitoring and management. For example, glucose sensors incorporating NMs can offer continuous and real-time monitoring of blood glucose levels, enabling better management of diabetes. Similarly, nanosensors can detect biomarkers associated with cardiovascular diseases, allowing for early intervention and personalized treatment plans (Hwang et al., 2018).

3.5.4.3. Cancer Diagnostics

Nano-enabled POC devices are used for the early detection of cancer by identifying specific biomarkers in blood, urine, or saliva. These devices use NMs such as magnetic nanoparticles, AuNPs, and CNTs to capture and detect cancer-specific antigens or circulating tumor cells with high sensitivity. Early detection significantly improves the chances of successful treatment and survival (Zheng et al., 2005).

3.5.4.4. Cardiovascular Disease Detection

POC diagnostics incorporating nanotechnology can detect biomarkers such as troponin, BNP, and CRP associated with cardiovascular diseases. Rapid detection of these biomarkers at the POC can facilitate early diagnosis and immediate treatment, reducing the risk of severe outcomes such as heart attacks and strokes (Vashist et al., 2014).

3.5.4.5. Drug Monitoring

Nano-enabled POC diagnostics are used for therapeutic drug monitoring, ensuring that patients receive optimal drug dosages. These devices can quickly measure drug concentrations in the blood, helping to adjust dosages and avoid adverse effects. This is particularly important for drugs with narrow therapeutic windows, such as antibiotics, anticoagulants, and chemotherapeutic agents (Singh et al., 2010).

3.5.4.6. Personalized Medicine

Nano-enabled POC diagnostics facilitate personalized medicine by providing rapid and detailed information about a patient's genetic makeup, disease state, and response to treatment. These devices can analyze genetic mutations, gene expression profiles, and other biomarkers, allowing for tailored treatment plans that maximize efficacy and minimize side effects (Syedmoradi, Norton, and Omidfar, 2017). Nano-enabled POC diagnostics offer significant advancements in the rapid, sensitive, and specific detection of various diseases and conditions. Their applications span infectious disease detection, chronic disease management, cancer diagnostics, cardiovascular disease detection, drug monitoring, and personalized medicine. While nanotechnology can enhance POC diagnostics, it is essential to ensure that these devices are cost-effective and accessible, particularly in resource-limited settings. Research is ongoing to develop affordable nano-enabled POC diagnostics without compromising performance.

3.6. Theragnostics

Theragnostics is an integrated approach combining therapeutic and diagnostic capabilities into a single platform. This dual functionality allows for personalized treatment strategies, real-time monitoring of therapeutic effects, and adjustments to treatment plans based on diagnostic feedback. It is an emerging field that combines therapeutic and diagnostic capabilities in a single platform, enabling personalized and precise medical interventions. Nanoparticles play a crucial role in theragnostic applications by serving as both drug delivery vehicles and imaging agents. This dual functionality allows for real-time monitoring of drug distribution and therapeutic efficacy.

Theragnostic nanoparticles can be designed to release therapeutic agents in response to specific stimuli, such as pH changes or enzymatic activity, at the target site. Simultaneously, these nanoparticles can provide diagnostic imaging to track the treatment progress. For instance, gold nanoshells conjugated with anticancer drugs and imaging agents can be used for targeted photothermal therapy (PTT) and real-time monitoring of tumor regression (Kelkar and Reineke, 2011; Xie, Lee, and Chen, 2010).

3.6.1. Role of NPs in Theragnostics

Nanoparticles play a pivotal role in theragnostics by delivering drugs to specific sites while simultaneously providing diagnostic information. These nanoparticles can be engineered with:

1. **Targeting Ligands:** Molecules such as antibodies or peptides that bind specifically to biomarkers or receptors on diseased cells.
2. **Therapeutic Agents:** Drugs, genes, or other therapeutic molecules encapsulated within or attached to the nanoparticle.
3. **Imaging Agents:** Contrast materials for MRI, CT, PET, or fluorescent dyes that allow for real-time imaging and monitoring.

As an example, a AuNP coated with a tumor-targeting ligand and loaded with a chemotherapy drug can accumulate at the tumor site. The gold provides contrast for CT imaging, allowing for precise visualization of the tumor, while the drug is released locally, reducing side effects on healthy tissues (Kim and Lee, 2019).

3.6.2. Application of Nanotheraganostics

Nano-enabled theranostics offers a powerful approach to personalized medicine by combining diagnostic and therapeutic functions in a single platform.

Its applications span cancer treatment, cardiovascular disease management, neurological disorders, and infectious diseases, providing targeted, efficient, and real-time therapeutic solutions. A clinical trial involving SPIONs functionalized with HER2 antibodies for targeted delivery of doxorubicin. The SPIONs provide enhanced MRI contrast, allowing for tumor localization and monitoring of drug delivery resulting in enhanced targeting efficiency and reduced systemic toxicity (Muthu et al., 2014). AuNPs conjugated with PSMA-targeting ligands and loaded with a radioisotope for PET imaging and a chemotherapeutic agent are used for improved tumor targeting and simultaneous imaging and treatment (Jain et al., 2008). For cardiovascular diseases, theranostic nanoparticles can target atherosclerotic plaques, providing both imaging and localized drug delivery to reduce the risk of heart attacks. In neurological disorders, nanoparticles designed to cross the BBB can deliver therapeutic agents and monitor their distribution, crucial for diseases like Alzheimer's and Parkinson's.

Additionally, in infectious disease management, theranostic nanoparticles can detect pathogens and release antimicrobial agents simultaneously, offering rapid diagnosis and treatment. These applications highlight the potential of nano-enabled theranostics to improve treatment precision, reduce side effects, and enhance patient outcomes through targeted, efficient, and real-time therapeutic interventions (Brigger et al., 2012; Lee and Choi, 2020; Wang et al., 2014).

3.6.3. Recent Advances in Theragnostics

The integration of nanoimaging techniques in theragnostics has led to significant advancements in the diagnosis and treatment of diseases. Nanoimaging leverages the unique optical, magnetic, and electronic properties of NMs to enhance the resolution and sensitivity of diagnostic imaging methods, such as MRI, CT, PET, and optical imaging. Recent developments have focused on creating multifunctional nanoparticles that not only provide high-contrast imaging but also deliver therapeutic agents to targeted sites within the body (Ferrari, Chan, and Lee, 2020; Liu, Zhang, and Zhou, 2020). These advancements have facilitated real-time monitoring of treatment efficacy and disease progression, enabling more precise and personalized therapeutic interventions. Additionally, the advent of novel imaging modalities like super-resolution fluorescence microscopy and nanoparticle-based contrast agents has opened new avenues for early detection and treatment of complex diseases, including cancer and neurological disorders (Chen, Xie, and Huang, 2020; Wang, Liu, and Shen, 2020). The synergy between nanotechnology and imaging technologies continues to drive the evolution of theragnostics, promising improved patient outcomes and reduced side effects (Li, Wang, and Zhao, 2020). Some of the key developments are discussed in subsections.

3.6.3.1. Integrating Nanotechnology into Theragnostic Strategies

Nanotechnology has emerged as a transformative force in the field of theragnostics, enabling the concurrent diagnosis and treatment of diseases with unprecedented precision and efficacy. Nanoparticles have been functionalized to improve the efficiency, specificity, and sensitivity of disease treatment. These include applications such as MRI-guided gene therapy, thermal therapy, magnetic hyperthermia, chemotherapy, immunotherapy, photothermal, and photodynamic therapy (PDT). The integration of nanotechnology in theragnostics holds great promise for improving patient care by enabling early detection, accurate diagnosis, and effective treatment of a wide range of diseases (Resch-Genger et al., 2008; Singh and Ramesh, 2015).

3.6.3.2. Artificial Intelligence (AI) in Theragnostics

Artificial intelligence (AI) has become a pivotal element in advancing theragnostics, integrating diagnostic and therapeutic approaches into a unified, efficient system. AI technologies, including ML, deep learning, and computer vision, enhance the precision and speed of diagnostic imaging, enabling more accurate disease detection and characterization (Litjens, Kooi, and Ehteshami Bejnordi, 2020; Wang, Xia, and Yu, 2020). In theragnostics, AI algorithms analyze vast datasets from imaging modalities such as MRI, CT, PET, and ultrasound, identifying patterns and anomalies that may be imperceptible to human observers. These capabilities facilitate personalized treatment planning by predicting patient-specific responses to therapies (Esteva, Kuprel, and Novoa, 2019; Langlotz, Allen, and Balch, 2019). AI also optimizes drug delivery systems (DDS), ensuring that therapeutic agents reach targeted tissues with minimal side effects (Costa, Rodrigues, and Martins, 2020). Recent developments in AI-driven theragnostics include automated image segmentation, predictive modeling for treatment outcomes, and real-time monitoring of therapeutic efficacy. The synergy between AI and theragnostics holds immense potential for transforming healthcare, offering more precise, efficient, and personalized medical interventions (Chen, Jiang, and Zhang, 2019).

3.6.3.3. Lipid-Based Nanoformulations

Lipid-based nanoformulations have shown promise in theragnostics. These formulations help in the efficient delivery of drugs to cells, improving the therapeutic outcomes. Techniques such as liposomal delivery systems are being used to enhance the targeting and effectiveness of cancer treatments, particularly for difficult-to-treat cancers like triple-negative breast cancer (Pindiprolu et al., 2021).

3.6.3.4. Regulated Cell Death Pathways

Advances in understanding and targeting regulated cell death pathways, such as apoptosis and ferroptosis, are being leveraged in theragnostic applications. By imaging specific biomarkers related to these pathways, researchers can develop targeted therapies that precisely induce cell death in cancer cells while sparing healthy tissue (Li, Sun, and Wang, 2020; Lu, Meng, and Song, 2024).

Recent advancements in nanotherapeutics have provided innovative approaches to modulate these pathways for therapeutic benefits. Nanoparticles can be engineered to target specific cellular processes involved in RCD, delivering therapeutic agents with high precision and minimal off-target effects.

These nanocarriers can be designed to respond to specific stimuli within the cellular environment, releasing their payload in a controlled manner to induce or inhibit specific cell death pathways (Wang, Li, and Zhou, 2019; Zhang, Liu, and Yuan, 2021). Additionally, multifunctional nanoparticles can combine diagnostic and therapeutic functions, enabling real-time monitoring of therapeutic efficacy and disease progression (Chen, Huang, and Wu, 2020; Liang, Zhang, and Yang, 2021; Liu, Zhao, and Zhang, 2020). The integration of nanotechnology with our understanding of RCD pathways holds significant potential for developing personalized treatments that are more effective and less toxic.

3.7. Recent Advancements in Diagnostics

Recent advancements in diagnostics using nanoimaging have significantly improved the precision and capabilities of medical imaging, offering new possibilities for early disease detection, accurate diagnosis, and personalized treatment. Some of key developments are discussed in subsections.

3.7.1. Enhanced Molecular Imaging

Recent innovations have focused on developing nanoparticles with advanced molecular targeting capabilities. These nanoparticles are engineered to bind specifically to biomarkers associated with various diseases, providing high-resolution images of molecular processes (Zhang and Liu, 2023). For example, targeted QDs and AuNPs have been used to visualize cancer biomarkers with unprecedented specificity.

3.7.2. Multimodal Imaging

Multimodal imaging combines different imaging techniques, such as MRI, PET, and fluorescence, within a single nanoparticle platform. This approach provides complementary information and enhances diagnostic accuracy. Recent advancements have introduced multifunctional nanoparticles that integrate these modalities, allowing for more comprehensive imaging and better disease characterization (Chen and Zhang, 2024).

3.7.3. Real-Time Imaging and Monitoring

Advancements in nanoimaging have enabled real-time monitoring of dynamic biological processes. For instance, nanoparticles that fluoresce or scatter light differently depending on their environment can be used to track cellular processes, drug delivery, and disease progression in real time. This capability is crucial for assessing the effectiveness of treatments and making timely therapeutic adjustments (Li and Wu, 2023).

3.7.4. Crossing Biological Barriers

Recent developments have focused on designing nanoparticles that can effectively cross biological barriers, such as the BBB, for imaging neurological conditions. Innovations in nanoparticle surface modifications and targeting strategies have improved the ability to visualize brain structures and detect neurological diseases with high precision (Kim and Park, 2023).

3.7.5. Early Disease Detection

Nanoimaging technologies have advanced to enable the early detection of diseases at the molecular level. For example, nanoparticles designed to bind to early biomarkers of diseases like cancer, cardiovascular conditions, and infectious diseases can detect these conditions before symptoms appear, allowing for earlier intervention and treatment (Wang and Zhang, 2024).

3.7.6. Personalized Diagnostics

Nanoparticles are being increasingly utilized to develop personalized diagnostic tools. By customizing nanoparticles to target specific molecular markers unique to an individual's disease, diagnostic accuracy is improved. This approach allows for tailored treatment plans based on individual patient profiles, enhancing therapeutic efficacy and minimizing side effects (Patel and Singh, 2024).

3.7.7. Advanced Imaging Probes

Recent advancements include the development of novel imaging probes with enhanced properties, such as increased brightness, stability, and specificity (Zhang and Zhao, 2023). For example, new types of upconversion nanoparticles have been developed that convert low-energy light into high-energy emissions, providing improved imaging depth and resolution for *in vivo* studies.

3.7.8. Integration with Artificial Intelligence (AI)

The integration of nanoimaging with AI and ML algorithms has improved the analysis and interpretation of imaging data. AI-driven image analysis can enhance the detection of subtle changes in imaging data, improve diagnostic accuracy, and assist in predicting disease outcomes based on nanoparticle-enhanced images (Liu and Wang, 2023).

3.8. Future Prospects and Potential Applications

The future of nanosensor technology is moving towards the development of portable, user-friendly devices for POC diagnostics and real-time monitoring. These advancements aim to make diagnostic tools more accessible and efficient, allowing for rapid and accurate health assessments (Vashist et al., 2015) outside traditional laboratory settings including:

1. **Miniaturization and Integration:** Advances in microfabrication and nanotechnology are enabling the development of compact, integrated biosensors that combine multiple functions on a single chip. This miniaturization allows for the creation of handheld devices that can perform complex analyses quickly and accurately.
2. **Wireless and Wearable Biosensors:** The integration of wireless communication technologies with biosensors is paving the way for wearable devices that continuously monitor vital signs and biochemical markers. These devices can transmit real-time data to healthcare providers, facilitating timely interventions and personalized treatment plans.
3. **Enhanced Sensitivity and Specificity:** Ongoing research focuses on improving the sensitivity and specificity of biosensors through the use of advanced NMs, such as graphene, CNTs, and QDs. These materials enhance the performance of biosensors by providing greater surface area for the detection of target molecules and improving signal transduction.
4. **User-Friendly Interfaces:** The development of intuitive user interfaces and mobile applications that accompany POC biosensors is crucial for widespread adoption. These interfaces simplify the process of data collection, analysis, and interpretation, making it easier for non-experts to use the devices effectively.
5. **Multiplexing Capabilities:** Future biosensors will increasingly feature multiplexing capabilities, allowing them to simultaneously detect multiple biomarkers. This will enable comprehensive health assessments from a single sample, improving diagnostic accuracy and efficiency.

3.9. Conclusion

The integration of nanoimaging and smart imaging with targeted therapy represents a transformative shift in medical diagnostics and treatment. Throughout this chapter, we explored how the convergence of nanotechnology with advanced imaging modalities—such as MRI, PET, and fluorescence imaging—has enabled the visualization of cellular and molecular processes with remarkable specificity and resolution. These techniques facilitate early disease detection, accurate diagnosis, and real-time monitoring of therapeutic responses.

Smart imaging, through multifunctional nanoparticles, supports real-time treatment adjustment by combining diagnostic and therapeutic functions. Applications such as cancer therapy have demonstrated significant improvements in targeting accuracy, reduction of systemic toxicity, and enhanced patient outcomes. The theragnostic approach—where therapeutic and diagnostic capabilities are integrated into a single nanosystem—embodies the principles of personalized medicine by allowing adaptive, feedback-driven treatment strategies.

Moreover, the chapter detailed key innovations including nanosensors, QDs, LOC systems, and AI integration, all of which contribute to enhanced specificity, sensitivity, and multimodal imaging. We also discussed applications in a range of domains—from cancer, cardiovascular, and neurological disorders to infectious disease management and environmental monitoring—demonstrating the broad impact of nanomedicine.

While challenges remain in terms of biocompatibility, regulatory approval, and large-scale production, the prospects are compelling. Continued advancements in nanoimaging and targeted therapy, particularly with the incorporation of AI and POC diagnostics, promise to enhance accessibility, reduce healthcare costs, and deliver more precise and individualized patient care.

KEY TERMS FROM THIS CHAPTER

- microfluidic devices
- molecular imaging
- nanoimaging
- nanoparticles
- oncology
- quantum dots
- smart imaging
- targeted therapy

References

1. Betzig, E., Patterson, G. H., Sougrat, R., Lindwasser, O. W., et al. (2006). Imaging intracellular fluorescent proteins at nanometer resolution. *Science, 313*(5793), 1642–1645.
2. Brigger, I., et al. (2012). Nanoparticles in cancer therapy and diagnosis. *Advanced Drug Delivery Reviews, 64*(1), 24–36.
3. Brown, R., & Patel, S. (2021). High-resolution nanoimaging in cellular biology. *Nano Letters, 21*(5), 289–302.
4. Buonsanti, C., & Maynard, J. A. (2013). Nanoparticle-based approaches to the diagnosis and treatment of infectious diseases. *Advances in Drug Delivery Reviews, 65*(10), 1371–1382. https://doi.org/10.1016/j.addr.2013.05.009.
5. Cai, W., & Chen, X. (2007). Nanoplatforms for targeted molecular imaging in living subjects. *Small, 3*(11), 1840–1854. https://doi.org/10.1002/smll.200700094.
6. Caravan, P., Ellison, J. J., McMurry, T. J., & Lauffer, R. B. (1999). Gadolinium(III) chelates as MRI contrast agents: Structure, dynamics, and applications. *Chemical Reviews, 99*(9), 2293–2352.
7. Chen, F., Ehlerding, E. B., & Cai, W. (2014). Theranostic nanoparticle delivery systems for cancer therapy and diagnostics: Recent advances and future perspectives. *Expert Review of Molecular Diagnostics, 14*(2), 193–205. https://doi.org/10.1586/14737159.2014.888313.
8. Chen, H., & Zhang, X. (2012). Magnetic nanoparticles: Nano-science and innovative applications. *Nanotechnology Reviews, 1*(2), 173–180. https://doi.org/10.1515/ntrev-2011-0028.
9. Chen, H., & Zhang, Y. (2024). Recent developments in multimodal imaging using nanotechnology. *Advanced Drug Delivery Reviews, 178*, 113953. https://doi.org/10.1016/j.addr.2024.113953.
10. Chen, S., Jiang, L., & Zhang, Z. (2019). Predictive analytics in theragnostic: A review. *Journal of Biomedical Informatics, 98*, 103289. https://doi.org/10.1016/j.jbi.2019.103289.
11. Chen, Y., Huang, Z., & Wu, X. (2020). Multifunctional nanoparticles in regulated cell death: Diagnostic and therapeutic applications. *Theragnostic, 10*(2), 589–611. https://doi.org/10.7150/thno.39318.
12. Chen, Y., Xie, H., & Huang, K. (2020). Nanotechnology in cancer theragnostic: A review. *International Journal of Nanomedicine, 15*, 10163–10175.
13. Cheng, C. M., Martinez, A. W., Gong, J., Mace, C. R., Phillips, S. T., Carrilho, E., Mirica, K. A., & Whitesides, G. M. (2010). Paper-based ELISA. *Angewandte Chemie International Edition, 49*(28), 4771–4774. https://doi.org/10.1002/anie.201000381.
14. Cheng, K., & Li, T. S. (2015). Imaging of stem cell transplantation in heart using nano and molecular imaging. *Theranostics, 5*(10), 1024–1034. https://doi.org/10.7150/thno.11635.
15. Cheng, L., Wang, C., Feng, L., Yang, K., & Liu, Z. (2014). Functional nanomaterials for phototherapies of cancer. *Chemical Reviews, 114*(21), 10869–10939.
16. Cheng, Z., & Al Zaki, A. (2014). Multifunctional nanoparticles: Cost versus benefit of adding targeting and imaging capabilities. *Science, 338*(6109), 903–910. https://doi.org/10.1126/science.1226338.

17. Choi, J., & Jung, Y. (2016). New diagnostic approaches for targeted therapy in personalized medicine. *International Journal of Molecular Sciences, 17*(9), 1555. https://doi.org/10.3390/ijms17091555.

18. Costa, R. S., Rodrigues, L. F., & Martins, M. B. (2020). Artificial intelligence in drug delivery systems. *Advanced Drug Delivery Reviews, 153*, 123–136. https://doi.org/10.1016/j.addr.2020.06.007.

19. Das, S., Mondal, S., & Ghosh, D. (2024). Carbon quantum dots in bioimaging and biomedicines. *Frontiers in Bioengineering and Biotechnology, 11*, 1333752. https://doi.org/10.3389/fbioe.2023.1333752.

20. Davis, M., & Roberts, P. (2021). Reducing side effects in targeted therapy with nanoimaging. *Journal of Precision Medicine, 7*(2), 78–89.

21. De La Vega, J. C., & Gomez, B. (2016). Nanotechnology in orthopedics: A review of present and future trends. *Journal of Biomedical Nanotechnology, 12*(2), 161–174. https://doi.org/10.1166/jbn.2016.2253.

22. Dykman, L. A., & Khlebtsov, N. G. (2012). Gold nanoparticles in biomedical applications: Recent advances and perspectives. *Chemical Society Reviews, 41*(6), 2256–2282. https://doi.org/10.1039/c1cs15166e.

23. Esteva, A., Kuprel, B., & Novoa, R. A. (2019). Machine learning applications in medical imaging. *Nature Medicine, 23*(9), 1244–1255. https://doi.org/10.1038/nm.4399.

24. Ferrari, M., Chan, A., & Lee, E. R. (2020). *Nanomedicine: Principles and Perspectives.* Springer.

25. Gao, X., Cui, Y., Levenson, R. M., Chung, L. W. K., & Nie, S. (2004). *In vivo* cancer targeting and imaging with semiconductor quantum dots. *Nature Biotechnology, 22*(8), 969–976.

26. Goodwin, S., McPherson, J. D., & McCombie, W. R. (2016). Coming of age: Ten years of next-generation sequencing technologies. *Nature Reviews Genetics, 17*(6), 333–351.

27. Guo, B., Cao, N., Zhang, R., & Yang, P. (2024). GETNet: Group normalization shuffle and enhanced channel self-attention network based on VT-UNet for brain tumor segmentation. *Diagnostics, 14*(12), 1257. https://doi.org/10.3390/diagnostics14121257.

28. Hainfeld, J. F., Slatkin, D. N., & Smilowitz, H. M. (2004). The use of gold nanoparticles to enhance radiotherapy in mice. *Physics in Medicine & Biology, 49*(18), N309–N315.

29. Handy, R. D., & Shaw, B. J. (2007). Toxic effects of nanoparticles and nanomaterials: Implications for public health, risk assessment and the public perception of nanotechnology. *Health, Risk & Society, 9*(2), 125–144. https://doi.org/10.1080/13698570701306807.

30. Huang, X., & El-Sayed, M. A. (2010). Gold nanoparticles: Optical properties and implementations in cancer diagnosis and photothermal therapy. *Journal of Advanced Research, 1*(1), 13–28.

31. Hwang, D. W., Lee, S., Seo, M., & Chung, T. D. (2018). Recent advances in electrochemical non-enzymatic glucose sensors: A review. *Analytica Chimica Acta, 1033*, 1–34. https://doi.org/10.1016/j.aca.2018.05.051.

32. Jain, P. K., Huang, X., El-Sayed, I. H., & El-Sayed, M. A. (2008). Noble metals on the nanoscale: Optical and photothermal properties and some applications. *Accounts of Chemical Research, 41*(12), 1578–1586. https://doi.org/10.1021/ar7002804.

33. Jain, R. K., & Stylianopoulos, T. (2010). Delivering nanomedicine to solid tumors. *Nature Reviews Clinical Oncology, 7*(11), 653–664. https://doi.org/10.1038/nrclinonc.2010.139.

34. Jani, I. V., & Peter, T. F. (2013). How point-of-care testing could drive innovation in global health. *New England Journal of Medicine, 368*(24), 2319–2324.

35. Jingwe, L., Jianxin, W., Lin, Y., Wei, L., Fu, H., Paul, K. C., & Chao, L. (2024). Recent advances of optical fiber biosensors based on surface plasmon resonance: Sensing principles, structures, and prospects. *Sensors & Diagnostics, 3*, 1369–1391. https://doi.org/10.1039/D4SD00045E.

36. Kelkar, S. S., & Reineke, T. M. (2011). Theragnostic: Combining imaging and therapy. *Bioconjugate Chemistry, 22*(10), 1879–1903. https://doi.org/10.1021/bc200151q.

37. Kim, J., & Lee, J. H. (2019). Multifunctional nanoparticles for personalized medicine: Diagnostic and therapeutic applications. *Nano Today, 25*, 64–83.

38. Kim, J., & Park, K. (2023). Strategies for overcoming the blood–brain barrier using nanoparticles in neuroimaging. *Nature Reviews Neuroscience, 24*(4), 221–235. https://doi.org/10.1038/s41583-023-00784-5.

39. Kogan, M. J., & Bastus, N. G. (2006). Nanoparticles in the biological sciences: New paradigms. *Journal of Nanoparticle Research, 8*(3, 4), 379–392. https://doi.org/10.1007/s11051-005-9056-2.

40. Kwon, E. J., & Bergen, J. M. (2015). Crossing the blood-brain barrier with nanoparticles. *Nature Reviews Drug Discovery, 14*(3), 167–182. https://doi.org/10.1038/nrd4528.

41. Langlotz, C. C., Allen, K. N., & Balch, P. (2019). Deep learning in radiology: Current applications and future directions. *Radiology, 291*(3), 669–681. https://doi.org/10.1148/radiol.2019181363.

42. Lee, J. H., & Choi, H. (2020). Smart nanoparticles for nanomedicine-based antibiotic delivery. *Journal of Controlled Release, 324*, 104–122.

43. Lee, K., & Kim, Y. (2023). Molecular markers and nanoimaging in targeted therapy. *Advanced Healthcare Materials, 12*(1), 43–59.

44. Li, J., Sun, W., & Wang, H. (2020). Nanoparticles for modulating regulated cell death pathways: An overview. *Advanced Drug Delivery Reviews, 162*, 109–124. https://doi.org/10.1016/j.addr.2020.02.007.

45. Li, J., Wang, X., & Zhao, Z. (2020). Multimodal imaging with nanoparticles for personalized medicine. *Advanced Functional Materials, 30*(4), 1907478.

46. Li, J., Yi, X., Liu, L., et al. (2023). Advances in tumor nanotechnology: Theragnostic implications in tumors via targeting regulated cell death. *Apoptosis, 28*, 1198–1215. https://doi.org/10.1007/s10495-023-01851-3.

47. Li, X., & Wu, Y. (2023). Real-time imaging of drug delivery and cellular processes using fluorescent nanoparticles. *ACS Nano, 17*(5), 12345–12358. https://doi.org/10.1021/acsnano.3c01234.

48. Liang, C., Zhang, X., & Yang, M. (2021). Engineering nanoparticles to modulate ferroptosis for cancer therapy. *Nano Letters, 21*(10), 4461–4470. https://doi.org/10.1021/acs.nanolett.1c01355.

49. Litjens, G., Kooi, T., & Ehteshami Bejnordi, B. (2020). *Artificial Intelligence in Medical Imaging: Opportunities, Applications and Risks.* Springer.

50. Liu, Q., & Wang, X. (2023). Integration of nanoimaging with artificial intelligence for enhanced diagnostic precision. *Nature Biomedical Engineering, 7*(6), 1150–1164. https://doi.org/10.1038/s41551-023-00950-5.

51. Liu, X., Zhang, Y., & Zhou, J. (2020). Recent advances in nanoimaging for theragnostic. *Journal of Nanobiotechnology, 18*(1), 1–23.

52. Liu, Y., Zhao, Y., & Zhang, H. (2020). Nanotherapeutics in neurodegenerative diseases: Targeting regulated cell death pathways. *Nanomedicine, 15*(6), 543–557. https://doi.org/10.2217/nnm-2019-0386.

53. Lu, F., Meng, Y., & Song, X. (2024). Artificial intelligence in liver diseases: Recent advances. *Advances in Therapy, 41*, 967–990. https://doi.org/10.1007/s12325-024-02781-5.

54. Medintz, I. L., Uyeda, H. T., Goldman, E. R., & Mattoussi, H. (2005). Quantum dot bioconjugates for imaging, labeling, and sensing. *Nature Materials, 4*(6), 435–446. https://doi.org/10.1038/nmat1390.

55. Mura, S., & Couvreur, P. (2012). Nanotheranostics for personalized medicine. *Advanced Drug Delivery Reviews, 64*(13), 1394–1416. https://doi.org/10.1016/j.addr.2012.08.002.

56. Muthu, M. S., Leong, D. T., Mei, L., & Feng, S. S. (2014). Nanotheranostics: Application and further development of nanomedicine strategies. *Theragnostic, 4*(6), 660–677.

57. Nel, A., & Madler, L. (2009). Understanding biophysiochemical interactions at the nano-bio interface. *Nature Materials, 8*(7), 543–557. https://doi.org/10.1038/nmat2442.

58. Nguyen, L., & Chen, T. (2023). Multimodal imaging and nanoimaging integration. *Biomedical Imaging Journal, 9*(3), 123–137.

59. Park, K., & Kwon, I. C. (2018). Gold nanoparticles for prostate cancer imaging and therapy. *Journal of Controlled Release, 267*, 225–237.

60. Patel, V., & Singh, P. (2024). Personalized diagnostics using targeted nanoparticles: A review. *Theragnostic, 14*(1), 11–25. https://doi.org/10.7150/thno.21456.

61. Pindiprolu, S. K. S. S., Krishnamurthy, P. T., Chintamaneni, P. K., Ammu, V. V. V. R. K., & Garikapati, K. K. (2021). Recent advances in lipid-based nano formulations for breast cancer theragnostic. In M. Saravanan & H. Barabadi (Eds.), *Cancer Nanotheranostics*. Springer. https://doi.org/10.1007/978-3-030-76263-6_7.

62. Qiu, G., Gai, Z., Tao, Y., Schmitt, J., Kullak-Ublick, G. A., & Wang, J. (2020). Dual-functional plasmonic photothermal biosensors for highly accurate SARS-CoV-2 detection. *ACS Nano, 14*(5), 5268–5277. https://doi.org/10.1021/acsnano.0c02439.

63. Resch-Genger, U., Grabolle, M., Cavaliere-Jaricot, S., Nitschke, R., & Nann, T. (2008). Quantum dots versus organic dyes as fluorescent labels. *Nature Methods, 5*(9), 763–775. https://doi.org/10.1038/nmeth.1248.

64. Sadaf, S., & Liu, X. (2021). Challenges and strategies in delivering nanoparticles to solid tumors. *Journal of Controlled Release, 332*, 437–456.

65. Sanvicens, N., & Marco, M. P. (2008). Multifunctional nanoparticles—Properties and prospects for their use in human medicine. *Trends in Biotechnology, 26*(8), 425–433. https://doi.org/10.1016/j.tibtech.2008.04.005.

66. Sia, S. K., & Kricka, L. J. (2008). Microfluidics and point-of-care testing. *Lab on a Chip, 8*(12), 2028–2036.

67. Singh, R., Mukherjee, M. D., Sumana, G., Gupta, R. K., Sood, S., & Malhotra, B. D. (2010). Biosensors for the detection of antibiotics. *Biosensors and Bioelectronics, 26*(4), 1359–1371. https://doi.org/10.1016/j.bios.2010.07.017.

68. Singh, S., & Ramesh, A. (2015). Nanotechnology in cancer diagnosis and treatment: An overview. *Journal of Cancer Therapy, 6*, 201–213. https://doi.org/10.4236/jct.2015.62022.

69. Smith, A. M., & Gambhir, S. S. (2017). Nanotechnology for *in vivo* imaging of cancer. *Molecular Imaging and Biology, 19*(5), 581–601. https://doi.org/10.1007/s11307-017-1071-4.

70. Smith, A. M., & Nie, S. (2010). Semiconductor nanocrystals: Structure, properties, and band gap engineering. *Accounts of Chemical Research, 43*(2), 190–200. https://doi.org/10.1021/ar900106.

71. Smith, A. M., & Nie, S. (2017). Semiconductor nanocrystals: Structure, properties, and band gap engineering. *Accounts of Chemical Research, 50*(3), 557–565.

72. Smith, J., & Jones, A. (2022). Advances in nanoimaging techniques for early disease detection. *Journal of Nanomedicine, 14*(3), 101–115.

73. Syedmoradi, L., Norton, M. L., & Omidfar, K. (2017). Point-of-care cancer detection with nano-enabled biosensors. *Analytical and Bioanalytical Chemistry, 409*(29), 6803–6817. https://doi.org/10.1007/s00216-017-0608-6.

74. Theranostics and AI—The next advance in cancer precision medicine. https://datascience.cancer.gov/news-events/blog/theranostics-and-ai-next-advance-cancer-precision-medicine (accessed on 7 May 2025).

75. Tinkle, S., & McNeil, S. E. (2014). Nanomedicines: Addressing the scientific and regulatory gap. *Nature Reviews Drug Discovery, 13*(8), 628–642. https://doi.org/10.1038/nrd4368.

76. Vashist, S. K., Luppa, P. B., Yeo, L. Y., Ozcan, A., & Luong, J. H. T. (2015). Emerging technologies for next-generation point-of-care testing. *Trends in Biotechnology, 33*(11), 692–705. https://doi.org/10.1016/j.tibtech.2015.09.001.

77. Vashist, S. K., van Oordt, T., Schneider, E. M., Zengerle, R., & von Stetten, F. (2014). Highly-sensitive and rapid detection of cardiac troponin I using a novel immunoassay. *Analytica Chimica Acta, 848*, 78–83. https://doi.org/10.1016/j.aca.2014.08.022.

78. Veiseh, O., Sun, C., & Fang, C. (2010). Iron oxide nanoparticles for brain tumor imaging and therapy: Recent advances and challenges. *Journal of Controlled Release, 146*(2), 194–203.

79. Wang, C., et al. (2014). Multifunctional theragnostic redox-responsive nanoparticles. *Nanoscale, 6*(14), 8497–8504.

80. Wang, J. (2005). Carbon-nanotube based electrochemical biosensors: A review. *Electroanalysis, 17*(1), 7–14. https://doi.org/10.1002/elan.200403113.

81. Wang, J., & Liu, G. (2008). Recent advances in nano sensors for bioanalysis. *Chemical Reviews, 108*(2), 814–825. https://doi.org/10.1021/cr068102g.

82. Wang, J., Xia, H., & Yu, M. (2020). AI-driven theragnostic: Transforming diagnosis and therapy. *Nature Reviews Drug Discovery, 19*(8), 573–590. https://doi.org/10.1038/s41573-020-0073-5.

83. Wang, L., & Zhang, H. (2024). Early detection of cancer and cardiovascular diseases using nanoparticle-based imaging. *Journal of Biomedical Nanotechnology, 20*(2), 365–378. https://doi.org/10.1166/jbn.2024.13456.

84. Wang, S., Liu, R., & Shen, L. (2020). Theragnostic nanoparticles for biomedical applications. *ACS Nano, 14*(3), 2585–2596.

85. Wang, X., & Zhao, H. (2022). Real-time monitoring of targeted therapy using nanoimaging. *Journal of Clinical Imaging Science, 10*(4), 215–228.

86. Wang, X., Li, Z., & Zhou, Z. (2019). Stimuli-responsive nanoparticles for controlled modulation of cell death pathways. *Nano Today, 25*, 85–104. https://doi.org/10.1016/j.nantod.2019.01.010.

87. Wang, Y., & Irudayaraj, J. (2010). A SERS DNAzyme biosensor for lead ion detection. *Chemical Communications, 46*(12), 2261–2263.

88. Wang, Y., & Zhang, L. (2021). Stimuli-responsive nanoparticles for personalized therapeutic delivery. *Advanced Functional Materials, 31*(4), 2007491.

89. Williams, D., & Johnson, R. (2022). Theragnostic: Combining diagnostics and therapy with nanoimaging. *Theragnostic, 8*(6), 152–167.

90. Winter, P. M., & Caruthers, S. D. (2014). Advances in molecular imaging of atherosclerosis with targeted nanoparticles. *Journal of Cardiovascular Translational Research, 7*(5), 694–700. https://doi.org/10.1007/s12265-014-9596-2.

91. Xie, J., Lee, S., & Chen, X. (2010). Nanoparticle-based theragnostic agents. *Advanced Drug Delivery Reviews, 62*(11), 1064–1079. https://doi.org/10.1016/j.addr.2010.07.009.

92. Yager, P., Domingo, G. J., & Gerdes, J. (2008). Point-of-care diagnostics for global health. *Annual Review of Biomedical Engineering, 10*, 107–144. https://doi.org/10.1146/annurev.bioeng.10.061807.160524.

93. Yih, T. C., & Al-Fandi, M. (2006). Engineered nanoparticles as precise drug delivery systems. *Journal of Cellular Biochemistry, 97*(6), 1184–1190. https://doi.org/10.1002/jcb.20796.

94. Zhang, L., & Gu, F. X. (2008). Nanoparticles in medicine: Therapeutic applications and developments. *Clinical Pharmacology & Therapeutics, 83*(5), 761–769. https://doi.org/10.1038/clpt.2008.31.

95. Zhang, P., Liu, W., & Yuan, S. (2021). Nanotechnology approaches to targeting regulated cell death pathways in cancer therapy. *Journal of Controlled Release, 330*, 158–174. https://doi.org/10.1016/j.jconrel.2021.01.030.

96. Zhang, X., & Zhao, Y. (2023). Up conversion nanoparticles for deep-tissue imaging: Recent advances and applications. *Advanced Functional Materials, 33*(9), 2208934. https://doi.org/10.1002/adfm.202208934.

97. Zhang, Y., & Liu, T. (2023). Advances in molecular imaging using quantum dots for cancer detection. *Journal of Nanobiotechnology, 21*(1), 45. https://doi.org/10.1186/s12951-023-01526-0.

98. Zhang, Y., & Ma, Y. (2021). Nanotheranostics for cancer: Personalized approaches and future directions. *Theragnostic, 11*(7), 3452–3471.

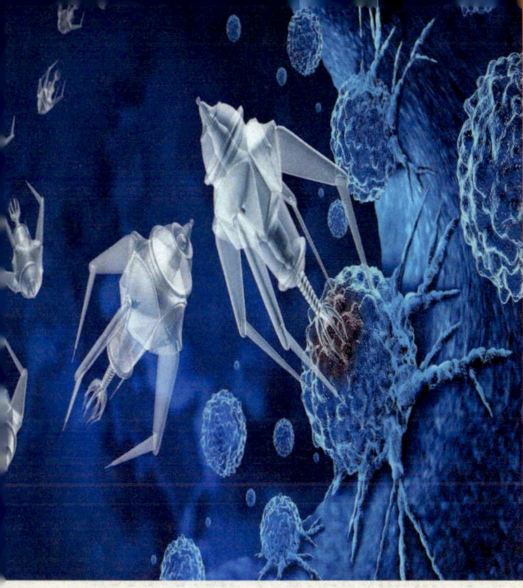

Chapter 4

NANOMEDICINE IN CANCER: ADVANCEMENTS AND PROMISING APPLICATIONS

Contents

Shweta Tripathi*

Department of Biology, Tuskegee University, Tuskegee, Alabama, USA

*Corresponding author.

Abstract

Cancer is still considered as one of the most difficult challenges in modern medicine and therefore new ways of diagnosing, treating, and managing it must be found. Nanomedicine offers an opportunity to modernize cancer treatment. This chapter is aimed at giving a brief description of the present state of nanomedicine application in oncology with accentuation on the major achievements and promising areas.

Traditional cancer therapy has been known to have many shortcomings thus the need for new strategies using nanotechnology which can help overcome these limitations. The use of nanoscale drug delivery systems (DDS) like liposomes, polymeric nanoparticles or lipid-based carriers among others has led to increased specificity towards target cells while minimizing systemic toxicity associated with conventional drugs delivery methods (Akbarzadeh et al., 2013; Danhier et al., 2012; Torchilin, 2014). Such modifications not only improved patients' life quality but also raised their chance survival rates significantly.

Moreover, apart from being used as carriers for drugs, nanoparticles play vital roles in cancer imaging as well as diagnostics. For example, quantum dots (QDs) and iron oxide particle sizes enable creation highly sensitive and specific imaging modalities such MRI or CT scan, among others (Jokerst and Gambhir, 2011). These techniques provide early detection of tumors, accurate localization during surgery and monitoring response to therapy in real time.

Additionally, breakthroughs within nanomedicine field were witnessed even in immunotherapy against cancers. Nanoparticle vaccines coupled with immunomodulators can be designed to 'awaken' the immune system so that it recognizes cancer cells thereby attacking them thus opening doors for personalized treatments which are directed specifically towards an individual patient's tumor type (Hua et al., 2018).

This abstract also discusses the potential of theranostic nanomedicine, where nanoparticles are designed to simultaneously diagnose, treat, and monitor cancer (Chu and Dupuy, 2014). These multi-functional nanocarriers are expected to provide patients holistic care by fighting cancer.

Development of nanomedicine for cancer still faces some challenges despite the outstanding progress made so far. Issues touching on scalability, safety, and regulatory approval should be continuously addressed during its creation and clinical translation.

In conclusion, nanomedicine is seen as a ray of hope in dealing with cancer. Drug delivery, diagnostics, and immunotherapy have been the major areas where it has influenced care for cancer patients greatly, but further studies can lead to more revolutionary discoveries. If we keep our focus on understanding what these small particles can do, they will remain an important weapon in our fight against this disease.

4.1. Nanomedicine

4.1.1. Introduction to Nanomedicine

In cancer treatment, nanomedicine is revolutionizing the field by using molecular precision for diagnosis and therapy. This chapter will investigate how nanomedicine has changed the way we think about fighting cancer. It is divided into different sections which cover the following topics:

1. **Targeted Cancer Therapies:** This section will discuss the molecular precision of therapy. For example, it will address nanoscale interventions—the design principles and working mechanisms of targeted therapies (Peer et al., 2007).
2. **Photothermal and Photodynamic Therapy (PDT):** The use of light in medicine is not new but its application as a therapeutic agent against tumors is a recent development. The part

also covers how nanoparticles can produce heat under light exposure or react chemically with oxygen when illuminated thereby killing nearby cells selectively (Hirsch et al., 2003).

3. **Nanoparticle-based Radiotherapy:** Nanoparticles are being integrated into the field of radiotherapy. There will be a discussion on this, as well as the synergistic effects with radiation and potential enhancements in treatment efficacy while reducing collateral damage (Zhang et al., 2008).
4. **Enhancements:** This section talks about how nanotechnology can improve conventional methods for fighting cancer. From drug delivery optimization to overcoming biological obstacles, there are various ways through which therapeutic outcomes may be improved by nanomedicine (Shi et al., 2017).
5. **Recent Advancements in Cancer Therapy:** This reviews the cutting-edge research in cancer, providing the latest breakthroughs. From novel drug formulations to advanced imaging techniques, this section summarizes the forefront of cancer therapeutics (Davis and Chen, 2008).
6. **Personalized Nanomedicine:** This discusses modifying personalized treatments based on individual patient profiles. From molecular profiling to customized nanoparticle formulations, this section discusses these modifications for individual patient characteristics (Li, Pu, and Semenza, 2019).
7. **Immunomodulatory Nanoparticles:** This discusses the intersection of nanotechnology and immunotherapy. Utilizing the potential of nanoparticles in modulating immune responses, this section describes the prospects of synergistic approaches in cancer treatment (Irvine and Dane, 2020).

This chapter discusses the interplay between nanomedicine and cancer therapeutics, their advancements, and promising applications.

4.1.2. Nanomedicine in Targeted Cancer Therapies: Precision, Innovation, and Beyond

Cancer is uncontrolled and abnormal growth of cells, a process controlled by genetic mutations. These cells can invade adjacent tissues and spread to other parts of the body, making cancer a high danger and metastatic disease (Hanahan and Weinberg, 2011). The growth of new blood vessels through angiogenesis supports the tumor's development and progression (Carmeliet and Jain, 2011). Cancer cells often evade the body's immune system and demonstrate heterogeneity, with diverse genetic and molecular characteristics (Binnewies et al., 2018). Dysregulation of cellular signaling pathways contributes to this uncontrolled cell division (Manning and Cantley, 2007). Tumor staging and grading help indicate how advanced the cancer is (Edge and Compton, 2010), while treatment options range from surgery to chemotherapy, radiation therapy, immunotherapy, and targeted drug treatments (Schirrmacher, 2019). Despite challenges that persist, ongoing research aims at broadening our knowledge base on all fronts concerning this disease to develop more effective therapies which can be specifically tailored for individual patients (Visvader and Lindeman, 2008).

Nanomedicine presents an innovative approach towards diagnosis and treatment of cancer. It refers to the use of tiny materials and devices at molecular levels to interact with biological systems, in relation to cancer. For example, nanoparticles may be designed in such a way that they specifically target cancer cells, hence delivering therapeutic agents directly to the tumor site while minimizing damages on healthy tissues (Blanco, Shen, and Ferrari, 2015). Consequently, this method of drug delivery increases treatment efficiency while reducing side effects associated with traditional modes of therapy. Furthermore, it allows for accurate imaging and early detection of malignant cells which facilitates timely intervention (Jokerst and Gambhir, 2011). Additionally, nanomaterials (NMs) possess unique characteristics that create room for development of new diagnostic methods and monitoring treatment response (Saha et al., 2012). The integration of conventional cancer therapy with nanomedicine boosts overall treatment efficacy thereby representing a breakthrough in the fight against cancer (Peer et al., 2007).

Nanodevices are tools that perform their functions on the scale of nanometers, usually between 1 and 100 nm (Ferry, 2009). Physical characteristics and behaviors of substances can be different at the nanoscale as compared to macroscale level due to which, nanodevices are created with an intention to possess specific features, manipulate matter at atomic or molecular level and frequently manage materials' distinct properties displayed at this size range (Cao, 2018; Shi et al., 2017). Medicine, electronics (Avouris, Chen, and Perebeinos, 2007), energy (Chu and Majumdar, 2012), and so on, are some of the areas where these devices find application.

For instance, in cancer therapy targeting drugs delivery imaging diagnostics may be done by nanodevices. Various types of nanodevices include but not limited to (Figure 4.1):

1. **Nanoparticles:** These are small particles having sizes within nanometer ranges which can be modified for drug delivery systems (DDS) among others like imaging agents used during diagnosis processes (Dreaden et al., 2012).
2. Nanotubes: Tubular structures of nanosize dimensions such as carbon nanotubes (CNTs) (Kam and Dai, 2005) have been employed in different applications, for example, delivering drugs into cells or creating electronic devices with high efficiency.
3. **Nanorobots:** Miniature robots meant specifically for carrying out tasks at the level of nanometer, for instance, targeted drug delivery or precise surgery (Liang et al., 2021).
4. **Nanowires:** These very thin wires existing at nanoscales can be utilized for various purposes including electronic sensors development even acting as carriers of therapeutic agents within biological systems (Patolsky et al., 2006).
5. **Quantum Dots (QDs):** They are semiconductor nanocrystals possessing special optical properties which make them suitable materials in high resolution imaging and diagnostics (Michalet et al., 2005).
6. **Nanocapsules:** These are tiny empty structures at the nanoscale that can hold active drugs to deliver them to their specific site of action (Kreuter, 2001).
7. **Nanocarriers:** Nanosized carriers designed for conveying drugs, genes, or imaging agents to body locations (Blanco, Shen, and Ferrari, 2015).
8. **Nanogels:** Cross-linked polymer networks capable of trapping medicines within them and releasing them slowly for therapeutic purposes (Blanco, Shen, and Ferrari, 2015). Due to their ability to target specific cells, improve bioavailability and lower toxicity, nanomedicines have become an attractive option in cancer therapy.

Nanoparticles which usually have diameters measured in nanometers provide an excellent delivery system for anti-cancer drugs because they can be engineered to deliver the drug to only the cancer cells while sparing the normal cells. Their targeting mechanisms can be broadly classified into passive and active approaches.

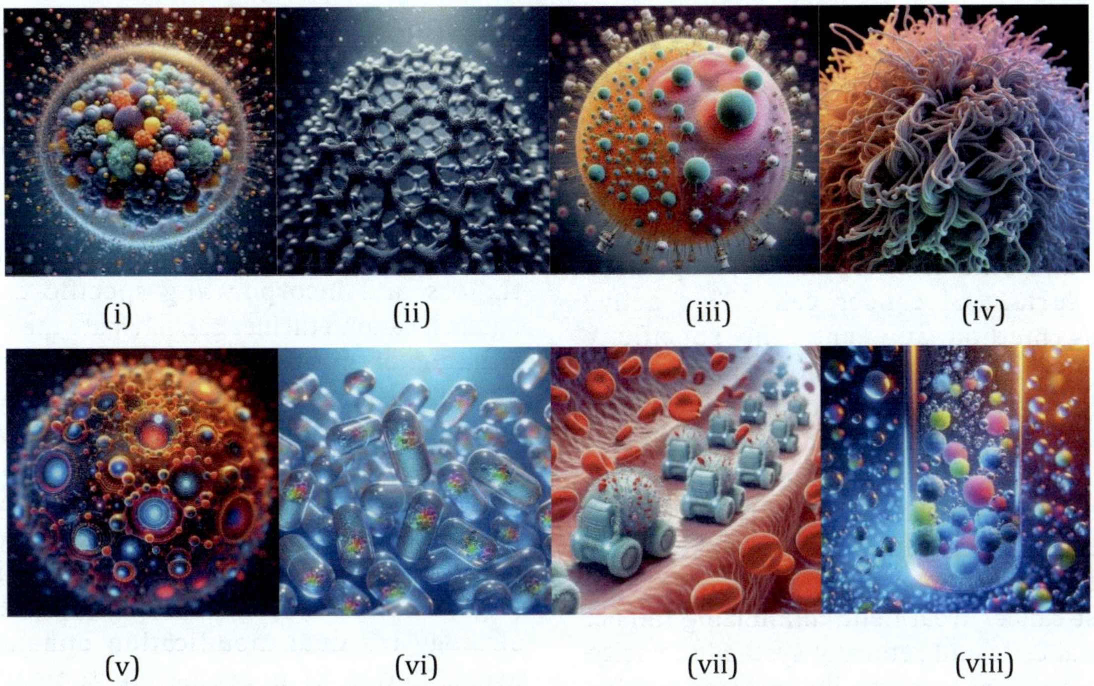

Figure 4.1. Various types of nanodevices, including: (i) nanoparticle; (ii) nanotube; (iii) nanorobots; (iv) nanowires; (v) quantum dots; (vi) nanocapsules; (vii) nanocarriers; and (viii) nanogels.

4.1.3. Passive Targeting

4.1.3.1. Enhanced Permeability and Retention (EPR) Effect

Nanoparticles exploit the EPR effect in tumors. Due to this effect, liposomal doxorubicin formulations such as Doxil accumulate in tumor tissue. Lymphatic drainage becomes inefficient because of this phenomenon, causing nanoparticles to be deposited within the neoplastic tissue, thus, advances drug delivery to cancer cells while minimizing exposure to normal tissues.

They can be used to encapsulate the drugs and deliver them selectively to cancer cells while sparing exposure of normal tissues. This will however depend on nature of the particles themselves (Greish, 2007).

Passive targeting takes advantage of some biological properties of cancer, so that nanoparticles may be preferentially retained within malignant neoplasm rather than normal tissue. For active targeting, Ligands or antibodies that are specific can be attached onto the surface of nanoparticle which will recognize and bind with receptors overexpressed by cancer cell. Nanoparticles take advantage of the EPR effect observed in tumors. Tumors often exhibit leaky blood vessels and impaired lymphatic drainage, leading to the accumulation of nanoparticles in the tumor tissue.

Liposomal doxorubicin formulations, like Doxil, accumulate in tumor tissues due to this effect. This improves drug delivery to cancer cells while minimizing exposure to normal tissues (Maeda et al., 2000).

4.1.4. Active Targeting

4.1.4.1. Surface Functionalization

Nanoparticles can be engineered with specific ligands or antibodies on their surface that identify and bind to receptors overexpressed on the surface of cancer cells. This active targeting method augments the specificity of drug delivery. Herceptin, a monoclonal antibody targeting HER2-overexpressing breast cancer cells, is integrated into nanoparticles like liposomes. These nanoparticles with Herceptin, selectively bind to HER2 receptors, concentrating therapeutic agents at the tumor site. This targeted approach increases precision in breast cancer treatment, minimizing impact on normal cells and reducing systemic toxicity. The potential of nanomedicine in advancing cancer therapies is improved efficacy with fewer side effects (Peer et al., 2007).

4.1.4.2. Cellular Internalization

Ligand-receptor interactions enable the internalization of nanoparticles into cancer cells, ensuring that the therapeutic payload is delivered precisely to the target site. Folate receptors are often overexpressed in certain cancer cells. Nanoparticles with folate ligands (Folate-targeted liposomal formulations for delivering anticancer agents) can actively target and deliver drugs to these cancer cells (Torchilin, 2007).

4.1.4.3. Subcellular Targeting

Some advanced nanomedicines are designed for subcellular targeting, to deliver drugs to specific organelles within cancer cells for ideal therapeutic effects. In acidic tumor microenvironments, pH-sensitive micelles can be designed for targeted delivery of chemotherapeutic drugs in cancer treatment. This is because the pH in tumor tissues is often lower compared to normal tissues (Wang, Zhang, and Zhang, 2016).

The combination of active and passive targeting strategies provides a comprehensive approach to address the heterogeneity of tumors and increase the precision of cancer treatment. By exploiting the unique microenvironment of tumors and incorporating specific targeting ligands, nanomedicines can navigate the complex situation of the body with remarkable accuracy. This dual-targeting approach increases the accumulation at the target site and improves the specificity of drug delivery. Liposomes modified with both passive (PEGylating for prolonged circulation by minimizing immune recognition) and active components like targeting ligands (e.g., antibodies) (Wilhelm et al., 2016). The strategy for dual modification enhances the accumulation of liposomes in tumor tissues through the effect of enhanced permeability and retention (EPR) hence their prolonged circulation as well as accurate targeting. In cancer treatment, these liposomes have been used to deliver drugs more effectively to the cancer cells while at the same time reducing systemic toxicity and improving therapeutic efficacy (Torchilin, 2011).

When handling solid tumors, it becomes very critical to consider primary targeting, secondary targeting, localized delivery, and intravascular delivery mechanisms in DDS for solid tumors because they are complex types of cancers with different cell populations within them.

4.1.4.4. Primary Targeting in Solid Tumors

In solid tumors, primary targeting methods are essential since interactions between drug carriers and cancerous cells happen mostly at this level compared to any other place. It is possible for ligands on nanoparticles to facilitate specific DDS by recognizing receptors overexpressed on tissues of certain types of cancers (Zhang, Chan, and Leong, 2013). Folate ligand-modified liposomes can be used as an example where they bind selectively with high affinity due to their conjugation with folate molecules onto them thus enabling such particles enter into cells which express more receptor number than usual amounts found outside these types of malignancies (Sawant and Torchilin, 2012).

4.1.4.5. Secondary Targeting in Solid Tumors

Most adaptable secondary targeting techniques become quite useful in such environments where conditions keep on changing from time to time especially inside living organisms like humans who may have been infected by diseases causing solid tumors such as carcinoma among others very dangerous if not treated at early stages. Therefore, it means that there should be responsive nanoparticles designed in such a way that they release their content under different conditions prevailing within these organs to ensure maximum benefit towards therapy against malignancies having solid tumor structures. pH-responsive nanoparticles will serve this purpose effectively since the majority, if not all, drug-loaded carriers must reach acidic microenvironment where most parts of these growths are located thereby making drugs available for action only at places where needed most thus sparing healthy cells (Gu et al., 2008).

4.1.4.6. Localized Delivery in Solid Tumors

Local delivering ways are frequently needed for strong tumors to enhance therapeutic effects and restrict systemic influence. Direct drug or nanoparticle introduction into the tumor—such as intratumoral injection—can concentrate medicines directly at the cancer site. Nanoparticles like liposomes or polymeric carriers may contain chemotherapeutic drugs (e.g., cisplatin, paclitaxel or 5FU) and offer accurate drug delivery platforms. For instance, oncolytic viruses can be injected directly into solid tumors with the goal of providing localized and targeted treatment for cancer. Talimogene laherparepvec (T-VEC) is an engineered oncolytic *herpes simplex* virus designed to infect and destroy only melanoma cells by replicating within them. Through direct injection into melanoma lesions, T-VEC exerts its oncolytic effect locally, causing the destruction of cancer cells while sparing normal tissues. Furthermore, T-VEC stimulates an anti-tumor immune response, enhancing the body's ability to recognize and attack melanoma cells (Miao et al., 2015). Local cancer care has shown effectiveness in treating unresectable cutaneous, subcutaneous, and nodal lesions of patients with melanoma who have had a recurrence following initial surgery. By directly injecting the virus, it reduces the systemic exposure but also applies the oncolytic virus potential for precise and efficient cancer treatment paradigms (Andtbacka et al., 2011).

4.1.4.7. Intravascular Delivery in Solid Tumors

The importance of intravascular delivery increases with solid tumors as it requires nanoparticle systemic circulation. Passive targeting strategies such as EPR effect should be used to help nanoparticles accumulate in tumor vessels which will in turn enhance drug delivery efficacy to solid tumors (Fang, Nakamura, and Maeda, 2011). For example, PEGylated liposomes accumulate passively within solid tumor through EPR effect thereby improving drug delivery to tumor site. Doxil liposomes are coated with polyethylene glycol (PEG) (Allen and Cullis, 2013) and being able to concentrate its chemotherapy payload specifically at the tumor site lowers systemic toxicity levels while improving therapeutic outcomes across various cancers including ovarian cancer, breast cancer, and Kaposi's sarcoma (Gabizon and Patil, 2021). These personalized nanomedicine control strategies for solid tumors illustrate how they can be applied to precision drug delivery optimization, implying better treatment results of therapies against cancer.

Two different approaches in the field of medicine are the polymeric and non-polymeric delivery systems, each with its own unique features and uses (Figure 4.2). Biocompatible polymers that can be easily broken down within the body are used to encase drugs during polymeric delivery systems. PLGA nanoparticles are one example, which are famed for their ability to regulate drug release while polycaprolactone (PCL) microparticles offer prolonged delivery (Danhier et al., 2012). These serve as ideal matrices since they release drugs at a localized site over time—a characteristic shared by hydrogels made from PEG (Hoffman, 2012). Intravascular delivery assumes heightened importance when addressing solid tumors, as it involves the systemic circulation of nanoparticles. Passive targeting mechanisms, such as the EPR effect, are harnessed to facilitate the accumulation of nanoparticles in the tumor vasculature, contributing to the overall efficacy of drug delivery to solid tumors (Fang, Nakamura, and Maeda, 2011). For instance, PEGylated liposomes passively accumulate in solid tumors through the EPR effect, improving drug delivery to the tumor site. The liposomes in Doxil are coated with PEG (Allen and Cullis, 2013), passively targeting through the EPR effect enables Doxil to concentrate its chemotherapy payload specifically at the tumor site, reducing systemic toxicity and improving the therapeutic outcome in various cancers, including ovarian cancer, breast cancer, and Kaposi's sarcoma (Gabizon and Patil, 2021).

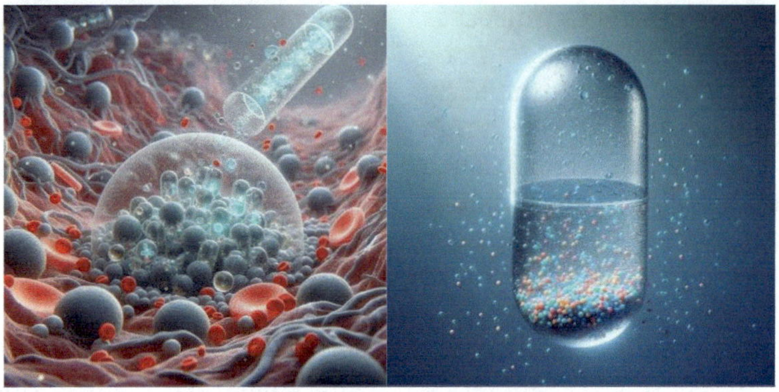

(i) (ii)

Figure 4.2. Examples of (i) polymeric delivery systems (biocompatible polymers such as PLGA nanoparticles); and (ii) non-polymeric delivery systems (polycaprolactone [PCL] microparticles).

These examples show how these strategies, modified specifically for solid tumors, control nanomedicine to optimize drug delivery precision, improve therapeutic outcomes, and advance the frontiers of cancer treatment.

Polymeric and non-polymeric delivery systems are two distinct approaches in the field of drug delivery, each offering unique characteristics and applications. Polymeric delivery systems involve the utilization of biocompatible and biodegradable polymers to encapsulate therapeutic agents. Examples include PLGA nanoparticles, known for their controlled drug release capabilities, and PCL microparticles, providing sustained drug delivery (Danhier et al., 2012). Hydrogels, such as those based on PEG, offer three-dimensional networks for localized drug release (Hoffman,

2012). Chitosan (CH) nanoparticles, sourced from crustacean shells, enhance drug bioavailability, and find applications in gene delivery and wound healing (Sarwar et al., 2015). Hyaluronic acid (HA) nanogels, derived from human connective tissues, show promise for targeted drug delivery, especially in cancer therapy. Alginate nanoparticles, extracted from seaweeds, enable controlled drug release, and have diverse applications (Choi and Park, 2019). Gelatin nanoparticles, originating from collagen, are biocompatible and adaptable for various drug delivery routes (Draget, Smidsrød, and Skjåk-Bræk, 2005). Silk fibroin nanoparticles, from silkworm silk, is particularly useful in drug delivery, wound healing, and tissue engineering (Mandal and Kundu, 2009). Natural polymers extend to DNA and protein-based nanocarriers, such as albumin nanoparticles, offering sustainable and biocompatible options (Kratz, 2008). Overall, natural polymers in nanomedicine present exciting prospects for advancing DDS with improved efficacy and reduced side effects. On the other hand, non-polymeric delivery systems include diverse carriers that do not rely on polymers. Liposomes, like liposomal doxorubicin, represent lipid-based vesicles with applications in cancer therapy (Torchilin, 2011). Micelles, exemplified by Pluronic micelles, are formed by the self-assembly of amphiphilic molecules, offering solubilization of hydrophobic drugs (Li, Lokitz, and McCormick, 2006). Inorganic nanoparticles, such as gold nanoparticles (AuNPs), showcase the versatility of non-polymeric carriers for drug delivery and imaging. These systems exhibit versatility, allowing for a range of options, including lipid-based and inorganic carriers, and can be designed for targeted drug delivery (Dreaden et al., 2012). Poly(lactic-co-glycolic acid) (PLGA) nanoparticles offer controlled release capabilities, widely applied in cancer therapy and vaccine delivery (Danhier et al., 2012). PEG modification enhances nanoparticle stability and circulation time, particularly in PEGylated liposomes for drug delivery (Gref et al., 1994). Poly(ethyleneimine) (PEI) is crucial in gene delivery, forming complexes with nucleic acids for efficient transfection (Fischer et al., 1999). PCL nanoparticles provide sustained drug release and find applications in tissue engineering (Labet and Thielemans, 2009). Poly(alkyl cyanoacrylate) (PACA) nanoparticles are explored for drug delivery to the central nervous system (CNS). Additionally, pH-sensitive poly(ortho esters) enables controlled drug release in response to physiological changes (Koffie et al., 2011; Tawfeek et al., 2017). These synthetic polymers offer personalized solutions, improving drug delivery efficiency and advancing the precision of therapeutic interventions. However, the choice between polymeric and non-polymeric systems pivots on specific therapeutic requirements, emphasizing the role of both approaches in advancing drug delivery technologies to enhance therapeutic outcomes while minimizing side effects.

Table 4.1 provides a summary of various cancer types, their corresponding molecular targets, and representative therapeutic agents that have demonstrated efficacy in the treatment of these malignancies. Each entry highlights the specific molecular target associated with a particular cancer type and the therapeutic agent designed to act on that target. Trastuzumab (Herceptin) stands as a primary anti-breast cancer therapeutic agent, addressing HER2-positive tumors and demonstrating its efficacy in improving patient outcomes (Slamon et al., 2001). Cetuximab, a monoclonal antibody inhibiting EGFR (epidermal growth factor receptor), has proven valuable in the treatment of colorectal cancer, shows the importance of targeting specific molecular pathways (Cunningham et al., 2004). In non-small cell lung cancer, Erlotinib, an EGFR inhibitor, has emerged as a targeted therapy, particularly effective in cases with EGFR mutation (Shepherd et al., 2005). The androgen receptor inhibitor Enzalutamide demonstrates precision medicine in advanced prostate cancer, offering a targeted approach with notable therapeutic benefits (Scher et al., 2012). Imatinib, targeting the BCR-ABL fusion protein, represents an innovative advancement in the management of chronic myeloid leukemia (Druker et al., 2001). Brentuximab vedotin, addressing CD30-positive lymphoma cells, has transformed Hodgkin's lymphoma therapy with enhanced efficacy and reduced toxicity (Younes et al., 2010). Vemurafenib, a BRAF inhibitor, showed the potential of targeting specific mutations in melanoma, leading to improved patient outcomes (Chapman et al., 2011). Olaparib, an inhibitor of poly(ADP-ribose) polymerase (PARP), has shown success in treating ovarian cancer with BRCA mutations, underscoring the significance of personalized therapies (Ledermann et al., 2014). Nab-paclitaxel (Abraxane) addresses the challenges posed by KRAS mutations in pancreatic cancer, providing a targeted and effective therapeutic option (Von Hoff et al., 2013). Bevacizumab, an anti-VEGF agent, has become a basis in renal cell carcinoma therapy, highlighting the pivotal role of angiogenesis inhibition (Escudier et al., 2007). Daratumumab, targeting CD38 in multiple myeloma, has significantly improved treatment outcomes, with the impact of precision medicine in hematological malignancies (Palumbo et al., 2016). Imatinib's success in gastrointestinal stromal tumors (GIST), through KIT inhibition, represents the transformative potential of targeted therapies. Lastly, thyroid cancers with precise modifications, including RET, BRAF, or NTRK, use tailored therapies such as Vandetanib (Wells et al., 2012), Dabrafenib (Hauschild et al., 2012), and Larotrectinib (Drilon et al., 2018), respectively, highlighting the evolution of precision medicine in oncology.

Table 4.1. Molecular Targets and Therapeutic Agents Across Various Cancer Types

Cancer Type	Molecular Target	Therapeutic Agent
Breast cancer	HER2	Trastuzumab (Herceptin)
Colorectal cancer	EGFR	Cetuximab
Lung cancer (non-small cell)	EGFR	Erlotinib
Prostate cancer	Androgen receptor	Enzalutamide
Leukemia (chronic myeloid)	BCR-ABL	Imatinib
Lymphoma (Hodgkin's)	CD30	Brentuximab vedotin
Melanoma	BRAF	Vemurafenib
Ovarian cancer	PARP	Olaparib
Pancreatic cancer	KRAS	Nab-paclitaxel (Abraxane)
Renal cell carcinoma	VEGF	Bevacizumab
Multiple myeloma	CD38	Daratumumab
Gastrointestinal stromal tumor (GIST)	KIT	Imatinib
Thyroid cancer	RET, BRAF, NTRK	Vandetanib, Dabrafenib, Larotrectinib

Table 4.1 compiles the precision and diversity of targeted therapies in cancer treatment, highlighting the importance of identifying specific molecular targets for designing effective and personalized therapeutic interventions. Each therapeutic agent signifies an important advancement in the pursuit for more targeted and less lethal cancer treatments. In addition to targeting, nanomedicines propose advantages in terms of bioavailability and low toxicity:

1. **Bioavailability:** Nanoparticles can encapsulate both hydrophobic and hydrophilic pharmaceuticals that enhance the solubility and stability of curative agents. This improves

drug bioavailability thus achieving more efficient delivery to the desired target (Torchilin, 2006; Wilhelm et al., 2016).

2. **Low Toxicity:** Nanomedicines minimize side effects by reducing the exposure of healthy tissues to therapeutic agents. This kind of delivery also helps bring down general toxicity levels which is something that often worries people about traditional forms of chemotherapy; it makes patients more capable of enduring treatment (Hare et al., 2017; Mura, Nicolas, and Couvreur, 2013).

4.2. Nanomedicine in Photothermal and Photodynamic Therapy (PDT): Enlightening the Future of Cancer Treatment

4.2.1. Introduction

In the development of cancer treatment towards amplified effectiveness and precision, nanomedicine has ascended as a potential game-changer. This section discusses the transformative role of nanotechnology in photothermal therapy (PTT) and photodynamic therapy (PDT), focusing on how these innovative approaches could transform the field of cancer treatment.

4.2.2. Photothermal Therapy (PTT): A Precision Heat Source

Photothermal therapy (PTT) therapy uses nanoparticles that have been designed to absorb and convert light in the near-infrared (NIR) range into heat. This localized hyperthermia provides a focused and precise approach, selectively targeting cancer cells inducing apoptosis and necrosis, while protecting the surrounding healthy tissue (Chen et al., 2010; Hirsch et al., 2003). AuNPs possess excellent biocompatibility making them good agents for PTT where they may be engineered with specific ligands on their surface enabling selective binding to target cells among other applications. The plasmonic properties of gold nanorods can be adjusted to control the amount of heat generated thus optimizing therapeutic outcomes while also minimizing adverse effects on normal tissues. There are many possibilities for combining different treatments with photothermal ablation such that synergy occurs between these two modalities leading into improved overall efficacy against malignant diseases but at the same time reducing toxicities associated with most current chemotherapeutic or radiation approaches used singly or in combination. Consequently, nanomedicine offers great promise for revolutionizing current standard cancer care by providing curative solutions hitherto unattainable finality (Dreaden et al., 2012; Huang et al., 2006). Other types of photo thermal agents include carbon-based materials like graphene or CNTs which exhibit high thermal conductivity and can therefore effectively induce hyperthermia when subjected to NIR light while remaining compatible with diverse therapeutic platforms due to their adjustable nature coupled with low systemic toxicity levels brought about by efficient elimination from body tissues after completion of treatment regimen (Liu et al., 2008; Robinson et al., 2011).

Moreover, copper sulfide nanoparticles can be used for PTT. They absorb strongly in the NIR region which enables efficient light-to-heat conversion. Adjusting the size and composition increases the potentiality of these particles to generate localized heat for PTT applications (Song et al., 2015; Tian et al., 2011).

Furthermore, combination of PTT with different NMs like magnetic nanoparticles or nanocomposites enhances targeted cancer therapy. These materials have various functions that can be utilized in multimodal treatments leading to better therapeutic results.

4.2.3. Photodynamic Therapy (PDT): Harnessing Light for Targeted Destruction

The utilization of Photosensitizer-Loaded Nanoparticles emerges as a sophisticated strategy, predominantly in the context of PDT. This advanced approach works on the unique properties of nanocarriers carrying photosensitizers, providing a targeted and controlled means to induce cell death upon contact with specific light wavelengths.

At its core, PDT includes a precise interaction of Light, Photosensitizer, and Oxygen. The process begins with the administration of Photosensitizer-Loaded Nanoparticles to the patient. These nanoparticles, designed to condense photosensitizing agents, navigate through the bloodstream and selectively accumulate in cancer cells, driven by active targeting mechanisms.

Upon attaining the target site, the next critical element comes into play is the Light. When exposed to light of specific wavelengths, the encapsulated photosensitizers within the nanoparticles experience photo activation.

This activation sets off a cascade of reactions leading to the generation of reactive oxygen species (ROS). These ROS, predominantly singlet oxygen, display potent cytotoxicity, inducing apoptosis and necrosis in the cancer cells. The selectivity of PDT is noticeably enhanced by the precise localization of photosensitizers within the cancer cells, confirming that the therapeutic effects are concentrated precisely where needed (Ethirajan et al., 2011; Lucky, Soo, and Zhang, 2015).

Crucially, the involvement of Oxygen is essential to the PDT mechanism. Molecular oxygen in the cellular environment participates in the generation of ROS during the photo activation process. This dependency on oxygen also contributes to the selectivity of PDT, as the generation of cytotoxic ROS is confined to the illuminated areas where both photosensitizer and oxygen are present in abundance. AuNPs serve as carriers for the photosensitizer Chlorin e6 (Ce6), creating a targeted Photosensitizer-Loaded Nanoparticle system (Dreaden et al., 2012; Huang, El-Sayed, Qian, and El-Sayed, 2006). Mesoporous silicon nanoparticles MSNPs can also be used as carriers for photosensitizers in PDT, offering a platform for targeted and controlled drug delivery (Chou, Ming, and Chan, 2011; He and Shi, 2011).

Furthermore, the Dual-Functionality exhibited by certain nanoparticles not only accommodates photosensitizers but also serve as carriers for therapeutic agents. This combined approach represents a complete and personalized approach to cancer treatment, showcasing the adaptability of nanomedicine in optimizing therapeutic outcomes (Lee et al., 2012; Wang et al., 2010).

In principle, the integration of Photosensitizer-Loaded Nanoparticles into PDT signifies a precision-guided revolution in cancer therapy. By addressing challenges related to selectivity, harnessing dual-functionality, and leveraging the unique properties of nanoparticles, this approach focuses on advancing the intricacies of targeted and multifaceted cancer Treatments, encouraging a more refined and effective therapeutic landscape.

4.2.4. Nanoparticles Bridging PTT and PDT: Integrating Photothermal and Photodynamic Effects

The key revolution lies in the ability to engineer nanoparticles with dual functionality, integrating both photo thermal and photodynamic elements (Wang et al., 2018). Nanoparticles achieve photothermal effects by absorbing light which is then converted into heat causing localized hyperthermia that destroys cancer cells at that specific site. At the same time, these very particles have also got photosensitizers for photodynamic effects (Lucky, Soo, and Zhang, 2015). These photosensitizers when exposed to light, produce ROS, inducing cytotoxicity and cell death. The dual action of photo thermal and photodynamic effects produces a stimulating effect on cancer cells, enhancing their therapeutic efficacy (Rengan et al., 2014).

4.2.4.1. Multimodal Imaging

Along with therapeutic benefits, these nanoparticles help monitoring of treatment responses through Multimodal Imaging. By integrating imaging agents into the nanoparticle structure, real-time visualization becomes possible.

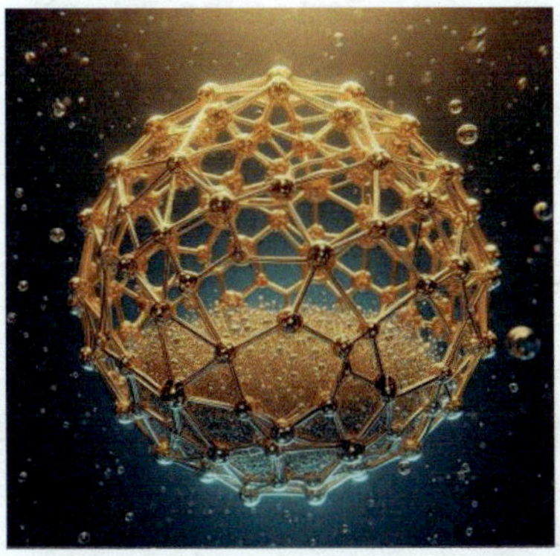

Figure 4.3. Gold nanocages showcasing their distinctive plasmonic properties, efficiently absorbing light and inducing photothermal effects by converting the absorbed light into heat.

This integration allows clinicians to monitor the distribution of nanoparticles within the body and assess their therapeutic response. Multimodal imaging techniques, such as fluorescence or photoacoustic imaging, provide detailed understanding of the nanoparticle's location, confirming targeted delivery to cancerous tissues. This real-time monitoring improves the precision of treatment, permitting for modifications and optimizations based on dynamic therapeutic responses (Chen et al., 2015; Jokerst and Gambhir, 2011). A prominent example illustrating nanoparticles that integrate PTT and PDT is the development of gold nanocages loaded with the photosensitizer Chlorin e6 (Ce6). Gold nanocages, with their characteristic plasmonic properties, efficiently absorb light, inducing Photothermal Effects by adapting the absorbed light into heat (Figure 4.3).

Simultaneously, the embedded Ce6 serves as a potent photosensitizer for PDT. This dual-functional nanoplatform not only arranges hyperthermia through PTT but also initiates ROS generation via PDT, a synergistic and potent therapeutic approach. Furthermore, the gold nanocages also, enable Multimodal Imaging, allowing for real-time tracking of their distribution and therapeutic effects in the targeted cancerous region (Jokerst, Cole, and Van de Sompel, 2012).

In crux, the incorporation of photothermal and photodynamic effects within engineered nanoparticles stands as a transformative approach in cancer treatment. The combination of these modalities holds potential for sensitive therapeutic outcomes, offering a multifaceted approach to fighting cancer with precision and versatility.

4.2.5. Overcoming Challenges with Nanotechnology: Advancements in Biocompatible Nanoparticle Design

One important way to treat cancer is by developing biocompatible nanoparticles, which help to reduce side effects and improve treatment.

4.2.5.1. Biocompatible Nanoparticle Design

The source of this approach is the comprehensive design of nanoparticles with biocompatibility (Blanco, Shen, and Ferrari, 2015). This includes selecting materials that are naturally safe for biotic systems. Superficial modifications play a crucial role in representing nanoparticles biocompatible.

The addition of biocompatible coatings, such as PEG, enhances stability, reducing the probability of immune recognition, following clearance. Moreover, these alterations contribute to prolonged circulation time in the bloodstream, ensuring that nanoparticles reach their proposed targets with efficacy (Wilhelm et al., 2016). Liposomes with PEGylation, lipid-based nanoparticles, signify the application of biocompatible design. PEGylation, the method of attaching PEG chains to liposome surfaces, imparts biocompatibility. This modification averts rapid clearance by the immune system and extends circulation time. PEGylated liposomes have been used in DDS, confirming enhanced stability, reduced toxicity, and enhanced overall therapeutic efficacy.

4.2.5.2. Targeting Strategies

Active targeting signifies a sophisticated strategy to improve treatment precision. Nanoparticles can be modified with specific ligands or antibodies on their surfaces, enabling recognition of unique receptors on cancer cells.

This active targeting approach ensures that therapeutic cargos are delivered accurately to cancerous tissues, minimizing side effects, and optimizing therapeutic outcomes. Folate-targeted nanoparticles have been explored in various cancer treatments, showcasing the potential of active targeting for enhanced efficacy (Albanese and Chan, 2011).

4.2.6. Clinical Implications and Future Directions of Nanomedicine in PTT and PDT

4.2.6.1. Translational Potential

Noticeably, gold-based nanoparticles, especially gold nanorods, have shown great promise in preclinical PTT studies (Dreaden et al., 2012). This translation potential is being exemplified in a variety of cancers such as breast and prostate through clinical trials evaluating the use of gold particles for treatment. These experiments are important because they help bridge the gap between successful preclinical tests and real-world applications.

4.2.6.2. Personalized Nanotherapeutics

The ability of nanomedicine to be used in treatments that can be tailored to individual patients has been established with the creation of tumor-specific nanoparticles. An example is liposomes modified using targeting ligands like antibodies or peptides which overexpress receptors on different tumors thereby enabling personalized nanotherapeutics. Clinical trials have been carried out with this kind of medication adjustment; one such case study includes targeted liposomal doxorubicin formulations showing efficacy rate when tested against non-targeted ones for treatment of breast cancer patients, among others. Consequently, customization not only aids precision treatment but also reduces systemic side effects since drugs concentrate more on affected areas than normal tissues.

During nanomedicine development ongoing experimental validations will have to be carried out to confirm its clinical applicability. In cancer therapy for example, targeted liposomal formulations demonstrate a shift from generic drugs towards precise medicine thereby indicating potentiality of personalized nanotherapeutics. This is where innovation meets individualization, and it is expected that these two combined together will bring about better results than before thus creating hope within future cancer care delivery systems which encompass efficient therapeutic strategies designed specifically according to each patient's needs and conditions (Jokerst and Gambhir, 2011; Matsumura and Maeda, 2011).

4.3. Nanoparticle-Based Radiotherapy: A Radiant Revolution in Cancer Treatment

4.3.1. Introduction

With continuous adjustment of cancer treatment strategies, nanotechnology has introduced a revolution in the field of radiotherapy. This section scientifically studies this transformative aspect of nanoparticles in radio therapeutic interventions, explaining how these minute carriers have the ability to elevate precision, efficacy, and safety, contributing to the advancement of cancer treatment.

4.3.2. Enhancing Radiation Dose Delivery

Nanotechnology offers an exciting avenue for enhancing dose delivery to cancer cells. This detailed study focuses on two key mechanisms—increased tumor uptake controlling the EPR effect, and the integration of high atomic number elements into NMs.

Nanoparticles can be engineered to attain the EPR effect, a phenomenon where leaky vasculature around tumors permits nanoparticles to selectively accumulate. This selective accumulation in tumor tissues significantly intensifies the delivery of radiation doses specifically to cancer cells, enhancing the therapeutic impact while minimizing collateral damage to surrounding healthy tissues. Considering an example, Liposomes, nanoscale lipid-based vesicles, represent this strategy. By modifying liposomes for extended circulation and surface functionality, they exploit the EPR effect, improving tumor-specific uptake. This approach has been explored in various cancers, such as breast and ovarian, indicating the potential of EPR-mediated nanoparticle delivery in radiation therapy.

Combining high atomic number (Z) elements into NMs significantly increases their ability to interact with ionizing radiation. These elements show strong interactions, leading to enhanced absorption and scattering of radiation. This strengthening improves the efficacy of radiation delivery to tumor sites, increasing the local dose and, subsequently, the therapeutic response. Example for such High Z elements are AuNPs (Hainfeld, Slatkin, and Smilowitz, 2004). Owing to their high atomic number and biocompatibility, they serve as classic agents. When presented into tumor tissues, they effectively absorb ionizing radiation, amplifying the local radiation dose (Matsumura and Maeda, 1986). This strategy has been investigated in preclinical and clinical studies for various cancers, including prostate and head and neck cancers, showcasing the potential of AuNPs in improving radiation therapy (Liu et al., 2015).

Both these strategies present a targeted approach to improve precision and efficacy. The examples provided highlight the potential of these strategies in evolving the field of radiation oncology.

4.3.3. Radio Sensitization for Improved Efficacy

Nanoparticles play a vital role in enhancing radiotherapy through their distinct capabilities.

One significant feature is their function as radio sensitizers, with gold nanoparticles (GNPs) serving as an important example (Figure 4.4). GNPs enhance therapeutic outcomes by increasing the local radiation dose through absorption and scattering, permitting lower radiation doses, and reducing damage to healthy tissues. Extensive studies, particularly in prostate and head and neck cancers, validate the potential of GNPs in improving radiotherapy precision.

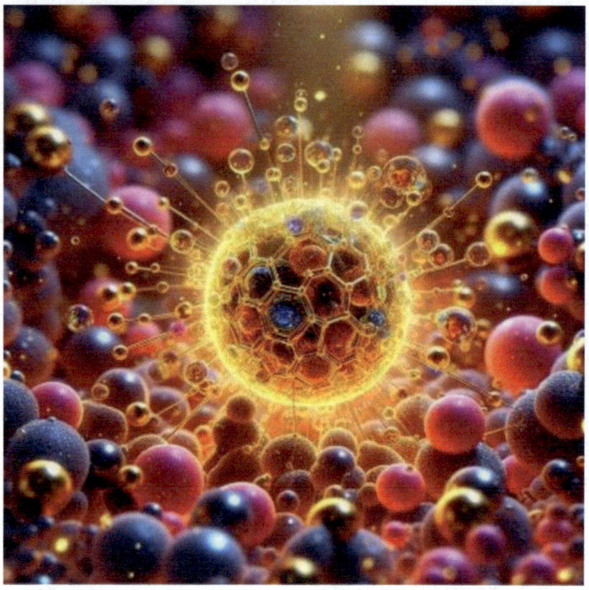

Figure 4.4. Gold nanoparticles (GNPs).

Simultaneously, addressing the challenge of tumor hypoxia, certain nanoparticles, such as perfluorocarbon-based NMs, contribute pointedly. These nanoparticles enable oxygen delivery to hypoxic tumor regions, overcoming the restrictions imposed by reduced oxygen levels. Preclinical studies in pancreatic and breast cancers determine the efficacy of perfluorocarbon nanoparticles in enhancing oxygen levels within tumors, increasing the impact of ionizing radiation. The combined functionalities of nanoparticles in radio sensitization and oxygen enhancement mark a progressive approach in refining radio therapeutic intrusions. This dual strategy not only improves the accuracy of radiation delivery but also tackles the life-threatening problem of tumor hypoxia (Hainfeld et al., 2008). Ongoing research promises further insights, for transformative progressions in the precision and efficacy of cancer radiotherapy.

4.3.4. Targeted Radiotherapy with Nanocarriers

Recent research has shown how important Nanocarriers are for cancer treatment. They have been described as "smart bombers" against tumors—because they are able to specifically target only cancerous cells within the human body. High levels of success were achieved with targeted liposomes in the treatment of glioblastoma multiforme (GBM), where the incorporation of ligands permitted most accurate radiation delivery yet known. Based on different writings, nanocarriers go a step further than conventional methods; besides acting singly, they facilitate combined therapies. AuNP loaded nanocarriers have been found to enhance the treatment outcomes for pancreatic cancer through their ability to make tumors more sensitive to radiation. Also, it should be noted that these agents allow for personalized medicine approaches tailored around specific types of malignant disease, molecular profiles, and patient characteristics alike. Therefore, nanocarriers form part and parcel of any radiotherapy that seeks to be precise enough while also surmounting various biological obstacles present in and around a tumor site with a view of even distribution therapeutic payloads there (Wilhelm et al., 2016). According to various investigations, these vehicles at different levels ranging from cellular through tissue up entire system can basically be considered as artificial organelles. Multiple benefits extend beyond this point; with ongoing studies promising even more unique advantages which herald an era characterized by refined individualized therapies (Jokerst, Cole, and Van de Sompel, 2012).

4.3.5. Imaging and Monitoring

Multimodal imaging, one of the key features of sophisticated cancer therapy, involves embedding imaging agents within nanoparticles to enable real-time monitoring of both nanocarrier distribution and radiation delivery.

This approach is necessary for treatment planning and evaluation as it provides important information about how treatments work. An example where this has been used is when iron oxide nanoparticles were used as contrast agents for magnetic resonance imaging (MRI) while at the same time acting as carriers for therapeutic substances. These dual-purpose nanoparticles allow treatment and imaging to be carried out concurrently leading to more accurate treatment (Jokerst and Gambhir, 2011). Furthermore, Theranostic Nanoparticles were devised following the same concept, specifically made for imaging and therapy at once.

This provides a complete solution in cancer care by offering both diagnostic information and treatment hence complete management of cancer. They include GNPs which have been widely studied because of their ability to act as contrast agents in CT scans besides possessing radiosensitizer effects. The radio enhancing property coupled with dual modality imaging capabilities enables real time imaging of the tumor site as well as improving radiation therapy outcomes (Jokerst, Cole, and Van de Sompel, 2012). Integration of imaging agents into nanoparticles along with design of theranostic NMs represents a new frontier for cancer treatment strategies. These techniques give clinicians instant data that they can use in planning and carrying out treatments with great precision which indicates what lies ahead in terms of personalized medicine for effective cancer control (Cormode, Naha, and Fayad, 2014).

4.3.6. Mitigating Side Effects and Improving Biocompatibility

Nanoparticles reduce systemic toxicity associated with conventional methods mostly by being able to aim specifically for certain things, this makes it possible for them to send radiation directly into the tumor but not affect any nearby normal tissues. GNPs exemplify this potential by being designed to accumulate preferentially in tumor tissues, facilitating a more focused and less toxic delivery of radiation (Hainfeld et al., 2004).

The development of nanoparticles with inherent biocompatibility ensures compatibility with the human body, mitigating the risk of adverse reactions. Liposomes, as lipid-based nanoparticles, are significantly biocompatible and have been explored for drug delivery in radiotherapy. Surface modifications further enhance stability, reduce the likelihood of degradation, and contribute to an overall improved safety profiles (Dreaden et al., 2012) and liposomes discussed earlier; various other nanoparticles exhibit the potential to reduce systemic toxicity in radiotherapy. Iron oxide nanoparticles, with their biocompatibility and imaging capabilities, enable real-time visualization of tumor sites during MRI, aiding in precise treatment planning and minimizing side effects (Liu et al., 2015). Silica nanoparticles, known for their tunable properties and ability to encapsulate therapeutic agents, are promising candidates for reducing systemic toxicity in radiotherapy. Polymeric nanoparticles, such as PLGA, contribute to reduced toxicity by enhancing drug stability and controlled release (Jokerst and Gambhir, 2011; Zhang et al., 2009). CNTs, with unique physicochemical properties, have been investigated for enhancing radiotherapy through their ability to absorb and convert NIR light into heat, selectively targeting tumor cells. Dendrimers, highly branched nanoparticles with customizable structures, offer controlled drug delivery in radiotherapy, concentrating therapeutic agents at the tumor site. Together, these examples emphasize the diverse applications of nanoparticles in mitigating systemic toxicity, contributing to the development of safer and more effective cancer treatment strategies.

4.3.7. Future Perspectives and Clinical Translations

Clinical trials are involved in advancing the field of nanoparticle-based radiotherapy, providing essential insights into the safety and efficacy of this innovative approach. Ongoing trials, such as the clinical trial NCT04137536 exploring the use of GNPs in combination with radiation therapy for head and neck cancers, contribute valuable data to validate the translational potential of nanoparticle-based radiotherapy (https://clinicaltrials.gov/ct2/show/NCT04137536).

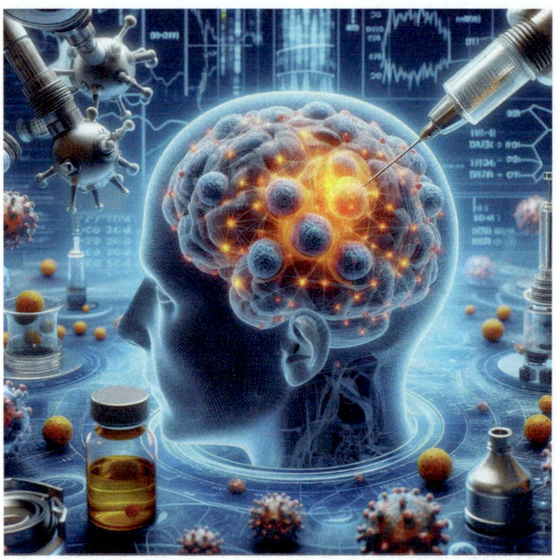

Figure 4.5. Iron oxide nanoparticles in radiotherapy for glioblastoma multiforme (GBM).

Personalized liposomal formulations for breast cancer radiotherapy represent another descriptive example. In this approach, liposomes are designed to encapsulate specific therapeutic agents based on the molecular characteristics of the patient's tumor, demonstrating the potential for custom made treatments to individual patient profiles. Furthermore, the clinical trial NCT02770475 investigates the use of iron oxide nanoparticles in GBM radiotherapy (Figure 4.5).

This trial explores the safety and efficacy of these nanoparticles for enhancing the precision of radiation therapy in treating brain tumors. This revolution at the nanoscale promises a brighter and more targeted future for cancer therapy (https://clinicaltrials.gov/ct2/show/NCT02770475).

4.4. Nanoparticles and Enhancements in Therapeutic Applications: Unlocking the Potential of the Microscopic Marvels

4.4.1. Introduction

In our attempt to study Nanoparticles, we further explore the several ways in which nanoparticles serve as agents of enhancement across various medical domains, from drug delivery to diagnostics and beyond.

4.4.2. Drug Delivery Revolution

Currently, nanoparticles are considered the best option in targeted drug delivery, represented by the development of antibody-conjugated liposomes. These nanocarriers, loaded with chemotherapy drugs, precisely target cancer cells, minimizing damage to healthy tissues. Another innovative example involves nanoparticles functionalized with peptides, facilitating the selective delivery of anti-inflammatory drugs to inflamed tissues. These advancements emphasize the potential of nanoparticles to treat cancer with unprecedented precision.

Solid lipid nanoparticles (SLNs) significantly improve the bioavailability of poorly water-soluble drugs such as *fenofibrate*, thereby amplifying their therapeutic effectiveness. Additionally, nanoemulsions suggest a solution to bioavailability challenges by encapsulating hydrophobic compounds, ensuring enhanced oral absorption. These examples highlight how nanocarriers address crucial issues related to drug solubility, stability, and overall efficacy. Nanoparticles also contribute to sustained release systems, for prolonged therapeutic effects (Torchilin, 2006). PLGA nanoparticles provide a prime instance by gradually releasing insulin over an extended period. This controlled release mechanism offers a sustained therapeutic effect and is particularly valuable in the management of conditions like diabetes (Danhier et al., 2012). Hydrogel-based nanoparticles represent another innovation, warranting the sustained release of antibiotics. This not only improves treatment convenience but also helps patient compliance by reducing the frequency of administration. The detailed exploration of these aspects reveals the transformative potential of nanoparticles in drug delivery, leading to personalized and highly effective therapeutic interventions (Wilhelm et al., 2016).

4.4.3. Imaging Advancements

Nanoparticles play a vital role as contrast agents, improving the visibility of tissues and structures in diverse imaging modalities. For instance, in MRI, superparamagnetic iron oxide nanoparticles (SPIONs) aid as effective contrast agents. These nanoparticles modify the relaxation times of nearby water protons, creating contrasting signals that enhance the clarity of the images. In computed tomography (CT), GNPs exhibit high X-ray absorption, enhancing contrast for better delineation of anatomical structures (Lee and Hyeon, 2012). Additionally, ultrasound benefits from the use of gas-filled nanoparticles that enhance acoustic signals, improving imaging precision.

The integration of different imaging agents into nanoparticles helps imaging abilities to a new level, enabling multimodal imaging. An exemplary application is the development of silica-coated gold nanorods, as contrast agents for both photoacoustic imaging and CT. This dual functionality provides an inclusive view of anatomical structures and enhances diagnostic accuracy (Boote et al., 2015). Similarly, the combination of iron oxide nanoparticles with fluorescent dyes allows real-time magnetic resonance and fluorescence imaging. Such multimodal approaches not only facilitate early disease detection but also provide a more comprehensive understanding of pathological conditions.

Thus, exploring contrast agents and multimodal imaging highlights the versatility and transformative potential of nanoparticles in the field of medical imaging (Thakor and Gambhir, 2013). These advancements not only improve the visibility of anatomical structures but also contribute to the development of more precise and comprehensive diagnostic tools.

4.4.4. Theranostics

Nanoparticles engineered for theranostics characterize a pioneering standard in healthcare by integrating diagnostic functionalities with therapeutic abilities. This complex approach enables real-time monitoring of treatment responses, developing a dynamic and adaptive treatment basis. QDs loaded with both imaging agents and therapeutic drugs allow for simultaneous tracking of the nanoparticles and delivery of therapeutic contents. This theranostic system provides valuable insights into treatment efficacy through imaging while actively engaging in targeted therapy. Also, iron oxide-based nanoparticles, when functionalized with both imaging probes and therapeutic agents, exhibit a dual role in MRI and drug delivery (Jokerst and Gambhir, 2011). This theranostic platform enables precise localization of the therapeutic content and facilitates on-demand treatment adjustments based on imaging feedback. Theranostic nanoparticles also play an important role in advancing future of personalized medicine (Jokerst, Cole, and Van de Sompel, 2012). By modifying treatments to individual patient characteristics, these nanoparticles contribute to optimized therapeutic outcomes and minimized side effects. The liposomes modified with patient-specific targeting ligands, guided by molecular profiling, enhance the selectivity of drug delivery. This personalized approach ensures that therapeutic agents are precisely directed to cancer cells, maximizing treatment efficacy (Cormode, Naha, and Fayad, 2014). Gold nanorods functionalized with imaging agents capable of identifying specific biomarkers enable a personalized theranostic strategy. This approach allows for the customization of treatment plans based on the unique molecular signature of each patient's disease.

4.4.5. Photothermal and Photodynamic Therapy (PDT)

GNPs, used in PTT, exhibit selectivity for cancer cells, distributing specific thermal ablation, as evidenced by studies on breast and prostate cancers. Furthermore, nanoparticles loaded with photosensitizers enable targeted PDT, inducing cell death upon exposure to specific light wavelengths (Hirsch et al., 2003). Clinical trials have established the potential of PDT with photosensitizer-loaded nanoparticles in treating skin and lung cancers (Lucky, Soo, and Zhang, 2015). Beyond individual modalities, the engineering of nanoparticles for combined PTT and PDT creates synergistic effects, enhancing treatment efficacy and mitigating the risk of resistance. Experimental studies with multimodal nanoparticles showcase improved outcomes in the treatment of high-grade tumors, highlighting their versatility in elevating therapeutic precision (Li et al., 2010).

4.4.6. Radio Sensitization in Radiotherapy

Nanoparticles surface as potent radiosensitizers, increasing the sensitivity of cancer cells to radiation. This heightened response allows for the administration of lower radiation doses, markedly reducing side effects to neighboring normal tissues (Hainfeld, Dilmanian, Slatkin, and Smilowitz, 2004). Notably, GNPs have exhibited significant radio sensitization effects in preclinical studies targeting prostate and head and neck cancers, underscoring their potential to elevate therapeutic outcomes. Simultaneously, surface modifications allow nanoparticles to selectively target cancer cells, increasing the precision of radiotherapy. With specific receptors or distinctive characteristics of cancer cells, nanoparticles contribute to an elevated specificity in radiation delivery, thereby minimizing undesired side effects (Butterworth et al., 2013; Chithrani et al., 2010).

4.4.7. Immunotherapy Augmentation

Nanoparticles serve as carriers for immune-stimulating agents, promoting an anti-cancer immune response. An illustrative example involves the use of liposomes loaded with immunomodulatory agents, demonstrating the potential to activate and amplify immune responses against cancer cells (Anselmo and Mitragotri, 2016). Furthermore, nanoparticles play a crucial role in antigen presentation, initiating a targeted immune response against cancer. For instance, polymeric nanoparticles carrying tumor-specific antigens have shown efficacy in stimulating antigen-presenting cells (APCs) and eliciting a targeted immune response against cancer cells (Irvine et al., 2015). This integration of nanoparticles into immunotherapeutic approaches signifies ground-breaking advancement in cancer treatment, benefitting from their ability to modify the immune system for improved therapeutic outcomes (Silva et al., 2017).

4.4.8. Biosafety and Biocompatibility

The safety of nanoparticles is an important concern in therapeutic applications, and ongoing research uses various strategies to confirm their biocompatibility and minimize their potential risks. Biodegradable polymers, such as PLGA, are frequently chosen as nanoparticle materials due to their ability to breakdown into non-toxic by products, reducing concerns about long-term buildup and potential adverse effects. These polymers undergo systematic degradation, allowing for the controlled release of therapeutic agents without compromising protection. Surface alterations play an essential role in enhancing safety by changing the interaction of nanoparticles with biological entities. Coating nanoparticles with biocompatible materials, such as PEG, decreases the probability of immune recognition and clearance, contributing to extended circulation times and minimizing unintended immune responses.

Detailed long-term safety studies include rigorous assessments of nanoparticle behavior in biological systems. Researchers conduct complete analyses to assess the persistence of nanoparticles, their distribution in various tissues, and potential impacts on organ function over prolonged durations. For example, GNPs, extensively studied for therapeutic applications, experience careful analysis to understand their long-term destiny within the body, ensuring that they do not cause unexpected adverse effects (Dreaden et al., 2012).

Furthermore, researchers focus on elucidating the mechanisms of nanoparticle-cell interactions, with cellular uptake, intracellular trafficking, and potential alterations in cellular functions (Albanese and Chan, 2011). By gaining insights into these aspects, scientists can improve nanoparticle designs to maximize therapeutic benefits while minimizing risks. Overall, the multifaceted approach to nanoparticle safety involves a vigilant selection of materials, considerate surface engineering, and comprehensive long-term studies (Blanco, Shen, and Ferrari, 2015).

4.4.9. Clinical Translation and Future Directions

To achieve clinical translation, researchers must modify drug treatments to the individual characteristics of patients, including their molecular profiles and genetic variations. Personalized nanomedicine protocols should be continuously improved through ongoing clinical trials so that they conform with strict safety requirements and provide measurable advantages in different patient populations (Ferrari, 2005). It is important for personalized nanomedicine to become part of routine clinical practice that its scalability can be addressed as well as questions of reproducibility and standardization in manufacture (Peer et al., 2007). Future aspects of clinical translation should concentrate on next generation NMs having enhanced functionality. Treatment personalization may be facilitated through advanced imaging techniques like molecular imaging and theranostic approaches which offer real time visualization and monitoring capabilities. Furthermore, the utilization of artificial intelligence (AI) within personalized drug therapies promises to optimize treatment algorithms, predict patient responses, and identify new therapeutic targets (Nie and Xing, 2008).

4.5. Immunomodulatory Nanoparticles: Orchestrating Precision in Cancer Immunotherapy

In the field of cancer immunotherapy, immunomodulatory nanoparticles have actively established in harnessing the body's immune system to combat cancer. This segment explores how immunomodulatory nanoparticles, create precise and targeted immune responses in the fight against cancer.

4.5.1. Enhancing Immune Activation

Immunomodulatory nanoparticles are involved in stimulating antigen presentation, a critical process for activating the immune system against cancer cells. Their role includes facilitating the recognition of tumor antigens by immune cells, thus introducing a strong and targeted immune response (Irvine et al., 2015).

One key mechanism employed by immunomodulatory nanoparticles is the use of antigen-loaded nanocarriers. These nanoparticles assist as efficient vehicles for transporting tumor antigens, ensuring their effective delivery to APCs. This targeted delivery improves the presentation of cancer-specific antigens to immune cells, setting off a series of immune responses against malignant cells (Sahdev, Ochyl, and Moon, 2014).

For example, liposomes loaded with tumor antigens can be considered to specifically target APCs. Upon reaching these cells, the liposomes release the antigens, facilitating their presentation to T cells and initiating an immune response against cancer. Similarly, polymeric nanoparticles can encapsulate tumor antigens, contributing protection throughout transport and controlled release within APCs, increasing the antigen presentation process (Cruz et al., 2012).

Immunomodulatory nanoparticles, through their utilization of antigen-loaded nanocarriers, strategically boosts antigen presentation. This targeted approach contributes to the precision and effectiveness of the immune response against cancer.

4.5.2. Modulating Immune Cells

The process of activating T cells and influencing regulatory T cells using immunomodulatory nanoparticles is complex in cancer immunotherapy.

By interaction with immune cell receptors, nanoparticles are meant to trigger cytotoxic T cells specifically. In this scenario, antigen-presenting nanoparticles like liposomes or polymeric ones can carry tumor-specific antigens. Such focused activation leads to an enhanced immune response against cancer cells. Antigen Loaded Nanoparticles are perfect example for T Cell Activation. These antigens which are specific for cancer if loaded into the particles will effectively activate T cells. For instance, lipid-based particles containing neo-antigens may be engineered to target cytotoxic T cells for specific activation (Irvine et al., 2015).

Immunomodulatory nanoparticles also modulate regulatory T cells, regulating the immune system. These nanoparticles check over activity and promote targeted anti-cancer responses. GNPs functionalized with immune-modulating agents, for instance, can impact the behavior of regulatory T cells. This modulation helps create an environment favorable to robust anti-cancer immune responses while avoiding excessive immunosuppression (Moon, Huang, and Irvine, 2012). Mesoporous silica nanoparticles (MSNs) functionalized with immunomodulatory molecules can impact the behavior of regulatory T cells. These nanoparticles can selectively target Tregs, modifying their function for an immune response. This helps create an immune microenvironment that shows more effective anti-cancer responses (Tang et al., 2016).

4.5.3. Cytokine Delivery and Immune Signaling

Nanoparticles can carry cytokines, allowing correct and partial release of immune-signaling molecules within the tumor microenvironment, reducing systemic side effects (Anselmo and Mitragotri, 2016). One example involves the use of liposomes with interleukin-2 (IL-2). IL-2 is a strong cytokine that proliferates and activates the T cells. Within liposomes, IL-2 can be sent directly to the tumor, causing a robust immune response against cancer cells. This specific cytokine release strategy makes sure that the immune-activating signals are concentrated at the tumor site, with maximum anti-cancer effects while reducing the risk of nonspecific target effects.

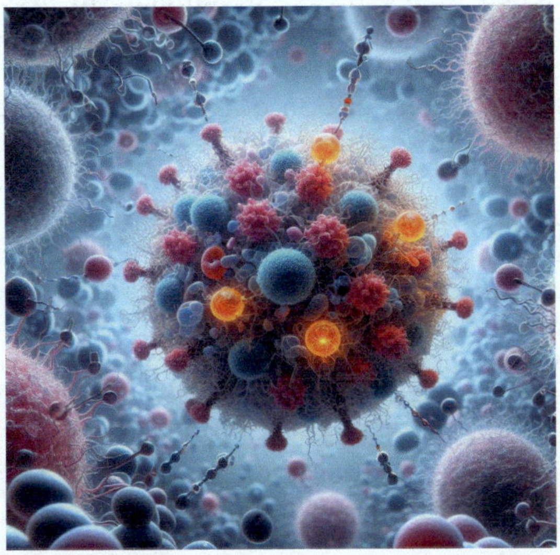

Figure 4.6. Nanoparticles conjugated with antibodies against PD-1 or CTLA-4.

Engineered nanoparticles inhibit immune checkpoint pathways. Immune checkpoints are regulatory proteins which can reduce the immune system's ability to attack cancer cells (Shi and Kantoff, 2017). These nanoparticles are composed of polymers or lipids, which can carry immune checkpoint inhibitors (ICIs) directly to the tumor. For instance, nanoparticles with antibodies against programmed cell death protein 1 (PD-1) or cytotoxic T-lymphocyte-associated protein 4 (CTLA-4) can generate a potent immune attack on cancer cells by interrupting these inhibitory pathways (Figure 4.6). This approach has shown promise in overcoming the tumor's immune evasion mechanisms and has thus, increase the use of cancer immunotherapy (Havel, Chowell, and Chan, 2019).

4.5.4. Personalized Immunotherapies

Immunomodulatory nanoparticles give a personalized approach depending on the unique molecular profile of each patient's tumor. For example, nanoparticles engineered to carry patient-specific antigens or antigens derived from the tumor can increase the immune system's response against cancer cells. This technique makes sure that the treatment is in line with the unique biological features of each patient's cancer (Li et al., 2018). These immunomodulatory nanoparticles may be useful for combination therapies. For example, nanoparticles carrying ICIs can be combined with traditional chemotherapy or radiotherapy. This combination favors the increased immune response while also sensitizing the cancer cells to other therapeutic involvements (Liu et al., 2016). In melanoma treatment, immunomodulatory nanoparticles with anti-PD-1 antibodies (checkpoint inhibitors) can be joint with PTT. The nanoparticles, when exposed to NIR light, induce limited hyperthermia, increasing the immune response. This integrated approach shows how well these immunomodulatory nanoparticles can manage complex anti-cancer approaches (Chen et al., 2016).

4.5.5. Overcoming Immunotherapy Challenges

Immunomodulatory nanoparticles play a key role in overcoming the challenge of resistance to immunotherapy. For instance, in cases where tumors show resistance to ICIs, nanoparticles can carry these inhibitors directly to the tumor site (Chen et al., 2019). This targeted delivery increases the local concentration of inhibitors overcoming resistance and restoring the efficiency of immunotherapy. In lung cancer with resistance to PD-1/PD-L1 checkpoint inhibitors, immunomodulatory nanoparticles carrying small interfering RNA (siRNA) against resistance associated pathways can be useful (Figure 4.7) (Deng et al., 2018).

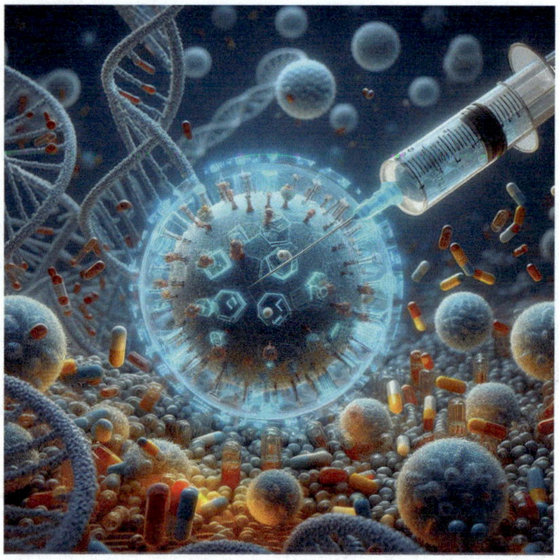

Figure 4.7. Immunomodulatory nanoparticles delivering siRNA.

These nanoparticles, silence genes related with resistance, stimulating the anti-cancer immune response. Thus, immunomodulatory nanoparticles stand as novel solutions in both altering the tumor microenvironment and overcoming resistance to immunotherapy (Ovais et al., 2019).

4.5.6. Imaging-Guided Immunotherapy

Immunomodulatory nanoparticles with imaging agents, also, play an important role in the real-time monitoring of treatment responses. These nanoparticles with imaging agents, such as fluorescent dyes or contrast agents for various imaging system allows clinicians to monitor the circulation of nanoparticles, their interaction with immune cells, and fluctuations in the tumor microenvironment in real time. In case, immunotherapy-induced immune cell infiltration is an anticipated response, real-time imaging with these nanoparticles affords a complete assessment of the treatment's effectiveness (Jokerst, Gambhir, and Peeters, 2019). In melanoma immunotherapy, immunomodulatory nanoparticles with both ICIs and NIR fluorophores can be used. The nanoparticles carry therapeutic agents and permit real-time fluorescence imaging. Clinicians can use this imaging to observe the influx of immune cells into the tumor, evaluate the activation of the immune response, and alter the treatment approach based on the observed situation.

Imaging-guided nanoparticles can be designed to specifically accumulate in precise immunosuppressive locations (Weissleder and Pittet, 2008). This targeted approach recovers the local concentration of immunomodulatory agents where they are needed and thus, affects their therapeutic impact. In breast cancer, where tumor heterogeneity shows challenges, immunomodulatory nanoparticles with MRI contrast agents can be used. These nanoparticles, guided by real-time MRI, travel through the tumor, concentrating in high immunosuppressive signal zones. This accuracy overcomes the challenges posed by the various microenvironment of the breast tumor (Kaittanis, Bolaender, and Shaffer, 2018).

4.5.7. Future Directions and Clinical Translation

These improvements in cancer immunotherapy increases the value of immunomodulatory nanoparticles for clinical applications. Researchers are exploring NMs with greater biocompatibility to address alarms of potential toxicity. For instance, we discussed the biodegradable polymers such as PLGA are being designed into nanoparticles. These polymers offer improved biocompatibility along with exact degradation, warranting the safe and gradual release of immunomodulatory agents. PLGA nanoparticles with immune-stimulating agents, such as toll-like receptor agonists, represent the next cohort of NMs (Figure 4.8).

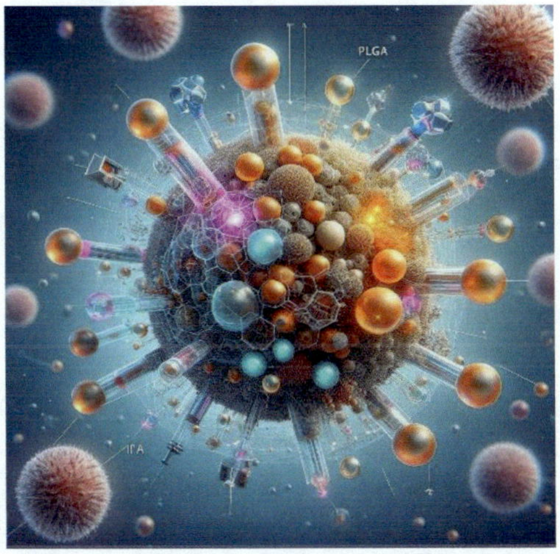

Figure 4.8. PLGA nanoparticles with toll-like receptor agonists.

The unique properties of PLGA allow for customization to optimize therapeutic outcomes (Irvine et al., 2015). Clinical trials are needed in assessing the safety and efficacy of immunomodulatory nanoparticles. These trials require administering these nanoparticles to human subjects, observing their responses, and evaluate any side effects. In a clinical trial studying melanoma immunotherapy, immunomodulatory nanoparticles with a combination of ICIs have been confirmed (Maeda, Nakamura, and Fang, 2013). The trial assessed the safety of nanoparticle-mediated immunotherapy and assess its efficiency in increasing anti-tumor immune responses. The patient outcomes provide important data to decide integrating immunomodulatory nanoparticles into melanoma treatment.

Converging next-generation NMs and the development of immunomodulatory nanoparticles through tough clinical trials means an important chapter in cancer immunotherapy. The assurance to biocompatibility, tunable attributes and validating real-world efficiency underlines the commitment of researchers and clinicians to immunotherapeutic strategies leading cancer treatment (Sun et al., 2019).

Nanoparticles from laboratories to clinical applications signifies greater therapeutic solutions for several diseases, bringing a change in medical interventions. With these microscopic agents, the prospect of medical options expands, offering hope to patients and clinicians for improved and personalized treatments.

KEY TERMS FROM THIS CHAPTER

- biosafety
- gene silencing
- immune checkpoint inhibitors
- immunotherapy
- radiotherapy
- cancer
- immune cell interaction
- immunomodulatory nanoparticles
- nanomedicine

References

1. Akbarzadeh, A., Rezaei-Sadabady, R., Davaran, S., Joo, S. W., Zarghami, N., Hanifehpour, Y., & Samiei, M. (2013). Liposome: Classification, preparation, and applications. *Nanoscale Research Letters, 8*, Article 102. https://doi.org/10.1186/1556-276X-8-102.
2. Albanese, A., & Chan, W. C. W. (2011). Effect of gold nanoparticle aggregation on cell uptake and toxicity. *ACS Nano, 5*(7), 5478–5489.
3. Allen, T. M., & Cullis, P. R. (2013). Liposomal drug delivery systems: From concept to clinical applications. *Advanced Drug Delivery Reviews, 65*(1), 36–48.
4. Andtbacka, R. H. I., Kaufman, H. L., Collichio, F., Amatruda, T., Senzer, N., Chesney, J., Delman, K. A., Spitler, L. E., Puzanov, I., Agarwala, S. S., Milhem, M., Cranmer, L., Curti, B., Lewis, K., Ross, M., Guthrie, T., Linette, G. P., Daniels, G. A., Harrington, K., & Kaufman, D. R. (2011). Durable complete responses in heavily pretreated patients with metastatic melanoma using T-cell transfer immunotherapy. *Clinical Cancer Research, 17*(13), 4550–4557.
5. Anselmo, A. C., & Mitragotri, S. (2016). Nanoparticles in the clinic: An update. *Bioengineering & Translational Medicine, 1*(1), 10–29.
6. Avouris, P., Chen, Z., & Perebeinos, V. (2007). Carbon-based electronics. *Nature Nanotechnology, 2*(10), 605–615.
7. Binnewies, M., Roberts, E. W., Kersten, K., Chan, V., Fearon, D. F., Merad, M., & Coussens, L. M. (2018). Understanding the tumor immune microenvironment (TIME) for effective therapy. *Nature Medicine, 24*(5), 541–550. https://doi.org/10.1038/s41591-018-0014-x.
8. Blanco, E., Shen, H., & Ferrari, M. (2015). Principles of nanoparticle design for overcoming biological barriers to drug delivery. *Nature Biotechnology, 33*(9), 941–951.
9. Boote, E., Fent, G., Kattumenu, R., Nakouti, I., & Vojnovic, B. (2015). Nanoparticles in medical imaging: Advances, opportunities, and challenges. *Journal of Materials Chemistry B, 3*(32), 6478–6485.
10. Butterworth, K. T., McMahon, S. J., Currell, F. J., & Prise, K. M. (2013). Physical basis and biological mechanisms of gold nanoparticle radio sensitization. *Nanoscale, 5*(21), 10103–10120.
11. Cao, G. (2018). *Nanomaterials and Devices: Fabrication and Applications*. Springer.
12. Carmeliet, P., & Jain, R. K. (2011). Principles and mechanisms of vessel normalization for cancer and other angiogenic diseases. *Nature Reviews Drug Discovery, 10*(6), 417–427. https://doi.org/10.1038/nrd3455.
13. Chapman, P. B., Hauschild, A., Robert, C., Haanen, J. B., Ascierto, P., Larkin, J., & McArthur, G. A. (2011). Improved survival with vemurafenib in melanoma with BRAF V600E mutation. *New England Journal of Medicine, 364*(26), 2507–2516.
14. Chen, F., Hong, H., Goel, S., Valdovinos, H. F., Hernandez, R., Shi, S., Barnhart, T. E., & Cai, W. (2015). The journey of a nanoparticle *in vivo*: From injection to site-specific biodistribution and targeting. *Accounts of Chemical Research, 48*(10), 2869–2877.
15. Chen, J., Glaus, C., Laforest, R., Zhang, Q., Yang, M., Gidding, M., & Welch, M. J. (2010). Gold nanocages as photothermal transducers for cancer treatment. *Small, 6*(7), 811–817.

16. Chen, Q., Chen, J., Yang, Z., Xu, J., Xu, L., Liang, C., & Liu, Z. (2016). Nanoparticle-enhanced radiotherapy to trigger robust cancer immunotherapy. *Advanced Materials, 28*(28), 10557–10564.

17. Chen, Q., Wang, C., Zhang, X., Chen, G., Hu, Q., Li, H., & Zhang, Y. (2019). *In situ* sprayed bio responsive immunotherapeutic gel for post-surgical cancer treatment. *Nature Nanotechnology, 14*(1), 89–97.

18. Chithrani, D. B., Jelveh, S., Jalali, F., van Prooijen, M., Allen, C., Bristow, R. G., & Hill, R. P. (2010). Gold nanoparticles as radiation sensitizers in cancer therapy. *Radiation Research, 173*(6), 719–728.

19. Choi, K. Y., & Park, K. (2019). Hyaluronic acid-based nanocarriers for intracellular targeting: Interfacial interactions with proteins in cancer. *Colloids and Surfaces B: Bio Interfaces, 177*, 28–34.

20. Chou, L. Y., Ming, K., & Chan, W. C. (2011). Strategies for the intracellular delivery of nanoparticles. *Chemical Society Reviews, 40*(1), 233–245.

21. Chu, K. F., & Dupuy, D. E. (2014). Thermal ablation of tumors: Biological mechanisms and advances in therapy. *Nature Reviews Cancer, 14*(3), 199–208. https://doi.org/10.1038/nrc3672.

22. Chu, S., & Majumdar, A. (2012). Opportunities and challenges for a sustainable energy future. *Nature, 488*(7411), 294–303.

23. ClinicalTrials.gov Identifier: NCT02770475. (n.d.). Iron oxide nanoparticles in radiation therapy for brain tumors (IRON-2). Retrieved from: https://clinicaltrials.gov/ct2/show/NCT02770475 (accessed on 8 May 2025).

24. ClinicalTrials.gov Identifier: NCT04137536. (2025). A study of gold nanoparticles in radiation therapy for head and neck cancer (GALEN). Retrieved from: https://clinicaltrials.gov/ct2/show/NCT04137536 (accessed on 8 May 2025).

25. Cormode, D. P., Naha, P. C., & Fayad, Z. A. (2014). Nanoparticle contrast agents for computed tomography: A focus on micelles. *Contrast Media & Molecular Imaging, 9*(1), 37–52.

26. Cruz, L. J., Rueda, F., Simón, L., Cordobilla, B., Albericio, F., & Domingo, J. C. (2012). Liposomes as immunoadjuvants in vaccine delivery: Current strategies and applications. *BioMed Research International, 2012*, 1–13.

27. Cunningham, D., Humblet, Y., Siena, S., Khayat, D., Bleiberg, H., Santoro, A., & Bleiberg, H. (2004). Cetuximab monotherapy and cetuximab plus irinotecan in irinotecan-refractory metastatic colorectal cancer. *New England Journal of Medicine, 351*(4), 337–345.

28. Danhier, F., Ansorena, E., Silva, J. M., Coco, R., Le Breton, A., & Préat, V. (2012). PLGA-based nanoparticles: An overview of biomedical applications. *Journal of Controlled Release, 161*(2), 505–522. https://doi.org/10.1016/j.jconrel.2012.01.043.

29. Davis, M. E., & Chen, Z. G. (2008). Nanoparticle therapeutics: An emerging treatment modality for cancer. *Nature Reviews Drug Discovery, 7*(9), 771–782. https://doi.org/10.1038/nrd2614.

30. Deng, H., Wang, H., Wang, M., Li, Z., Wu, T., Wu, X., & Zhang, H. (2018). Reducing PD-1 expression by plasmid DNA immunization augments anti-tumor efficacy of therapeutic HPV DNA vaccines. *Cancer Immunology, Immunotherapy, 67*(9), 1377–1388.

31. Draget, K. I., Smidsrød, O., & Skjåk-Bræk, G. (2005). Alginates from algae. In *Biopolymers Online*. Wiley-VCH Verlag GmbH & Co. KGaA.

32. Dreaden, E. C., Alkilany, A. M., Huang, X., Murphy, C. J., & El-Sayed, M. A. (2012). The golden age: Gold nanoparticles for biomedicine. *Chemical Society Reviews, 41*(7), 2740–2779.

33. Dreaden, E. C., Austin, L. A., Mackey, M. A., & El-Sayed, M. A. (2012). Size matters: Gold nanoparticles in targeted cancer drug delivery. *Therapeutic Delivery, 3*(4), 457–478.

34. Drilon, A., Laetsch, T. W., Kummar, S., DuBois, S. G., Lassen, U. N., Demetri, G. D., & Bauer, T. M. (2018). Efficacy of Larotrectinib in TRK fusion–positive cancers in adults and children. *New England Journal of Medicine, 378*(8), 731–739.

35. Druker, B. J., Talpaz, M., Resta, D. J., Peng, B., Buchdunger, E., Ford, J. M., & Sawyers, C. L. (2001). Efficacy and safety of a specific inhibitor of the BCR-ABL tyrosine kinase in chronic myeloid leukemia. *New England Journal of Medicine, 344*(14), 1031–1037.

36. Edge, S. B., & Compton, C. C. (2010). The American Joint Committee on Cancer: The 7th edition of the AJCC cancer staging manual and the future of TNM. *Annals of Surgical Oncology, 17*(6), 1471–1474. https://doi.org/10.1245/s10434-010-0985-4.

37. Escudier, B., Pluzanska, A., Koralewski, P., Ravaud, A., Bracarda, S., Szczylik, C., & Bukowski, R. M. (2007). Bevacizumab plus interferon alfa-2a for treatment of metastatic renal cell carcinoma: A randomized, double-blind phase III trial. *The Lancet, 370*(9605), 2103–2111.

38. Ethirajan, M., Chen, Y., Joshi, P., & Pandey, R. K. (2011). The role of porphyrin chemistry in tumor imaging and photodynamic therapy. *Chemical Society Reviews, 40*(1), 340–362.

39. Fang, J., Nakamura, H., & Maeda, H. (2011). The EPR effect: Unique features of tumor blood vessels for drug delivery, factors involved, and limitations and augmentation of the effect. *Advanced Drug Delivery Reviews, 63*(3), 136–151.

40. Ferrari, M. (2005). Cancer nanotechnology: Opportunities and challenges. *Nature Reviews Cancer, 5*(3), 161–171.

41. Ferry, D. K. (2009). *Transport in Nanostructures* (2nd ed.). Cambridge University Press.

42. Fischer, D., Bieber, T., Li, Y., Elsässer, H. P., & Kissel, T. (1999). A novel non-viral vector for DNA delivery based on low molecular weight, branched polyethyleneimine: Effect of molecular weight on transfection efficiency and cytotoxicity. *Pharmaceutical Research, 16*(8), 1273–1279.

43. Gabizon, A. A., & Patil, Y. (2021). Liposomal drug delivery: Current clinical applications. *Pharmaceutics, 13*(1), 1–31.

44. Gref, R., Minamitake, Y., Peracchia, M. T., Trubetskoy, V., Torchilin, V., & Langer, R. (1994). Biodegradable long-circulating polymeric nanospheres. *Science, 263*(5153), 1600–1603.

45. Greish, K. (2007). Enhanced permeability and retention (EPR) effect for anticancer nanomedicine drug targeting. In *Methods in Molecular Biology* (Vol. 624, pp. 25–37). Humana Press. https://doi.org/10.1007/978-1-59745-054-7_3.

46. Gu, F., Zhang, L., Teply, B. A., Mann, N., Wang, A., Radovic-Moreno, A. F., Langer, R., & Farokhzad, O. C. (2008). Precise engineering of targeted nanoparticles by using self-assembled bio integrated block copolymers. *Proceedings of the National Academy of Sciences, 105*(7), 2586–2591.

47. Hainfeld, J. F., Dilmanian, F. A., Slatkin, D. N., & Smilowitz, H. M. (2008). Radiotherapy enhancement with gold nanoparticles. *Journal of Pharmacy and Pharmacology, 60*(8), 977–985.

48. Hainfeld, J. F., Dilmanian, F. A., Slatkin, D. N., & Smilowitz, H. M. (2004). Radiotherapy enhancement with gold nanoparticles. *Journal of Pharmacy and Pharmacology, 60*(8), 977–985.

49. Hainfeld, J. F., Slatkin, D. N., & Smilowitz, H. M. (2004). The use of gold nanoparticles to enhance radiotherapy in mice. *Physics in Medicine & Biology, 49*(18), N309–N315.

50. Hanahan, D., & Weinberg, R. A. (2011). Hallmarks of cancer: The next generation. *Cell, 144*(5), 646–674. https://doi.org/10.1016/j.cell.2011.02.013.

51. Hare, J. I., Lammers, T., Ashford, M. B., Puri, S., & Storm, G. (2017). Challenges and strategies in anti-cancer nanomedicine development: An industry perspective. *Advanced Drug Delivery Reviews, 108*, 25–38.

52. Hauschild, A., Grob, J. J., Demidov, L. V., Jouary, T., Gutzmer, R., Millward, M., & Garbe, C. (2012). Dabrafenib in BRAF-mutated metastatic melanoma: A multicenter, open-label, phase 3 randomized controlled trial. *The Lancet, 380*(9839), 358–365.

53. Havel, J. J., Chowell, D., & Chan, T. A. (2019). The evolving landscape of biomarkers for checkpoint inhibitor immunotherapy. *Nature Reviews Cancer, 19*(3), 133–150.

54. He, Q., & Shi, J. (2011). Mesoporous silica nanoparticle based nano drug delivery systems: Synthesis, controlled drug release and delivery, pharmacokinetics, and biocompatibility. *Journal of Materials Chemistry, 21*(16), 5845–5855.

55. Hirsch, L. R., Stafford, R. J., Bankson, J. A., Sershen, S. R., Rivera, B., Price, R. E., & West, J. L. (2003). Nanoshell-mediated near-infrared thermal therapy of tumors under magnetic resonance guidance. *Proceedings of the National Academy of Sciences, 100*(23), 13549–13554. https://doi.org/10.1073/pnas.2232479100.

56. Hoffman, A. S. (2012). Hydrogels for biomedical applications. *Advanced Drug Delivery Reviews, 64*(Suppl), 18–23.

57. Hua, S., de Matos, M. B. C., Metselaar, J. M., & Storm, G. (2018). Current trends and challenges in the clinical translation of nanoparticulate nanomedicines: Pathways for translational development and commercialization. *Frontiers in Pharmacology, 9*, 790. https://doi.org/10.3389/fphar.2018.00790.

58. Huang, X., El-Sayed, M. A., Qian, W., & El-Sayed, M. A. (2006). Cancer cell imaging and photothermal therapy in the near-infrared region by using gold nanorods. *Journal of the American Chemical Society, 128*(6), 2115–2120.

59. Irvine, D. J., & Dane, E. L. (2020). Enhancing cancer immunotherapy with nanomedicine. *Nature Reviews Immunology, 20*(5), 321–334. https://doi.org/10.1038/s41577-019-0269-6.

60. Irvine, D. J., Hanson, M. C., Rakhra, K., & Tokatlian, T. (2015). Synthetic nanoparticles for vaccines and immunotherapy. *Chemical Reviews, 115*(19), 11109–11146.

61. Jokerst, J. V., & Gambhir, S. S. (2011). Molecular imaging with theragnostic nanoparticles. *Accounts of Chemical Research, 44*(10), 1050–1060. https://doi.org/10.1021/ar200106e.

62. Jokerst, J. V., Cole, A. J., & Van de Sompel, D. (2012). Gold nanoparticles for photoacoustic imaging. *Nanomedicine, 7*(6), 883–897.

63. Jokerst, J. V., Gambhir, S. S., & Peeters, R. (2019). Nanoparticles for imaging: top or flop? *Radiology, 292*(2), 416–417.

64. Kaittanis, C., Bolaender, A., & Shaffer, T. M. (2018). Visualization of immunomodulation by liposomal encapsulation using quantitative and conventional MRI. *Journal of Visualized Experiments,* (134), e57586.

65. Kam, N. W. S., & Dai, H. (2005). Carbon nanotubes as intracellular transporters for proteins and DNA: An investigation of the uptake mechanism and pathway. *Angewandte Chemie International Edition, 45*(4), 577–581.

66. Koffie, R. M., Farrar, C. T., Saidi, L. J., William, C. M., Hyman, B. T., & Spires-Jones, T. L. (2011). Nanoparticles enhance brain delivery of blood–brain barrier-impermeable probes for *in vivo* optical and magnetic resonance imaging. *Proceedings of the National Academy of Sciences, 108*(46), 18837–18842.

67. Kratz, F. (2008). Albumin as a drug carrier: Design of prodrugs, drug conjugates and nanoparticles. *Journal of Controlled Release, 132*(3), 171–183.

68. Kreuter, J. (2001). Nanoparticulate systems for brain delivery of drugs. *Advanced Drug Delivery Reviews, 47*(1), 65–81.

69. Labet, M., & Thielemans, W. (2009). Synthesis of polycaprolactone: A review. *Chemical Society Reviews, 38*(12), 3484–3504.

70. Ledermann, J., Harter, P., Gourley, C., Friedlander, M., Vergote, I., Rustin, G., & Matulonis, U. (2014). Olaparib maintenance therapy in platinum-sensitive relapsed ovarian cancer. *New England Journal of Medicine, 366*(15), 1382–1392.

71. Lee, D. E., Koo, H., Sun, I. C., Ryu, J. H., Kim, K., & Kwon, I. C. (2012). Multifunctional nanoparticles for multimodal imaging and theragnosis. *Chemical Society Reviews, 41*(7), 2656–2672.

72. Lee, N., & Hyeon, T. (2012). Designed synthesis of uniformly sized iron oxide nanoparticles for efficient magnetic resonance imaging contrast agents. *Chemical Society Reviews, 41*(7), 2575–2589.

73. Li, A. W., Sobral, M. C., Badrinath, S., Choi, Y., Graveline, A., Stafford, A. G., & Irvine, D. J. (2018). A facile approach to enhance antigen response for personalized cancer vaccination. *Nature Materials, 17*(6), 528–534.

74. Li, J., Pu, K., & Semenza, G. L. (2019). Nanomaterials-based strategies for personalized medicine. *Frontiers in Pharmacology, 10*, 621. https://doi.org/10.3389/fphar.2019.00621.

75. Li, X., Lovell, J. F., Yoon, J., Chen, X., & Zheng, G. (2010). Activatable molecular probes for cancer imaging. *Current Opinion in Biotechnology, 21*(5), 803–810.

76. Li, Y., Lokitz, B. S., & McCormick, C. L. (2006). Thermo-responsive micellization of amphiphilic block copolymers in water: A kinetic and mechanistic study. *Macromolecules, 39*(6), 1924–1933.

77. Liang, X., Chen, C., Zhao, Y., & Jia, L. (2021). Micro/nanorobots for biomedicine: Delivery, surgery, sensing, and detoxification. *Science Robotics, 6*(51), eabb2922.

78. Liu, Y., Maccarini, P., Palmer, G. M., Etienne, W., Zhao, Y., Lee, C. T., & Dewhirst, M. W. (2016). Synergistic immune photothermal nano therapy (SYMPHONY) for the treatment of unresectable and metastatic cancers. *Scientific Reports, 6*(1), 1–13.

79. Liu, Y., Zhang, P., Li, F., Jin, X., Li, J., Chen, W., & Tang, Y. (2015). Gold nanoparticles mediated detection and enhanced therapeutic capabilities in head and neck squamous cell carcinoma. *Journal of Materials Chemistry B, 3*(44), 8559–8568.

80. Liu, Z., Robinson, J. T., Sun, X., & Dai, H. (2008). PEGylated nanographene oxide for delivery of water-insoluble cancer drugs. *Journal of the American Chemical Society, 130*(33), 10876–10877.

81. Lu, W., Zhang, G., Zhang, R., Flores, L. G., Huang, Q., Gelovani, J. G., & Li, C. (2010). Tumor site-specific silencing of NF-κB p65 by targeted hollow gold nanosphere-mediated photothermal transfection. *Cancer Research, 70*(8), 3177–3188.

82. Lucky, S. S., Soo, K. C., & Zhang, Y. (2015). Nanoparticles in photodynamic therapy. *Chemical Reviews, 115*(4), 1990–2042.

83. Maeda, H., Nakamura, H., & Fang, J. (2013). The EPR effect for macromolecular drug delivery to solid tumors: Improvement of tumor uptake, lowering of systemic toxicity, and distinct tumor imaging *in vivo*. *Advanced Drug Delivery Reviews, 65*(1), 71–79.

84. Maeda, H., Wu, J., Sawa, T., Matsumura, Y., & Hori, K. (2000). Tumor vascular permeability and the EPR effect in macromolecular therapeutics: A review. *Journal of Controlled Release, 65*(1, 2), 271–284. https://doi.org/10.1016/S0168-3659(99)00248-5.

85. Mandal, B. B., & Kundu, S. C. (2009). Non-bioengineered silk fibroin protein 3D scaffolds for potential application in bone tissue engineering. *Macromolecular Bioscience, 9*(2), 119–130.

86. Manning, B. D., & Cantley, L. C. (2007). AKT/PKB signaling: Navigating downstream. *Cell, 129*(7), 1261–1274. https://doi.org/10.1016/j.cell.2007.06.009.

87. Matsumura, Y., & Maeda, H. (1986). A new concept for macromolecular therapeutics in cancer chemotherapy: Mechanism of tumor tropic accumulation of proteins and the antitumor agent smancs. *Cancer Research, 46*(12 Pt 1), 6387–6392.

88. Miao, L., Guo, S., Lin, C. M., Liu, Q., & Huang, L. (2015). Nano formulations for combination or cascade anticancer therapy. *Advanced Drug Delivery Reviews, 98*, 19–34.

89. Michalet, X., Pinaud, F. F., Bentolila, L. A., Tsay, J. M., Doose, S., Li, J. J., Sundaresan, G., Wu, A. M., Gambhir, S. S., & Weiss, S. (2005). Quantum dots for live cells, *in vivo* imaging, and diagnostics. *Science, 307*(5709), 538–544.

90. Moon, J. J., Huang, B., & Irvine, D. J. (2012). Engineering nano- and microparticles to tune immunity. *Advanced Materials, 24*(28), 3724–3746.

91. Mura, S., Nicolas, J., & Couvreur, P. (2013). Stimuli-responsive nanocarriers for drug delivery. *Nature Materials, 12*(11), 991–1003.

92. Nie, S., & Xing, Y. (2008). Nanotechnology applications in cancer. *Annual Review of Biomedical Engineering, 9*, 257–288.

93. Ovais, M., Mukherjee, S., Pramanik, A., Das, D., Mukherjee, A., Raza, A., & Panda, S. (2019). Designing stimuli-responsive upconversion nanoparticles that exploit tumor acidity for NIR light-triggered photodynamic therapy. *Chemistry–A European Journal, 25*(57), 13024–13035.

94. Palumbo, A., Chanan-Khan, A., Weisel, K., Nooka, A. K., Masszi, T., Beksac, M., & Röllig, C. (2016). Daratumumab, bortezomib, and dexamethasone for multiple myeloma. *New England Journal of Medicine, 375*(8), 754–766.

95. Patolsky, F., Timko, B. P., Yu, G., Fang, Y., Greytak, A. B., Zheng, G., & Lieber, C. M. (2006). Detection, stimulation, and inhibition of neuronal signals with high-density nanowire transistor arrays. *Science, 313*(5790), 1100–1104.

96. Peer, D., Karp, J. M., Hong, S., Farokhzad, O. C., Margalit, R., & Langer, R. (2007). Nanocarriers as an emerging platform for cancer therapy. *Nature Nanotechnology, 2*(12), 751–760.

97. Rengan, A. K., Jagtap, M., De, A., Banerjee, R., Srivastava, R., & Srivastava, R. (2014). Multifunctional gold-coated thermo-sensitive liposomes for multimodal imaging and photo-thermal therapy of breast cancer cells. *Nanoscale, 6*(2), 916–923.

98. Robinson, J. T., Tabakman, S. M., Liang, Y., Wang, H., Sanchez Casalongue, H., Vinh, D., & Dai, H. (2011). Ultrasmall reduced graphene oxide with high near-infrared absorbance for photothermal therapy. *Journal of the American Chemical Society, 133*(17), 6825–6831.

99. Saha, K., Agasti, S. S., Kim, C., Li, X., & Rotello, V. M. (2012). Gold nanoparticles in chemical and biological sensing. *Chemical Reviews, 112*(5), 2739–2779.

100. Sahdev, P., Ochyl, L. J., & Moon, J. J. (2014). Biomaterials for nanoparticle vaccine delivery systems. *Pharmaceutical Research, 31*(10), 2563–2582.

101. Sarwar, A., Katas, H., Samsudin, S. N., Zin, N. M., & Regenstein, J. M. (2015). Antimicrobial chitosan and chitosan derivatives: A review of the structure-activity relationship. *Chemistry Central Journal, 9*(1), 25.

102. Sawant, R. R., & Torchilin, V. P. (2012). Enhanced cytotoxicity of TATp-bearing paclitaxel-loaded micelles *in vitro* and *in vivo*. *International Journal of Pharmaceutics, 436*(1, 2), 25–31.

103. Scher, H. I., Fizazi, K., Saad, F., Taplin, M. E., Sternberg, C. N., Miller, K., & Small, E. J. (2012). Increased survival with enzalutamide in prostate cancer after chemotherapy. *New England Journal of Medicine, 367*(13), 1187–1197.

104. Schirrmacher, V. (2019). From chemotherapy to biological therapy: A review of novel concepts to reduce the side effects of systemic cancer treatment. *International Journal of Oncology, 54*(2), 407–419. https://doi.org/10.3892/ijo.2018.4661.

105. Shepherd, F. A., Rodrigues Pereira, J., Ciuleanu, T., Tan, E. H., Hirsh, V., Thongprasert, S., & Seymour, L. (2005). Erlotinib in previously treated non–small-cell lung cancer. *New England Journal of Medicine, 353*(2), 123–132.

106. Shi, J., & Kantoff, P. W. (2017). Tumor-associated macrophages as targets for cancer therapy. *Nature Reviews Clinical Oncology, 14*(7), 399–416.

107. Shi, J., Kantoff, P. W., Wooster, R., & Farokhzad, O. C. (2017). Cancer nanomedicine: Progress, challenges and opportunities. *Nature Reviews Cancer, 17*(1), 20–37. https://doi.org/10.1038/nrc.2016.108.

108. Silva, J. M., Duarte, A. R., Sousa, J. J., & Espina, M. (2017). Application of nanotechnology in the development of new strategies for cancer immunotherapy. *Advanced Healthcare Materials, 6*(10), 1700157.

109. Slamon, D. J., Leyland-Jones, B., Shak, S., Fuchs, H., Paton, V., Bajamonde, A., & Norton, L. (2001). Use of chemotherapy plus a monoclonal antibody against HER2 for metastatic breast cancer that overexpresses HER2. *New England Journal of Medicine, 344*(11), 783–792.

110. Song, J., Yang, X., Jacobson, O., Lin, L., Huang, P., Niu, G., & Chen, X. (2015). Sequential drug release and enhanced photothermal and photoacoustic effect of hybrid reduced graphene oxide-loaded ultrasmall gold nanorod vesicles for cancer therapy. *ACS Nano, 9*(9), 9199–9209.

111. Sun, Q., Barz, M., De Geest, B. G., Diken, M., Hennink, W. E., Kiessling, F., & Shi, Y. (2019). Nanomedicine and macroscale materials in immuno-oncology. *Chemical Society Reviews, 48*(7), 2018–2045.

112. Tang, L., Zheng, Y., Melo, M. B., Mabardi, L., Castaño, A. P., Xie, Y. Q., & Irvine, D. J. (2016). Enhancing T cell therapy through TCR-signaling-responsive nanoparticle drug delivery. *Nature Biotechnology, 34*(7), 648–654.

113. Tawfeek, H. M., Elnaggar, Y. S., Hebishy, E., Abbas, A. M., Jaleel, G. A., & Aldawsari, H. M. (2017). Enhanced oral bioavailability of the poorly water-soluble weak base ketoconazole using soluplus®-PEG 4000 binary mixed micelles: Design, optimization using D-optimal design and *in vitro–in vivo* evaluation. *International Journal of Nanomedicine, 12*, 709–725.

114. Thakor, A. S., & Gambhir, S. S. (2013). Nano oncology: The future of cancer diagnosis and therapy. *CA: A Cancer Journal for Clinicians, 63*(6), 395–418.

115. Tian, Q., Jiang, F., Zou, R., Liu, Q., Chen, Z., Zhu, M., & Yang, S. (2011). Hydrophilic Cu9S5 nanocrystals: A photothermal agent with a 25.7% heat conversion efficiency for photothermal ablation of cancer cells *in vivo*. *ACS Nano, 5*(12), 9761–9771.

116. Torchilin, V. (2006). Multifunctional nanocarriers. *Advanced Drug Delivery Reviews, 58*(14), 1532–1555.

117. Torchilin, V. P. (2006). Recent advances with liposomes as pharmaceutical carriers. *Nature Reviews Drug Discovery, 5*(2), 145–150.

118. Torchilin, V. P. (2007). Targeted pharmaceutical nanocarriers for cancer therapy and imaging. *The AAPS Journal, 9*(2), E128–E147.

119. Torchilin, V. P. (2011). Multifunctional, stimuli-sensitive nanoparticulate systems for drug delivery. *Nature Reviews Drug Discovery, 10*(9), 748–765.

120. Torchilin, V. P. (2014). Multifunctional, stimuli-sensitive nanoparticulate systems for drug delivery. *Nature Reviews Drug Discovery, 13*(11), 813–827. https://doi.org/10.1038/nrd4333.

121. Visvader, J. E., & Lindeman, G. J. (2008). Cancer stem cells in solid tumors: Accumulating evidence and unresolved questions. *Nature Reviews Cancer, 8*(10), 755–768. https://doi.org/10.1038/nrc2499.

122. Von Hoff, D. D., Ervin, T., Arena, F. P., Chiorean, E. G., Infante, J., Moore, M., & Chen, L. T. (2013). Increased survival in pancreatic cancer with nab-paclitaxel plus gemcitabine. *New England Journal of Medicine, 369*(18), 1691–1703.

123. Wang, S., Gao, R., Zhou, F., & Selke, M. (2018). Nanomaterials and singlet oxygen photosensitizers: Potential applications in photodynamic therapy. *Chemical Society Reviews, 47*(5), 1801–1817.

124. Wang, Y., Zhang, X., & Zhang, X. (2016). pH-sensitive polymeric micelles triggered drug release for extracellular and intracellular drug targeting delivery. *Asian Journal of Pharmaceutical Sciences, 11*(4), 381–389.

125. Wang, Y., Zhou, K., Huang, G., Hensley, C., Huang, X., Ma, X., & Nie, S. (2010). A nanoparticle-based strategy for the imaging of a broad range of tumors by nonlinear amplification of microenvironment signals. *Nature Materials, 13*(2), 204–212.

126. Weissleder, R., & Pittet, M. J. (2008). Imaging in the era of molecular oncology. *Nature, 452*(7187), 580–589.

127. Wells, S. A., Robinson, B. G., Gagel, R. F., Dralle, H., Fagin, J. A., Santoro, M., & Kreissl, M. C. (2012). Vandetanib in patients with locally advanced or metastatic medullary thyroid cancer: A randomized, double-blind phase III trial. *Journal of Clinical Oncology, 30*(2), 134–141.

128. Wilhelm, S., Tavares, A. J., Dai, Q., Ohta, S., Audet, J., Dvorak, H. F., & Chan, W. C. W. (2016). Analysis of nanoparticle delivery to tumors. *Nature Reviews Materials, 1*, 16014.

129. Younes, A., Bartlett, N. L., Leonard, J. P., Kennedy, D. A., Lynch, C. M., Sievers, E. L., & Forero-Torres, A. (2010). Brentuximab vedotin (SGN-35) for relapsed CD30-positive lymphomas. *New England Journal of Medicine, 363*(19), 1812–1821.

130. Zhang, G., Yang, Z., Lu, W., Zhang, R., Huang, Q., Tian, M., & Li, C. (2009). Influence of anchoring ligands and particle size on the colloidal stability and *in vivo* biodistribution of polyethylene glycol-coated gold nanoparticles in tumor-xenografted mice. *Biomaterials, 30*(10), 1928–1936.

131. Zhang, X., Xing, J. Z., Chen, J., & Ko, L. (2008). A novel therapeutic approach for treating cancer: Nanomaterials. *Reviews in Nanoscience and Nanotechnology, 8*(1), 63–84. https://doi.org/10.1166/rnn.2009.1002.

132. Zhang, Y., Chan, H. F., & Leong, K. W. (2013). Advanced materials and processing for drug delivery: The past and the future. *Advanced Drug Delivery Reviews, 65*(1), 104–120.

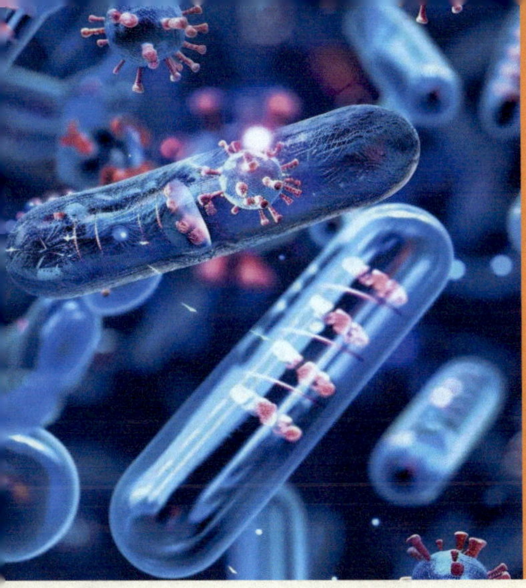

Chapter 5

NANOMEDICINE FOR NEUROLOGICAL DISORDER

Contents

Sheetal, Diksha, and Archana Gupta*

Department of Biotechnology and Microbiology, Faculty of Science and Humanities, SRM University Delhi-NCR, Sonepat, Haryana, India

*Corresponding author.

Abstract

Due to brain conditions such multiple sclerosis (MS), stroke, Parkinson's disease (PD), Alzheimer's disease (AD), where there are structural, biochemical, and electrical abnormalities affects the normal functioning of the nervous system which affects around 1.5 million individuals and account for 1% of global fatalities. Numerous conventional medications have been identified as possible treatments for neurological diseases. However, because of the brain's physical and biochemical dynamic barriers, such the blood–brain barrier (BBB), which block some chemicals and infections from entering the brain from the circulatory system, into the brain, the therapeutic success of these potential drugs is still limited. To overcome these challenges, we have to explore different strategies for bypassing and the BBB being crossed. The advent of Nanotechnology and the exploration of its principles and possibilities has brought a remarkable revolution in the field of neurology. Within this field, Nanomedicines, also referred to as nanotherapeutics medicines, have remarkably emerged as game-changers in neurological disease treatments by bypassing the various barriers. This chapter 'Nanomedicine for neurological disorder' explores the remarkable advancement made in the use of nanotechnology in the management of neurological conditions. This chapter delves into the groundbreaking research and potential of nanomedicines in revolutionizing the way we understand and treat brain disorders by overcoming the challenges imposed by the BBB and nanoparticles-based drug delivery systems (DDS). We are also going to explore the ethical and regulatory consideration along with the future perspective and challenges of nanomedicine in neurological disorder treatment. The objective is to guide and bring awareness about the immense scope of nanomedicines in treatments of neurological disease.

5.1. Introduction

The nervous system is a network of neurons, the primary role of which lies in the control and coordination of all bodily activities relating to internal and external stimuli. Major divisions include the peripheral nervous system, which consists of nerves outside the central nervous system (CNS), and the CNS, which includes the brain and spinal cord as the principal control unit. The PNS further divides into the somatic and autonomic nervous systems. Essential to its proper functioning are two main cell types: neurons, responsible for transmitting electrical signals and communicating with other cells, and glial cells, such as oligodendrocytes, microglia, and astrocytes, which support structure, control the chemical environment, and contribute to functions such as immune response and inflammation (Thau, Reddy, and Singh, 2022). Neurons possess unique structures, including a cell body housing the nucleus and organelles, as well as dendrites and axons for signal transmission. The myelin sheath, a white insulating substance, wraps around axons. Structural, electrical, and biochemical abnormalities can disrupt normal nervous system function, leading to several neurological conditions, including multiple sclerosis (MS), stroke, Parkinson's disease (PD), Alzheimer's disease (AD), tumor, and so on (Thakur et al., 2016). Despite the discovery of conventional drugs for CNS treatments, the BBB poses a challenge by limiting substance movement into and out of the brain, hindering effective drug delivery. Nanobiotechnology emerges as a potential game-changer, offering targeted therapy for neurological diseases (Ambesh and Angeli, 2015). Nanoparticles and nanocarriers can be created in a variety of sizes, shapes, and surface charges, including lipid, polymer, and inorganic based varieties. Functional group modifications enhance their ability to penetrate barriers and target specific areas. Nanobiotechnology finds applications in gene delivery, molecular imaging, tissue engineering, biosensors, biomarkers, and more (Mittal et al., 2022). While it holds promise as a potential cure for neurological diseases, concerns about possible toxicity and environmental impact have sparked debates among regulatory organizations in the field of nanotechnology.

5.2. Understanding Neurological Disorders and the Blood–Brain Barrier (BBB)

5.2.1. Blood–Brain Barrier (BBB)

The CNS is separated from the peripheral circulation by a barrier known as the BBB. Its physiological processes, structural integrity, and molecular mechanisms are all interactive to the control compounds' flow through it between the blood and the brain. BBB selectivity is due to the tight connections and adherents of the endothelium lining. Adherens junctions allow the interaction of endothelial cells, while tight junctions seal inter-endothelial clefts to form a continuous blood vessel lumen (Alahmari, 2021). In addition to endothelial cells, BBB consists of astrocytes, pericytes, and mural cells that are vascular smooth muscle cells (Kadry, Noorani, and Cucullo, 2020). In the molecular mechanism that controls substances' passage over the BBB, inflow and efflux mechanisms play a role.

While small molecules can pass past tight junctions, bigger macromolecules can be selectively uptake by receptor-mediated transcytosis. RMT is caused by a variety of ligands such as plasma proteins and growth factors, which form a link between receptors present on endothelial cells. There exists another inflow process known as adsorptive-mediated transcytosis (AMT), which is triggered by electrostatic interactions existing between the negatively charged surface of endothelial cells and the positively charged protein moieties (Pawar et al., 2022; Zhang et al., 2020). Efflux mechanisms, particularly the activity of ATP-binding cassette (ABC) transporters, are central for drugs to gain entry into the brain. The luminal membrane of the brain capillary endothelial cells contains P-glycoprotein (P-gp), also known as ABCB1 which is a most well-known ABC efflux transporter. P-gp, or protein 1 that is drug-resistant, pumps many drugs out of cells, thus making it difficult for the drugs to accumulate within the brain. Research has focused on blocking efflux transporters to enhance drug accumulation, with studies showing that inhibiting P-gp allows increased drug concentration in the brain, presenting a potential avenue for improved drug delivery (Schinkel, 1999).

5.2.2. Neurological Disorders

Table 5.1 summarizes common neurological disorders along with their causes, currently available drugs, and the associated limitations of these treatments. This overview highlights the ongoing need for more effective and targeted therapeutic strategies.

Table 5.1. Various Types of Neurological Disorders, Their Causes, Current Available Drugs, and Limitations of Current Treatments

SL. No.	Disease	Caused by	Current Drug(s)	Limitation(s)
1.	Alzheimer's disease	Buildup of amyloid-beta peptide (Aβ) in the medial temporal lobe and neocortical regions of the brain leads to neurofibrillary tangles and neuritic plaques	Donepezil, Rivastigmine, Galantamine, and Memantine	Diarrhea, muscle cramps, fatigue, nausea, vomiting, anorexia, and insomnia

2.	Parkinson's disease	Tremor, rigidity, and bradykinesia, with postural instability appearing in some patients as the disease progresses	Levodopa, Carbidopa	Nausea, vomiting, low blood pressure, and restlessness
3.	Multiple sclerosis	Autoimmune attack on the myelin—the protective layer around nerve fibers—leading to inflammation and lesions	Ocrelizumab, Ofatumumab, Natalizumab, Alemtuzumab	Fatigue, allergic reactions, headache, rash, nausea, and pyrexia
4.	Stroke	A sudden neurological episode caused by reduced blood circulation to the brain	Aspirin, Warfarin, Clopidogrel	Nausea, vomiting, dizziness, and hemorrhage
5.	Brain tumor	Abnormal cell growth within the brain	Chemotherapy, seizure medication	Tumor regrowth, nausea, and vomiting

5.3. Breaking Blood–Brain Barrier (BBB)

There are several phases involved in breaking down or altering the immunological, transport, and physical barriers in order to disrupt the BBB, which are discussed in subsections.

5.3.1. Breakdown of the Physical Barrier

Physical Barrier Breakdown: Agrin accumulation, a proteoglycan containing heparan sulfate, on the basal lamina of brain microvascular endothelial cells (BMECs) is essential for maintaining the integrity of the BBB. Agrin loss is a result of neuroinflammation, which also damages the BBB and causes cerebral edema. A lack of pericyte can inhibit the production of tight junction proteins, which weakens the integrity of the junction and encourages immune cells to infiltrate the susceptible CNS. In neurodegenerative diseases, proteins such as occludin, fibronectin, laminin, and heparan sulfate in the basal lamina are attacked by matrix metalloproteinases (MMPs), further impairing the integrity of tight junctions and adherens junctions (Alahmari, 2021).

5.3.2. Alteration/Breakdown of the Transport Barrier

Neuroimmune modulators cause alterations to the typical pattern of transporter expression. Examples include the upregulation of GLUT1 in starvation and hypoxia, and the differential regulation of P-gp in various conditions. Spinal cord injury, stroke, and neurodegenerative diseases affect transport rates of molecules like TNF, PACAP, and LIF-50 (Knox et al., 2022). Neurodegenerative illnesses cause alterations in the expression of certain receptors, including TfR, IR, LRP, LDLR, and DTR. Several substances can alter transporter function during illness, which frequently leads to more BBB disruption. DTR is especially prone to overexpression in inflammatory circumstances.

5.3.3. Invasion of the Immune Barrier

One typical sign of neuroinflammation is increased leukocyte trafficking into the CNS. Inflammatory mediators transiently open the BBB and upregulate adhesion molecules like vascular cell adhesion molecule-1 (VCAM-1), which promotes immune cell transendothelial migration. These cells are a diverse population that comprises pro-inflammatory and immunosuppressive cells (such as regulatory T cells and myeloid suppressor cells) (Haarmann et al., 2015). Clinical signs of diseases such glioblastoma multiforme (GBM), MS, encephalitis, meningitis, and HIV-1 are closely linked to immune cell invasion. When it comes to HIV-1, infected monocytes employ the "Trojan Horse" technique to sneak infections across the BBB (Pardridge, 2006). The disruption of these barriers highlights the complex interplay of molecular mechanisms involved in BBB compromise during various pathological conditions.

5.4. Nanotechnology a Game Changer to Overcome Challenges

Nanotechnology is revolutionizing the field of neurotherapeutics by offering a highly effective and innovative approach to bypass the BBB and deliver treatments.

Over the past few decades, nanomedicines have demonstrated significant potential in delivering drugs to the CNS. This may be because of their nanometer-size dimension, unique physical and chemical properties, and the capability of using biocompatible and biodegradable materials at their surface. Indeed, using nanotechnology, one can fine-tune drug transport and delivery precisely to the location within the brain. In fact, the drug itself, which is one of the most important components of the nanoengineered complex, can take many roles, being encapsulated to protect it from enzymes or providing the desired pharmacological effects (Soni, Ruhela, and Medhi, 2016).

Overall, encapsulation of the drug via nanotechnology certainly presents a new horizon within CNS drug delivery. It is the accurate and tailored solutions that will be required for treatment of those conditions involving the brain (Figure 5.1).

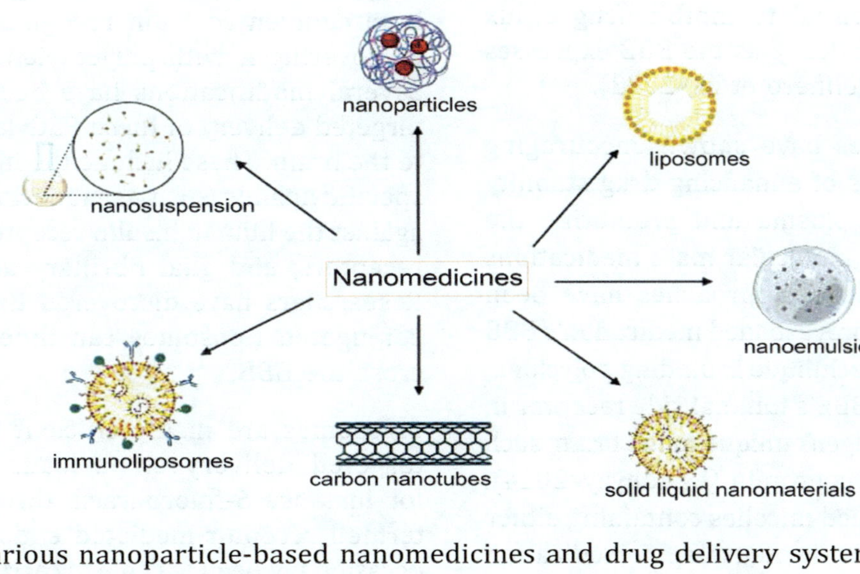

Figure 5.1. Various nanoparticle-based nanomedicines and drug delivery systems (DDS).

5.4.1. Nanoparticles-Based Drug Delivery Systems (DDS)

5.4.1.1. Micelles

Because of its effectiveness as drug delivery to the CNS, micelles of either amphiphilic surfactants or amphiphilic. These polymers, it appears, have become of much concern for researchers (Gerardos, Balafouti, and Pispas, 2023). Polymeric micelles are known to have a core-shell structure with diameters between 10 and 100 nm. It is comprised of the inner hydrophobic core containing phospholipids, fatty acids, and polycaprolactone (PCL) end. It, therefore, includes an interior hydrophobic layer, mainly made up of PEG and primarily composed of PEG on the exterior as a hydrophilic layer.

Drugs that are hydrophobic can be loaded effectively because of this specific layout. Additionally, the hydrophilic coating not only ensures micelle stability in aqueous environments but also lengthens their circulation duration in the bloodstream, protects them from the reticuloendothelial system (RES), and enhances their ability to cross barriers. An intriguing area of research focuses on *Pluronic* copolymers, more commonly known as poloxamers, due to their potential to inhibit drug efflux transporters, specifically as the BBB expresses P-gp (Naharros-Molinero et al., 2022).

These micelles have shown encouraging outcomes in terms of enhancing drug stability and solubility in plasma and promoting the absorption of low molecular mass medications into the brain. Novel approaches have been investigated to improve loaded medication's BBB penetration. One technique is binding polyclonal antibodies to the BBB's luminal side receptor in order to target antigens unique to the brain, such as insulin or 2-glycoprotein (Upadhyay, 2014). When these modified micelles containing either a fluorescent dye or the neuroleptic medication haloperidol are injected intravenously, the drug and fluorescent dye are efficiently carried across the BBB (Braga et al., 2021).

5.4.1.2. Liposome

In the 1970s, the initial colloidal nanocarriers' creation, referred to as liposomes, emerged and were put to the test as a revolutionary medicine delivery system. These minuscule, spherical vesicles consist of one or more phospholipid bilayers covering an interior compartment that is hydrophilic. Due to their similarities to cell membranes, known for their ability to transport medications, proteins, and peptides, liposomes have quickly gained recognition and usage. These vesicles come in three distinct forms: By size and number of bilayers, they are classified as tiny unilamellar (10–50 nm), enormous unilamellar (50–1000 nm), and multilamellar (20–100 nm). In addition, the bonding between molecules and non-covalent interactions like van der Waal forces and molecular bonding contribute to their structure. Furthermore, these structures have the flexibility to be manipulated. In their natural form, liposomes can circulate within the body (Seo and Park, 2021). Efforts have been devoted to creating liposomes that are specifically designed for long-term circulation and targeting. The RES is circumvented from recognizing liposomes by covering it with polyethylene glycol (PEG). Several modifications have been tried in the targeted delivery of these PEGylated liposomes to the brain. These include the incorporation of specific ligands, such as monoclonal antibodies against the human insulin receptors, transferrin receptors, and glial fibrillary acidic proteins. Researchers have discovered that transferrin-conjugated liposomes can indeed be able to cross the BBB.

Liposomes are highly efficient vectors in the targeted delivery of payloads to the brain, for instance 5-fluorouracil, through a process termed receptor-mediated endocytosis. It has occasionally been feasible to carry out successful immunoliposomes by integrating prednisolone-loaded liposomes with specific monoclonal antibodies which can bind to cell surface receptors expressed in the target tissue (Pandian et al., 2022).

5.4.1.3. Polymeric Nanoparticle

The area of application for polymeric nanoparticles ranges from the field of biodegradation to areas related to drug delivery and biocompatibility. In general terms, versatile particles consist of a hydrophobic core where lipophilic drugs are encapsulated along with an anchoring hydrophilic corona. Encapsulation is one of the delivery mechanisms whereby drugs get encapsulated within the nanoparticles. Drugs can also be adsorbed or chemically attached on the surface of the nanoparticles for drug delivery. Incorporation of hydrophilic polymers, such as PEG, in the formulation may improve the shelf-life of nanoparticles circulating in the body. This can be done by targeting with polysaccharides or other hydrophilic polymers. The conjugation of PS80-coated 1% poly(n-butyl cyanoacrylate) nanoparticles with conventional therapy also proves to increase the delivery of drugs targeted towards the brain, like rivastigmine or tacrine at reduced systemic concentration. Recently, scientists found that Dalargin nanoparticles coated with PS80 could freely pass through the BBB when given and achieved optimum pain relief upon oral administration. Further studies suggested that PS80-coated PACA nanoparticles can also bind with ApoE and B in the blood when administered intravenously (Zhang et al., 2021). This binding makes it possible for transcytosis to occur across the BBB via low-density lipoprotein receptors, which makes it a viable technique for effective and safe BBB drug administration. Furthermore, research employing hCMEC/D3 cells and *C57BL/6* mice showed that venlafaxine-loaded PLGA nanoparticles, which are able to pass across the BBB intact, had antidepressant properties. Remarkably, receptor-mediated PLGA nanoparticle distribution was unaffected by P-gP pump efflux, a frequent obstacle in intranasal administration, leading to enhanced biodistribution in the brain and after 24 hours of receptor binding, there were no variations in the P-gP pump concentration (Cunha et al., 2021) (Figure 5.2).

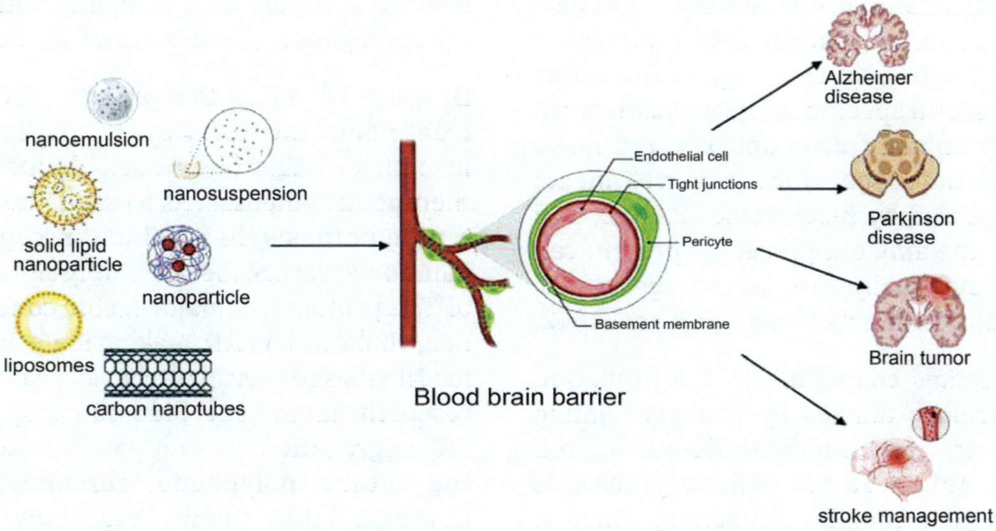

Figure 5.2. Nanomedicines used to cross the blood–brain barrier (BBB) for the treatment of various neurological disorders.

5.5. Nanomedicines for Alzheimer's Disease (AD)

A buildup of Aβ deposits outside of cells and an accumulation of tau protein inside of cells are the hallmarks of AD, a frequent type of dementia. Aβ clusters are created when pre amyloid protein breaks down abnormally. These clusters then form insoluble fibrils with a beta-sheet shape. These fibrils disrupt synaptic communication, causing neurotoxicity and subsequently, the development of dementia. To date, only five medications have been sanctioned by the FDA for the treatment of AD; these include galantamine, memantine, rivastigmine, donepezil, and tacrine (Alhazmi and Albratty, 2022). There are promising drugs that may be used in probably preventing or slowing down the onset and course of AD through pertinent factors such as cholinergic levels, amyloid aggregates, and tau protein. However, due to the complexity of the brain and its various barriers, a high dose of these drugs is required with their oral formulations in practice. This would lead to side effects due to off-target effects and also due to a very short half-life; hence, treatment of AD patients can be very challenging. The use of nanocarriers with specific functionalization can dramatically enhance drug delivery and make possible the improved efficacy of treatments for AD. Processed by β-secretase (BACE1) and γ-secretase, the amyloid precursor protein can be cleaved, eventually forming Aβ aggregates, with the major products being Aβ40 and Aβ42.

These aggregates contribute to the formation of neurofibrillary tangles by phosphorylating and cleaving the microtubule-associated protein tau. Moreover, tau pathology disrupts the nuclear pore complex's function, which is the source of neurotoxicity in the AD brain. As such, reversal of the AD pathophysiology may be attainable either through interference with cellular constituents involved in Aβ generation or through preventing neurofibrillary tangle formation. In order to do this, Aβ-binding substances have been linked to nanoparticles (NPs) for therapeutic applications; liposomes and PEG-PLA NPs have been the most popular options because of their documented safety profiles and capacity to completely disintegrate without inducing immunological responses (Poudel and Park, 2022). In lab experiments, the study discovered that liposomes associated with derivatives of curcumin had a considerable binding affinity (1–5 nM) for Aβ fibrils. Another research discovered that liposomes containing phosphatidic acid (PA) or cardiolipin (CL) were highly effective (22–60 nM) at preventing Aβ formation, with a specific focus on targeting GM1 ganglioside. Recently, researchers developed PLGA NPs functionalized with KLVFF to inhibit Aβ aggregation without causing harm to cells and potentially reverse Aβ-induced pathologies (Ghalandari et al., 2022; Trebesova et al., 2022). Additionally, D-FexCuySe NPs, made of chiral iron copper selenide and activated by light, were able to reduce Aβ aggregation and fibril formation and improve cognitive abilities in mice with AD. Remarkably, PLGA NPs conjugated with a substance were able to significantly decrease Aβ aggregation (Trebesova et al., 2022).

Despite Aβ being the primary focus for AD treatment, the efficacy of its interference in clinical trials has raised doubts about its therapeutic potential. As a result, the alternative tau hypothesis has gained recognition. As mentioned earlier, the misfolding and aggregation of Tau protein is a major factor contributing to neuronal death in AD, making it a primary target for NPs-based therapeutics. According to recent research, methylene blue can stop or reduce tau aggregation in tauopathies. Additionally, the natural polyphenol curcumin, found in Curcuma longa plants, has shown potential neuroprotective properties. In light of this, curcumin compounds, discovered by Okuda et al., function as dual inhibitors of tau and Aβ aggregation. Moreover, Gao et al. have reported on the development of neuron-targeting biomimetic nanoparticles (NPs) for effective delivery of curcumin, which has the potential to halt the progression of AD by inhibiting tau aggregation. In AD treatment, these tau-targeted NPs, such as FA-AuNPs and AuFeNPs, have demonstrated an impressive binding affinity for both tau and tubulin (Ghalandari et al., 2022). Furthermore, protein-capped metal NPs have been shown by Shweta et al. to suppress tau aggregation in AD models. *In vitro* tau aggregation has been inhibited by newly produced PC-Fe_3O_4 and PC-CdS NPs, offering important new insights into the potential of biological nanomedicine for treating AD using anti-tau aggregation medicines.

5.6. Nanomedicines for Parkinson's Disease (PD)

Parkinson's disease (PD) is linked to a buildup of α-synuclein protein, which forms Lewy bodies in the cytoplasm and lowers the amount of dopamine in the striatum by causing the destruction of dopaminergic neurons in the substantia nigra. Progress has been made in treating PD over the years, However, the best drug to treat its symptoms is still levodopa. Additional PD medications reduce cognitive impairment, target dopamine stimulation, and help with antidepressant and anti-tremor effects. Each patient's treatment should be personalized, and various medications besides levodopa can cause side effects such as the on/off effect and dyskinesia, which can be mitigated by combining dopamine agonists with dopamine precursors. Adding a CO medication can also help smooth out any adverse effects. Numerous factors contribute to the development of PD, such as the build-up of Lewy bodies and the protein α-Synuclein in the brain. Recent studies have shown that interactions between α-Synuclein and nanoparticles (NPs) can enhance the effectiveness of NP configurations in combating existing fibrils and α-Synuclein fibrillation. Researchers are testing a variety of NPs-such as metal, inorganic, polymeric, and lipid-based vesicles-for Parkinson's therapy (Hawthorne et al., 2016).

The function of dopamine systems has been explored on a wide scale in research studies, especially in respect to neuropsychiatric disorders such as PD and drug addiction. In PD, degeneration in the ventral tegmental area (VTA) affects dopamine production at the later stages of the disease. The number of dopaminergic neurons in the SNpc and VTA is reduced, thereby lowering dopamine concentration in the PFC and striatum. Presently, therapeutic intervention in PD targets the improvement of dopamine levels through the administration of dopamine precursors that are converted into dopamine in the brain (Hawthorne et al., 2016). A new approach utilizes polymeric scaffold technology as well as nanotechnology to release dopamine exclusively with precise delivery within the CSF in rat models. Improvement in the efficacy of dopamine replacement therapy is made with carboxylated carbon nanotubes (c-CNT), as these enhance the BBB permeability and can reduce any adverse effects (Rahamathulla et al., 2021). In addition, PEGylated PLGA nanoparticles are smart delivery systems, which overcome the barriers of solubility in delivering therapeutic agents across biological barriers. Nanoparticles based on polydopamine can regulate electrical activity reversibly in both neurons and cardiomyocytes, *in vitro* and *in vivo*. This might be a promising treatment for PD. Albumin/PLGA nanosystems also loaded with BBB showed an impressive improvement in the motor function when combined with dopamine in a model of PD in mice. The crucial factor in the treatment of PD is to visually observe the build-up of epigallocatechin gallate (EGCG) in targeted dopaminergic neurons. In a recent study, a specialized traceable nanoparticle (made up of DSPE-PEG-B6, DSPE-PEG-MA, DSPE-PEG-phenylboronic acid, and superparamagnetic iron oxide nanocubes) containing EGCG was administered intravenously to mice overexpressing human α-syncline (Li et al., 2018). This resulted in a significant reduction of αS aggregation and a notable increase in dopaminergic neurons, providing a promising avenue for the treatment of PD. Vitamins have shown promising potential in mitigating structural changes and cytotoxicity caused by NPs. For example, a study reported that vitamin K1 effectively reduced the build-up of α-synuclein when single-walled carbon nanotubes (SWCNTs) are present, which reduces cytotoxicity. Moreover, cellular investigations revealed that co-cultivating α-synuclein with vitamin K1 in the presence of SWCNTs resulted in decreased cytotoxicity in comparison to the absence of vitamin K1 (Rahamathulla et al., 2021; Xiang et al., 2020).

5.7. Nanomedicines for Stroke

One of the main causes of mortality and disability is stroke, making it a pressing concern. Fortunately, NPs (nanoparticles) offer a targeted approach to delivering stroke treatments and improving outcomes. In particular, liposomes have been utilized to transport hemoglobin (Hb) to ischemic brain cells and restore oxygen supply. Multiple studies have demonstrated that liposomal NPs can effectively reduce the required dosage of drugs by extending their circulation and concentrating them at the site of injury. For example, intravenously given liposomal FK506 was found to selectively lower oxidative stress in the ischemic striatum, while protecting the healthy cortical area in a rat model of transient middle cerebral artery occlusion (tMCAO). Moreover, it was demonstrated that liposomal CsA was more effective than empty carriers or a dosage equal to free CsA (Fukuta et al., 2022). Micelles have also been used in combination with thrombolysis in addition to liposomes. In particular, after tissue plasminogen activator (tPA) therapy, IA-administered poly(lactic-co-glycolic acid) (PLGA) micelles containing the antioxidants catalase and superoxide dismutase were given (Yan et al., 2023). In comparison to both untreated controls and those receiving tPA alone, this led to the mobilization of neural progenitor cells (NPC) from the subventricular zone, enabling higher neurogenesis. Furthermore, research has demonstrated the antioxidant properties of inorganic nanoparticles, which have been used in hemorrhagic stroke models. Most recently, the integration of LWX7 onto the surface of CeO_2-NPs has been found to enhance targeting to the ischemic penumbra in *tMCAO* rats by interaction with integrin $\alpha v\beta_3$, ultimately leading to reduced neuronal death and immune response.

5.8. Nanomedicine for Brain Tumor

Glioblastoma multiforme (GBM) is a prevalent type of brain tumor, making up nearly half of all primary malignant CNS tumors. One of the available treatments for GBM at the moment is a maximum surgical removal. This is succeeded by a combination chemotherapy and/or radiation therapy. However, due to the limited effectiveness of these treatments, there is a pressing need for new techniques and advancements in technology. As a result, DDS based on nanocarriers have been developed. One such system is nanoparticles (NPs), which have demonstrated promise in pre-clinical and clinical trials for the treatment of GBMs. For example, convection-enhanced delivery (CED) was used to successfully distribute poly(lactide-co-glycolide) (PLGA) NPs in an intracranial rat model with a *U87MG* xenograft, resulting in a considerably longer median survival compared to usual therapies (Su et al., 2021). Through the use of a liposomal nanoparticle (NP) carrying DOX and linked to atherosclerotic plaque-specific peptide-1 (AP-1), this treatment shows potential for specifically targeting IL-4 receptors and inducing endocytosis to enhance tumor killing in GBM tissue. Promising results have been seen in mouse models with the use of interleukin-13-conjugated liposomes and IL-4 receptor-targeted liposomal doxorubicin, resulting in a significant reduction in tumor size compared to unconjugated liposomes (Liang et al., 2022). Sun et al. also reported on the use of TfR-PEG polymeric micelles, which exhibited rapid absorption by tumor cells and effective traversal of the BBB. When paclitaxel was added to these micelles, *U87* GBM cell growth was successfully inhibited *in vitro*, extending the median survival time in GBM-afflicted nude mice (Zhao et al., 2023). An intriguing development in the delivery of siRNA to glioma cells is the innovative method of coating two distinct oncogenes with beta-cyclodextrin (β-CD) and silencing them using poly(amidoamine) (PAMAM) dendrimer-entrapped gold (Au) NPs (Zhao et al., 2023). This clever design not only effectively targets and silences specific genes but also enhances drug delivery via conjugating d-glucosamine with polyether-copolyester (PEPE) dendrimers (Dhanikula et al., 2008; Zhao et al., 2023). This specifically tailored design has shown promising results in killing methotrexate-resistant cells. In the realm of nanomedicine, gold nanoparticles (AuNPs) prove to be the optimal material for treating GBM (Zhao et al., 2023). Although numerous studies have demonstrated the potential of nanotechnology and nanocarriers for treating GBM, only a limited number of clinical trials have been conducted in this area (Figure 5.3).

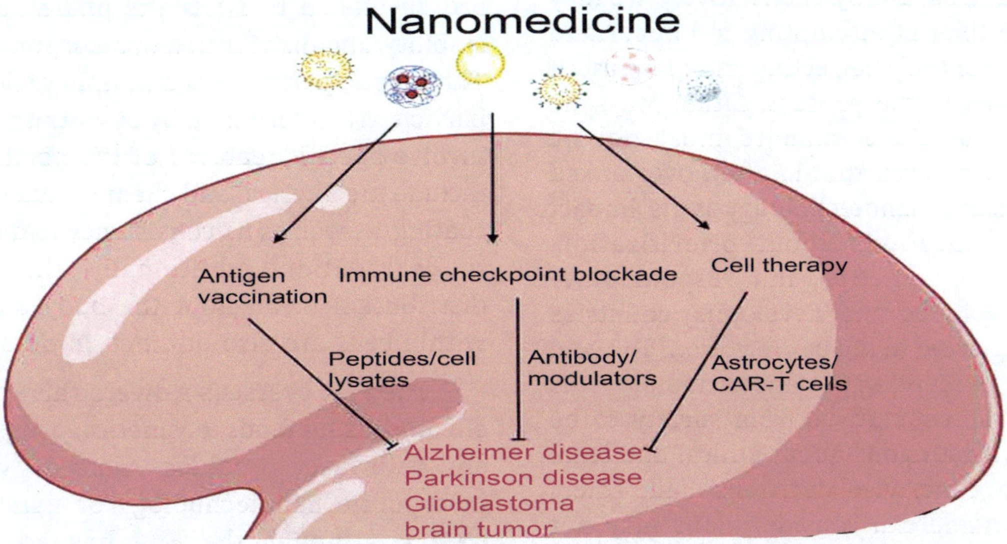

Figure 5.3. Nanomedicines act through various mechanisms as potential treatments for Alzheimer's disease (AD), Parkinson's disease (PD), and brain tumors.

5.9. Ethical and Regulatory Considerations

The term nanoethics arose from the ethical concerns stemming from a deeper understanding of nanotechnology. To establish the existence of a distinct ethical domain within nanotechnology, we must examine the unique ethical issues it presents, as well as consider its relation to established ethical problems. It is worth noting that nanotechnology shares similar ethical concerns with biotechnology, but its potential for creating extraordinary properties and rapidly advancing technology sets it apart as more powerful. As a result, we can conclude that nanotechnology poses comparable, yet more significant ethical concerns than biotechnology. Nanotechnology, like any other technology, will undoubtedly bring about significant changes in our lifestyles. However, what sets it apart is the incredibly rapid pace at which these changes will occur. The exponential growth rate of nanotechnological information, as highlighted by Ray Kurzweil, will have a profound impact on the speed of these changes. As this process accelerates, the time we have to understand and adapt to these changes decreases, leaving us with little choice but to embrace the "blessings" of nanotechnology without fully comprehending their consequences (Gökçay and Arda, 2015). Alternatively, we may invest more time in attempting to understand and adapt, potentially neglecting other important considerations in the process. Either way, the implications of these changes must not be overlooked. One area that is often overlooked when discussing nanotechnology is its impact on society. Questions about prioritization, distribution of benefits, and responsibility between developed and developing countries are often neglected in the conversation. To avoid a one-sided perception of nanotechnology, it is crucial for representatives from society to be included in discussions about ethical and legal implications. Otherwise, decisions made solely based on commercial considerations may not align with the best interests of humanity.

According to regulatory standards, the use of biological nanomedicines is governed by the European Medicines Agency (EMA). The EMA set out an integral framework related to the regulation of follow-on biological nanomedicines with guidelines for quality assessment and further non-clinical and clinical studies to ensure safety and efficacy. For nanomedicines with different surface coatings, including intravenous liposomal, block copolymer micelle, and iron-based nano-colloidal products, EMA has published a number of reflection papers previously. Articles published here are deemed to be of importance in the development of new nanomedicines and nanosimilars, bringing to developers useful advice in the development of applications for marketing permission (Soares et al., 2018).

All these products contain information of great wealth, including prerequisite knowledge on the topics of the complexity of nanosystems and block-copolymer micelle, "liposome-like" nanoparticle iron therapeutic development, and nonclinical preliminary clinical investigations. All these products are meant to impact the distribution, stability, and pharmacokinetics of integrated medications. These products are developed to affect the pharmacokinetics, stability, and distribution of incorporated drugs. The kinetic parameters and final toxicity of the particle are determined by essential factors that involve specific features of the particle. These include the physical and chemical makeup of the coating, as well as its consistency and resistance to degradation. Additionally, the product's distribution throughout the body and its fate within cells are also outlined in detail.

The FDA oversees a diverse array of goods, encompassing foods, cosmetics, drugs, devices, and veterinary products, some of which may incorporate nanotechnology or nanomaterials (NMs). Although the FDA has not officially released a of its own definition, it played a role in the creation of the National Nanotechnology Initiative (NNI) definition. Under this definition, potential areas of interest for the FDA could include the development of research and technology that aligns with the NNI criteria and pertains to a product under the FDA's jurisdiction. A recent analysis delves into the 51 medical products, composed of NMs, which have thus far received FDA approval and discusses noteworthy patterns in this burgeoning field of study.

5.10. Future Perspectives and Challenges

Undoubtedly, nanomedicine has emerged as an innovative and highly promising approach for targeted treatment of CNS disorders. By engineering carriers that can penetrate the BBB, diffuse throughout brain tissue, and specifically target desired cells and signaling pathways, nanomedicine has the potential to revolutionize therapeutic delivery. Because it has the capacity to carry larger quantities of drugs due to its large surface area, various biomaterial options, and inclusion of ionic surface charges such as PEGylation for further aiding drug binding and functionalization, nanomedicine has proven to have numerous benefits over the more traditional delivery means of drugs. Additionally, the use of the ligand binding coupled with antibody tagging allows it to target particular areas within the brain with even higher accuracy. In general, the scope of nanomedicine for CNS therapeutics is very exciting.

There are many hopes and optimisms related to personalized nanomedicine strategies for the treatment of CNS disorders. Even with all the promise, however, personalized nanomedicine still faces major obstacles to the practical application of CNS illness therapy, such as safety, efficacy, and regulatory compliance. According to Sanhai et al., there are seven primary challenges for future nanomedicines as identified by the FDA. The list of challenges includes the determination of the distribution of the administered nanocarriers by the body, their ability to transport diverse medications as well as diagnostic payloads and their ability to transverse the barriers involved, such as BBB. To accurately evaluate the disadvantages as well as advantages of nanocarriers, new computational and mathematical approaches must be produced. They shall ensure safety and efficiency by evaluation standards, preparation of fact sheets, and analytical tools for nanocarriers.

5.11. Conclusion

CNS illnesses are a major component to the overall global disease burden because they include a broad spectrum of brain abnormalities that can result in temporary as well as permanent disability. However, the promising field of nanomedicine has emerged as a new approach, using advanced nanoscale targeting techniques to deliver active agents with improved pharmacokinetics. These individualized nanomedicines have the potential to improve clinical outcomes by efficiently delivering therapeutic agents across the BBB and treating CNS illnesses.

Through careful design, nanomedicine has the ability to completely transform the way that CNS illnesses are treated. By extensively considering the end user's perspective during the formulation and laboratory experimentation stages, a clearer understanding of the necessary efforts and investments can be achieved. The success of CNS drug development has been hampered by the complexity of CNS disorders and the difficulties associated with AD neuropharmacology research. This can be addressed, though, by carrying out additional research on the pairing of novel nanocarriers with therapeutic targets, which may result in a synergistic effect for the treatment of CNS disorders. Because nanomedicine is biodegradable and biocompatible, it may be used as a therapeutic agent for brain disorders; nevertheless, it should be remembered that every nanocarrier has specific benefits and drawbacks. As we have discussed previously, it is important to take into account several worries related to nanomedicine. These include the possibility of buildup in essential organs including the liver, renal system, and the spleen as well as the danger of oxidative brain harm to the brain. These variables represent a serious risk to longevity of health after administering nanomedicines. The pharmacodynamics and pharmacokinetics of these medicines are also not well studied, and managing their possible adverse effects in a clinical context continues to be a major problem.

KEY TERMS FROM THIS CHAPTER

- biocompatible materials
- biodegradable materials
- carbon nanotubes
- inflammation
- nanocarriers
- nanomedicine
- neuropharmacology
- neurotoxicity
- polyethylene glycol

References

1. Alahmari, A. (2021). Blood-brain barrier overview: Structural and functional correlation. *Neural Plasticity, 2021*, 6564585. https://doi.org/10.1155/2021/6564585.

2. Alhazmi, H. A., & Albratty, M. (2022). An update on the novel and approved drugs for Alzheimer disease. *Saudi Pharmaceutical Journal, 30*(12), 1755–1764. https://doi.org/10.1016/j.jsps.2022.10.004.

3. Ambesh, P., & Angeli, D. G. (2015). Nanotechnology in neurology: Genesis, current status, and future prospects. *Annals of Indian Academy of Neurology, 18*(4), 382–386. https://doi.org/10.4103/0972-2327.169535.

4. Braga, C. B., Pilli, R. A., Ornelas, C., & Weck, M. (2021). Near-infrared fluorescent micelles from poly(norbornene) brush triblock copolymers for nanotheranostics. *Biomacromolecules, 22*(12), 5290–5306. https://doi.org/10.1021/acs.biomac.1c01196.

5. Cunha, A., et al. (2021). PLGA-based nanoparticles for neuroprotective drug delivery in neurodegenerative diseases. *Pharmaceutics, 13*(7), 1042. https://doi.org/10.3390/pharmaceutics13071042.

6. Dhanikula, R. S., Argaw, A., Bouchard, J. F., & Hildgen, P. (2008). Methotrexate-loaded polyether-copolyester dendrimers for the treatment of gliomas: Enhanced efficacy and intratumoral transport capability. *Molecular Pharmaceutics, 5*(1), 105–116. https://doi.org/10.1021/mp700086j.

7. Fukuta, T., et al. (2022). Application and utility of liposomal neuroprotective agents and biomimetic nanoparticles for the treatment of ischemic stroke. *Pharmaceutics, 14*(2), 361. https://doi.org/10.3390/pharmaceutics14020361.

8. Gerardos, A. M., Balafouti, A., & Pispas, S. (2023). Mixed copolymer micelles for nanomedicine. *Nanomanufacturing, 3*, 233–247. https://doi.org/10.3390/nanomanufacturing3020015.

9. Ghalandari, B., Asadollahi, K., Ghorbani, F., Ghalehbaghi, S., Rafiee, S., Komeili, A., Kamrava, S. K. (2022). Determinants of gold nanoparticle interactions with proteins: Off-target effect study. *Spectrochimica Acta Part A: Molecular and Biomolecular Spectroscopy, 269*, 120736. https://doi.org/10.1016/j.saa.2021.120736.

10. Gökçay, B., & Arda, B. (2015). Nanotechnology, nanomedicine; ethical aspects. *Revista Română de Bioetică, 13*(3). Retrieved from: http://www.bioetica.ro/index.php/arhiva-bioetica/article/view/829/pdf (accessed on 8 May 2025).

11. Haarmann, A., Nowak, E., Deiß, A., van der Pol, S., Monoranu, C. M., Kooij, G., Müller, N., van der Valk, P., Stoll, G., de Vries, H. E., Berberich-Siebelt, F., & Buttmann, M. (2015). Soluble VCAM-1 impairs human brain endothelial barrier integrity via integrin α-4-transduced outside-in signaling. *Acta Neuropathologica, 129*(5), 639–652. https://doi.org/10.1007/s00401-015-1417-0.

12. Hawthorne, G. H., Bernuci, M. P., Bortolanza, M., Tumas, V., Issy, A. C., & Del-Bel, E. (2016). Nanomedicine to overcome current Parkinson's treatment liabilities: A systematic review. *Neurotoxicity Research, 30*(4), 715–729. https://doi.org/10.1007/s12640-016-9663-z.

13. Kadry, H., Noorani, B., & Cucullo, L. (2020). A blood-brain barrier overview on structure, function, impairment, and biomarkers of integrity. *Fluids and Barriers of the CNS, 17*(1), 69. https://doi.org/10.1186/s12987-020-00230-3.

14. Knox, E. G., Aburto, M. R., Clarke, G., Cryan, J. F., & O'Driscoll, C. M. (2022). The blood-brain barrier in aging and neurodegeneration. *Molecular Psychiatry*, *27*(6), 2659–2673. https://doi.org/10.1038/s41380-022-01511-z.

15. Li, Y., et al. (2018). "Cell-addictive" dual-target traceable nanodrug for Parkinson's disease treatment via flotillin's pathway. *Theragnostic*, *8*(19), 5469–5481. https://doi.org/10.7150/thno.28295.

16. Liang, R., et al. (2022). Targeting interleukin-13 receptor α2 (IL-13Rα2) for glioblastoma therapy with surface functionalized nanocarriers. *Drug Delivery*, *29*(1), 1620–1630. https://doi.org/10.1080/10717544.2022.2075986.

17. Mittal, K. R., Pharasi, N., Sarna, B., Singh, M., Rachana, Haider, S., Singh, S. K., Dua, K., Jha, S. K., Dey, A., Ojha, S., Mani, S., & Jha, N. K. (2022). Nanotechnology-based drug delivery for the treatment of CNS disorders. *Translational Neuroscience*, *13*(1), 527–546. https://doi.org/10.1515/tnsci-2022-0258.

18. Naharros-Molinero, A., Caballo-González, M. Á., de la Mata, F. J., & García-Gallego, S. (2022). Direct and reverse Pluronic micelles: Design and characterization of promising drug delivery nano systems. *Pharmaceutics*, *14*(12), 2628. https://doi.org/10.3390/pharmaceutics14122628.

19. Pandian, S. R. K., et al. (2022). Liposomes: An emerging carrier for targeting Alzheimer's and Parkinson's diseases. *Heliyon*, *8*(6), e09575. https://doi.org/10.1016/j.heliyon.2022.e09575.

20. Pardridge, W. M. (2006). Molecular Trojan horses for blood-brain barrier drug delivery. *Discovery Medicine*, *6*(34), 139–143.

21. Pawar, B., Vasdev, N., Gupta, T., Mhatre, M., More, A., Anup, N., & Tekade, R. K. (2022). Current update on transcellular brain drug delivery. *Pharmaceutics*, *14*(12), 2719. https://doi.org/10.3390/pharmaceutics14122719.

22. Poudel, P., & Park, S. (2022). Recent advances in the treatment of Alzheimer's disease using nanoparticle-based drug delivery systems. *Pharmaceutics*, *14*(4), 835. https://doi.org/10.3390/pharmaceutics14040835.

23. Rahamathulla, M., et al. (2021). Carbon nanotubes: Current perspectives on diverse applications in targeted drug delivery and therapies. *Materials*, *14*(21), 6707. https://doi.org/10.3390/ma14216707.

24. Schinkel, A. H. (1999). P-Glycoprotein, a gatekeeper in the blood-brain barrier. *Advanced Drug Delivery Reviews*, *36*(2, 3), 179–194. https://doi.org/10.1016/s0169-409x(98)00085-4.

25. Seo, M. W., & Park, T. E. (2021). Recent advances with liposomes as drug carriers for treatment of neurodegenerative diseases. *Biomedical Engineering Letters*, *11*(3), 211–216. https://doi.org/10.1007/s13534-021-00198-5.

26. Soares, S., et al. (2018). Nanomedicine: Principles, properties, and regulatory issues. *Frontiers in Chemistry*, *6*, 360. https://doi.org/10.3389/fchem.2018.00360.

27. Soni, S., Ruhela, R. K., & Medhi, B. (2016). Nanomedicine in central nervous system (CNS) disorders: A present and future prospective. *Advanced Pharmaceutical Bulletin*, *6*(3), 319–335. https://doi.org/10.15171/apb.2016.044.

28. Su, Y., et al. (2021). PLGA-based biodegradable microspheres in drug delivery: Recent advances in research and application. *Drug Delivery*, *28*(1), 1397–1418. https://doi.org/10.1080/10717544.2021.1938756.

29. Thakur, K. T., Albanese, E., Giannakopoulos, P., Jette, N., Linde, M., Prince, M. J., Steiner, T. J., & Dua, T. (2016). Neurological disorders. In V. Patel, D. Chisholm, T. Dua, R. Laxminarayan, & M. E. Medina-Mora (Eds.), *Mental, Neurological, and Substance Use Disorders: Disease Control Priorities, Third Edition (Volume 4)* (Chapter 5). The International Bank for Reconstruction and Development/The World Bank. PMID: 27227247.

30. Thau, L., Reddy, V., & Singh, P. (2022). Anatomy, central nervous system. In *StatPearls* [Internet]. StatPearls Publishing. https://www.statpearls.com (accessed on 8 May 2025).

31. Trebesova, H., et al. (2022). The anti-aggregative peptide KLVFF mimics Aβ1-40 in the modulation of nicotinic receptors: Implications for peptide-based therapy. *Biomedicines, 10*(9), 2231. https://doi.org/10.3390/biomedicines10092231.

32. Upadhyay, R. K. (2014). Drug delivery systems, CNS protection, and the blood-brain barrier. *Biomedical Research International, 2014*, 869269. https://doi.org/10.1155/2014/869269.

33. Xiang, C., et al. (2020). Biomimetic carbon nanotubes for neurological disease therapeutics as inherent medication. *Acta Pharmaceutica Sinica B, 10*(2), 239–248. https://doi.org/10.1016/j.apsb.2019.11.003.

34. Yan, J., et al. (2023). The recent applications of PLGA-based nanostructures for ischemic stroke. *Pharmaceutics, 15*(9), 2322. https://doi.org/10.3390/pharmaceutics15092322.

35. Zhang, W., et al. (2021). Development of polymeric nanoparticles for blood-brain barrier transfer—Strategies and challenges. *Advanced Science, 8*(10), 2003937. https://doi.org/10.1002/advs.202003937.

36. Zhang, W., Liu, Q. Y., Haqqani, A. S., Leclerc, S., Liu, Z., Fauteux, F., Baumann, E., Delaney, C. E., Ly, D., Star, A. T., Brunette, E., Sodja, C., Hewitt, M., Sandhu, J. K., Stanimirovic, D. B. (2020). Differential expression of receptors mediating receptor-mediated transcytosis (RMT) in brain micro vessels, brain parenchyma, and peripheral tissues of the mouse and the human. *Fluids and Barriers of the CNS, 17*(1), 47. https://doi.org/10.1186/s12987-020-00209-0.

37. Zhao, Y., et al. (2023). Recent advances in drug delivery systems for targeting brain tumors. *Drug Delivery, 30*(1), 1–18. https://doi.org/10.1080/10717544.2022.2154409.

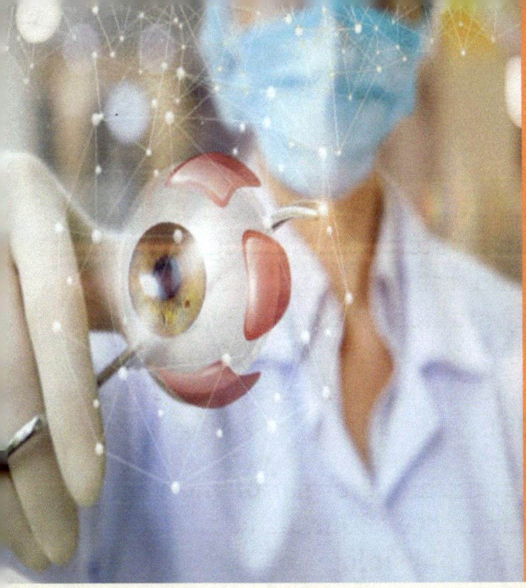

Chapter 6

NANOMEDICINE IN OPHTHALMOLOGY

Contents

Chanchal [1] and Ramendra Pati Pandey [1,*]

[1]School of Health Sciences and Technology (SoHST), University of Petroleum and Energy Studies (UPES), Dehradun, Uttarakhand, India

*Corresponding author.

Abstract

Ophthalmology could be greatly advanced by nanomedicine, which provides regulated and targeted drug delivery for a range of eye conditions. This chapter examines how nanotechnology can be used to treat eye diseases such diabetic retinopathy, glaucoma, and ocular cancer. It emphasizes how liposomes, dendrimers, and nanoparticles can improve therapeutic bioavailability and accuracy, reduce adverse effects, and increase patient compliance. The chapter also addresses the difficulties and opportunities that lie ahead in incorporating nanomedicine into standard ocular treatments, opening the door for novel, patient-focused treatments.

6.1. Introduction

Nanomedicines, a subfield of nanotechnology known as significantly improves the effectiveness of treatments for a number of illnesses, including eye ailments (Schnichels, Oellerich, and Kruse, 2020; Xie, Zhang, and Wu, 2023). Early on, the idea that small nanorobots and similar devices may be created, built, and inserted into the human body to carry out molecular-level cellular repairs gave rise to the concept of nanomedicine (Freitas, 2005). The goal of nanomedicine is to use designed nanostructures and nanodevices that work entirely in tandem at the single-cell level to monitor, regulate, construct, repair, protect, and enhance human biological mechanisms at the level of molecules in order to ultimately produce medical benefits (Morrow, Graham, and Ford, 2007). To create tiny tubes, spheres, wires, and films for particular purposes, including producing electricity or delivering medications throughout the body, each of the atoms and molecules can be manipulated. The use of nanoscale technology in medicine will significantly change how we approach illness prevention, diagnosis, and treatment (Pison, Poirier, and Ploquin, 2006). Since nanoparticles are more readily taken up by cells as instead of micromolecules, they may be employed as successful delivery and transportation vehicles. Medications can be embedded into the particle matrix or attached to the surface of the particles for medicinal purposes. The outcome of a medicine entering the biological environment must be regulated by a medication targeting mechanism. For the transport of drugs and genes, nanosystems exhibiting diverse compositions and biological properties have been thoroughly studied (Brannon-Peppas and Blanchette, 2004; Ma et al., 2019; Schätzlein, 2006; Stylios, McGetrick, and Stewart, 2005; Yokoyama, 2005).

A complicated and unique organ of the visual senses is the human eye (Bourlais et al., 1998). The anatomy and physiology of the eye are distinct. The two main parts of the eye's anatomy are the anterior and posterior segments. The eye's anterior portion makes up around a third of the total area, with the posterior portion taking up the remaining fraction. Many disorders that might impair vision affect both the anterior and posterior portions of the eye. Glaucoma, cataracts, anterior uveitis, and allergic conjunctivitis are among the conditions that affect the anterior segment. Diabetic retinopathy and age-related macular degeneration (AMD) are the two most common conditions harming the back of the eye (Barar et al., 2009; Gulsen and Chauhan, 2004). The stability of the cells and tissues in the anterior and posterior portion of the eye, where the particular limitations of the ocular tissues membranes and barriers regulate the movement of solutes to preserve the equilibrium of the eyes by flawless roles of biological barriers in the eyes, is largely responsible for the flawless functionality of the visual cells (Willoughby et al., 2010).

As a general rule in ocular pharmacotherapy, developed drug delivery systems (DDS) and equipment are frequently required for the treatment of ophthalmic diseases. Ideally, these devices will allow for the long-term, programmed release of drugs into the eye's anterior or posterior portions, increasing patient adherence to the treatment plan and, ultimately, the therapy's success (Fan et al., 2024).

Numerous therapeutic substances can be encapsulated in nanomedicines. Drug molecules are protected from degradation by their encapsulation in nanomedicine, which also improves their targeting capabilities through surface modification (Li et al., 2024; Nguyen, Luo, and Lai, 2020; Tan et al., 2018).

In the field of ophthalmology, a lot of work has been done to increase the retention and effective penetration of medications administered topically to the anterior portion of the eye. Chitosan (CH), hydroxypropyl methylcellulose (HPMC), gellan, gelatin, hyaluronic acid (HA), and carboxymethylcellulose are commonly used as mucoadhesive agents in the formulation of nanomedicines to prolong the retention time on the ocular surface due to the movement of flashing and the spontaneous generation of tears. They may also exhibit ophthalmic clearance limit (Gómez-Ballesteros et al., 2019; Tang et al., 2022; Tighsazzadeh and Boateng, 2024).

6.2. Compositions of Ocular Nanomedicine

The family of NMs, with their varied compositions and architectures, has enhanced a variety of nanomedical applications. In ocular nanomedicine, the most pertinent formulations consist of synthetic organic NMs (such as dendrimers, polyester, polymeric micelles, lipid-based nanoparticles, and natural biopolymers), inorganic NMs (such as metal [oxide] nanoparticles, QDs, carbonous and silica nanoparticles [SiNPs]), and biological components of purified biomolecules (such as exosomes) (Zhan et al., 2018). Highlights several ocular nanomedicines with distinctive structures, compositions, and qualities based on current representative research.

6.2.1. Lipid-Based Nanoparticles

Typical liposomes, solid lipid nanoparticles (SLNs), and nanostructured lipid carriers (NLCs) can all be used to create lipid-based nanoparticles that can be used as colloidal systems. Liposomes can encapsulate hydrophilic and/or lipophilic biopharmaceuticals since they are non-covalent aggregates made up of one or more phospholipid bilayer membranes (Chang et al., 2020). Liposomes have been extensively developed for topical instillation in the anterior eye segment. As a result, cationic liposomes create ionic bonds with the cornea, which increase drug absorption in the cornea by extending the duration of drug residence and lowering toxicity and antigenicity (Kim et al., 2020). However, because of the intricate ocular barriers, medication transport into the posterior eye segment—particularly the retina—remains difficult. Light-activated liposomes have been developed with time- and site-specific medication delivery into intraocular tissues to enhance cellular localization and retinal distribution (Kari et al., 2020; Paek et al., 2019). Furthermore, by targeting certain signals (such as the disease driver shared by various retinal illnesses) or by designing with a particular antibody to target the pathophysiological niche of diseased tissues, liposomal nanoparticles may provide targeted protection against ocular disorders (Vighi et al., 2018; Wong et al., 2022). Fascinatingly, numerous clinical investigations have confirmed that biocompatible liposomes for various drug delivery can effectively treat a number of eye conditions, such as retinoblastoma, metastatic malignant uveal melanoma (UM), and glaucoma (Sun and Hu, 2021). Important substitutes for liposomes are lipid nanoparticles, particularly SLNs and NLCs, which have a significant advantage over liposomes in terms of easy scale-up, less drug leakage, and cost-effective manufacture. Because SLNs are made of physiological and biocompatible solid lipids including triglycerides, steroids, and fatty acids, they are superior to liquid formulations because they do not contain organic solvents (Apaolaza et al., 2016). However, following SLN delivery via parenteral and topical administration, reports have indicated a short-term release window (3 hours to 2 weeks) and insufficient therapeutic concentrations of substrates in ocular tissues, including the retina, vitreous body, and tear film/cornea interface membrane (Liu et al., 2020; Morita et al., 2021). Both NLCs and SLNs have demonstrated the ability to carry small molecules into different ocular tissues thus far; however, more research is required to determine whether SLNs can deliver peptide- and protein-based biomacromolecules into ocular tissues (Zhan et al., 2018).

6.2.2. Polymeric Micelles

Block copolymers with amphiphilic components make up polymeric micelles (10–100 nm), which typically allow for self-assembly in aqueous environments to produce ordered supramolecular core–shell structures (Mandal et al., 2017). Polymeric micelles, particularly those made using poly(lactide), acrylic acid, and vinylpyrrolidone, have been widely employed as nanocarriers to enhance treatment results for various eye conditions in recent years (Schnichels et al., 2021). The ability of polymeric micelles to stabilize and solubilize hydrophobic substances is said to improve medication penetration by extending retention on the ocular surface (Begines et al., 2020). Additional benefits for polymeric nanoparticles used in ophthalmology include easy surface modification and tailored distribution to increase drug absorption (Weng et al., 2018). To create a customized DSPE-PEG2000-cRGD nanomicelle for encapsulating flurbiprofen, for example, 1,2-distearoyl-*sn*-glycero-3-phosphoethanolamine-*N*-[maleimide (polyethylene glycol)-2000] (DSPE-PEG2000-MAL) was made responsive with a cyclic peptide ligand (GRGDSPKC) (cRGD). When cRGD is combined with the corneal integrin receptors, the produced nanomicelle might precisely target the cornea, promoting strong and quick mucosal adhesion, excellent penetration through the cornea, and nanomicelle maintenance on the ocular surface (Qin et al., 2020). Before self-assembled polymeric micelles are widely used in ophthalmology, however, significant efforts should be made to overcome their limitations, which include limited entrapment of macromolecule agents, inadequate utilization in gene delivery, and inappropriate upscaling techniques.

6.2.3. Dendrimers

Dendrimers having branching and multilayer topologies that resemble trees, as opposed to linear polymers, can be classified into multiple generations according to the size and quantity of branches and functional gatherings at the terminal (Heredero-Bermejo et al., 2020). Throughout dendrimer production, these adaptable dendrimer topologies offer greater control over molecular weight, particular size, stability, distribution range, dispersion, ability to dissolve, and bioactivity. It is interesting to note that dendrimers with multivalent properties can carry larger payloads of imaging agents, biocompatible medications, and tiny biological molecules (Soiberman et al., 2017). The most popular and commercially available systems for ocular uses at the moment are dendrimers derived from poly(amidoamine) (PAMAM), which provide improved drug absorption, acceptability, and biological effect while also reducing drug removal from the human system after injection under the eye's conjunctiva (Sharma et al., 2020). In inflammatory areas, dendrimer-driven carriers also show strong inherent inflammation reducing and oxidation preventing properties. These vehicles may be able to efficiently transport treatment-based materials to the inflammatory ocular tissue for better healing results (Than et al., 2018). However, the development of dendrimers from laboratory to clinical settings is severely hampered by a number of fundamental drawbacks, including toxicological concerns, complicated multistep synthesis, insufficient assessments of *in vivo* quality assurance and meticulous planning costs.

6.2.4. Natural Polymers

Cell-induced protein breakdown, biological response, minimal or virtually no harmful effects, and increased membrane's selective transport ability are characteristics of naturally occurring polymers (Van Hoorick et al., 2020). Gelatin, CH, and its byproducts, such as HA, are the primary sources of natural biopolymer-based nanomedicines used to treat ophthalmic ailments. Among these, gelatin-based hydrogels are frequently utilized to promote the regeneration of ocular tissue because they closely mimic the extracellular matrix found in the skin naturally (Li et al., 2018).

The physical, environmentally degradable, and biological characteristics of the created cross-linkable gelatin can be easily altered by various technologies. For example, thiolated and acrylated gelatin with adjustable mechanical properties was used to create an injectable, photo-curable gelatin system. UV light did not appear to have any detrimental effects on the tissues of the eyes, and the developed system may be utilized as a framework that supports cells to help heal focal corneal lesions. By altering the light intensity, the proportion of acrylate to thiol groups, and the solid content, the mechanical properties of the produced hydrogels (0.3–22 kPa of the shear modulus after curing) could be easily changed. Furthermore, by changing the solid composition, the biodegradation times could be adjusted (Chun et al., 2021). Furthermore, a current study found that an injectable gelatin-tyramine hydrogel with positive charge adjustment and cross-linking capabilities was particularly successful in protecting and delivering siRNA. In a rabbit model, the carriers dramatically decreased subconjunctival scarring following filtration surgery for glaucoma without causing cell toxicity. A new delivery method on the basis of a gelatin hydrogel that can be charged exhibits excellent translational potential for epigenetic silencing therapy and is generally very scalable and easy to build (Chen et al., 2020).

There have been few passively targeted nanocarriers that are used for eye related therapeutic applications, despite the fact that a range of biodegradable organic polymers have been effectively employed in numerous preclinical investigations. Furthermore, the chemical synthesis, exact purity, and composition/structure identification of natural polymers, like ocular nanocarriers, continue to be difficult, resulting in batch-to-batch variability (Zhan et al., 2018).

6.2.5. Exosome-Based Nanomaterials (NMs)

Several common nanocarriers, including the previously mentioned dendrimers and inorganic nanoparticles, have made significant progress in creating viable and plentiful methods for a range of ocular applications; nevertheless, these artificially manufactured exogenous nanosystems may appear heterogeneous in different living organisms, potentially causing strong immunogenicity and toxicity (Zhang et al., 2018). Exosomes, on the other hand, are naturally endowed with a little toxicity, low possibility of immunological rejection, and enhanced target-homing selectivity, as they are many endogenous cell-derived nanovesicles (Mead and Tomarev, 2017). Mesenchymal stem cells (MSCs) have been found to produce a variety of exosome types, including adipose, bone marrow, and umbilical MSCs. Crucially, they have been shown to have significant beneficial impacts on the Ocular tissue healing, both anatomically and functionally, including the cornea, retina, and optic nerve. These effects are closely linked to a variety of mechanisms, such as immunomodulation, tissue regeneration, and the control of angiogenesis and inflammatory pathways (Deng et al., 2021; Samaeekia et al., 2018; Senturk et al., 2016). Rapid excretion from the body is still a major disadvantage, though. It has not been well investigated what happens to nanovesicles that are applied as eye drops or by intravitreal or subconjunctival channels, although it is possible that in some circumstances, a comparable quick exosome clearance could also take place.

Another issue that needs to be addressed is the production of vesicles with consistent high purity and quality, which is crucial for a sustained exosome-based delivery system on a large scale. However, given the aforementioned overwhelming advantages, exosome-based nanosystems offer special benefits for the logical development of next-generation nanomedicine, enabling research in the multidisciplinary fields of nanomedicine and ophthalmology throughout the coming decades.

6.3. Core Physicochemical Characteristics of Eye-Focused Nanomedicine

Due to the unmatched viability and excellence of nanotechnologies, the ophthalmologic sector has demonstrated a variety of nanoplatforms with a wide range of compositions and nanostructures to date. Determining how the basic physicochemical characteristics and associated biological consequences of eye-focused nanomedicine direct relationships with the surroundings is a recurring issue in theranostics in eye-related illnesses. Ocular nanomedicine's distinct basic physicochemical characteristics, primarily size, hydrophilia and/or hydrophobia, charge at the surface, and biodegradability, may have a substantial impact on its bioavailability, penetration, biodistribution, and elimination in targeted ocular cells/tissues. These properties must be investigated to attain optimal utilization (Zhan et al., 2018).

6.3.1. Hydrophilia and/or Hydrophobia

When nano-structured materials interact with the biological interface of several eye structures (cornea, sclera, and choroid), their intrinsic hydrophilic, lipophilic, or amphiphilic qualities have a significant impact on permeability, endocytosis, and diffusion. Enhanced hydrophilicity of the nanoparticle surface in the tear film/cornea biological interface membrane may enhance medication bioavailability at the ocular surface following injection (Morita et al., 2021). However, because of their long-term display of bioactive sequences and their capacity to stay at the place of interest for longer periods of time, amphiphilic nanocarriers—like peptide amphiphile nanofibers—have been found to be particularly advantageous for corneal administration (Wang et al., 2020). The combination of the choroid and Bruch's membrane provides a more difficult barrier for lipophilic nano-structured materials than for hydrophilic ones, as evidenced by the striking trend of reduced permeation due to increasing nanoparticle hydrophobicity in sclera–choroid–retinal pigmented epithelium (RPE) barriers compared to the relatively hydrophilic sclera alone (Mahaling et al., 2018). Amphiphilic core-shell-based nanocarriers, which feature a hydrophilic shell (like PEG) to give good water dispersity and a hydrophobic core (like polycaprolactone [PCL]) to encapsulate hydrophobic pharmaceuticals, have been proposed as a non-invasive way to transport drugs into intraocular tissues or cells. When applied topically, these techniques show great promise for treating posterior segment ocular disorders (Ogunjimi et al., 2017). Furthermore, by facilitating cellular membrane wrapping processes, the hydrophilic nature and/or hydrophobic nature of NMs is believed to be a crucial element influencing cellular internalization. The hydrophobic characteristic of nano-sized particles is the fundamental basis for biological interactions with cells; increased endocytosis and substrate combination are made possible by nanosystems that contain more hydrophobic substances as opposed to those found in cellular membranes. On the other hand, retinal cells can absorb NMs with hydrophilic surfaces the best (Tavakoli et al., 2020). Therefore, before being used, NMs with hydrophilic, lipophilic, or amphiphilic qualities must be carefully evaluated under particular circumstances for ocular distribution (Zhan et al., 2018).

6.3.2. Charge at the Surface

Another factor that affects phagocytosis, penetration, and biodistribution in ophthalmology is the surface charge of nanomedicines (Chaw et al., 2021). The influence of electrostatic characteristics on "nano-bio" interactions have been the focus of research. When positively charged nano-sized particles interact with negatively charged elements of membranes or surfaces between cells, they may enhance particle phagocytosis. This suggests that, in contrast to their negatively charged counterparts, positively charged nanoparticles may optimize cellular internalization (Liu et al., 2016). It is intriguing to observe that the possibility of targeted delivery even in the absence of ligands that are particularly targeted is demonstrated by the occurrence of cellular absorption and biological connections in reaction to the charge of particles. For instance, a nonbiodegradable cationic polymer that can pass through the cornea and into the retina thanks to static electricity-based contact with the retina has been designed to successfully deliver medicinal antisense oligonucleotides (ASO) or plasmid DNA (Lin et al., 2019). Additionally, through electrostatic interactions with ocular tissues, surface charges can affect the biodistribution of nanoparticles *in vivo*. Cationic nanoparticles, like triblock copolymeric micelles and chitosan/peptide-decorated polymeric, can interact electrically with the cornea and conjunctiva (which have a negatively charged mucin layer) in the anterior eye segment. This prolongs drug retention and increases the permeability of nanoformulations (Li et al., 2015; Schnichels et al., 2021). Conversely, negatively charged nanoparticles are said to prevent adherence to healthy or normal ocular cells or surfaces, extending the period that tears are retained (Han et al., 2020). A net negative charge exists in the vitreous, whereas the retinal cells' cellular membranes in the posterior eye segments are made of negatively charged phospholipids. As opposed to anionic particles frequently diffuse into the vitreous body, positively charged nano-sized particles are thought to attract negatively charged elements of the vitreous and stay confined until reaching targeted areas by slowing both diffusion and convection motion, taking into account electrostatic interactions (Jung et al., 2018). When using charged NMs in the ophthalmologic field, it is important to keep in mind that the electrostatic explanation might not be applicable to all types of NMs due to other factors like durability or introduced ligands that could disrupt or dynamically change the behavior of electrostatics (Zhan et al., 2018).

6.3.3. Size

Ocular nanomedicine usually spans at least one dimension, from 1 to 1000 nm. Corresponding nanomedicines for the eyes with comparable chemical makeups exhibit unique chemical/physical characteristics and biological consequences when compared to large-scale particulate systems (Robinson et al., 2011). The enhanced cellular absorption of nanoparticles is a clear advantage over their bigger counterparts. Mammalian cells typically have a diameter of a few micrometers in nature, and their organelles seem to be much smaller in the nanometer scale. Smaller particles are more readily absorbed by cells than larger ones, and Internalization of nanoparticles is a straightforward size-dependent process (Patel et al., 2019). Consequently, it is hypothesized that nanoparticles are more able to find themselves into particular cells and organelles than micron-sized systems. After being administered intraocularly, tiny particles enter particular cells or tissues by overcoming eye physiological barriers. Two weeks after a single intravitreal delivery, significantly more Nanoscale spheres with fluorescent markings were found in the vitreous than larger-scaled microspheres; only nanospheres were found at week four after management, indicating the critical role that size of biomaterials plays in better intraocular delivery (Robinson et al., 2011). While nanoparticles of 50 nm might pass through retinal barriers and gather in the retina, nano-sized particles between 100 and 200 nm in diameter were uniformly dispersed in the vitreous when taking nanoparticle biodistribution into account (Patel et al., 2019). Furthermore, in order to achieve long-term therapeutic effects, the rate constant of the *in vivo* circulating half-life has drawn a lot of attention, which may also have an impact on the size of the biomaterial (Taghe et al., 2020). While larger particles (ideally >100 nm) may escape quick clearance and allow for prolonged circulation inside ocular tissues, smaller nanoparticles are more likely through the lymphatic system, choroidal blood flow, or general circulation following systemic or topical injection (Apaolaza et al., 2016). By extending their exposure and residence time in surrounding surroundings, these phenomena demonstrate that biomaterials with comparatively large sizes are more advantageous for long-lasting release as an ocular delivery method (Hackett et al., 2020). Generally speaking, one crucial factor influencing the internalization, penetration, biological distribution, and removal of ocular biomaterials is their size.

6.3.4. Biodegradability

Because of their beneficial impacts on extending Holding and releasing cargo and reducing cell toxicity in ocular cells and tissues, many degradable nanoparticles have recently improved ocular medication delivery. The rate at which carriers degrade in the biological environment has a significant impact on the therapeutic window and bioavailability of the cargo delivered from biodegradable ocular nanomedicine, and the rate at which nanomedicine degrades is largely influenced by its molecular weight, composition, and mode of administration (Bochot and Fattal, 2012; Valencia et al., 2011). Low molecular weight NMs, for example, often degrade quickly; instability tends to disintegrate or agglomerate, which may result in burst cargo release and reduced therapeutic results. High molecular weight biomaterials, on the other hand, will degrade slowly *in vivo*, increasing the possibility of ocular tissue buildup. Therefore, to achieve greater drug availability without cytotoxicity, a controlled rate of degradation for ocular nanomedicine in regions of interest is still essential. Using rare-earth nanoparticles that are extremely tiny and have higher NIR-II luminescence, Li et al. created microenvironment-triggered degradable hydrogels that can release drugs in response to heat energy and glutathione in the tissues surrounding the tumor. The hydrogel composites' physiological degradability helps to reduce long-term biological toxicity and promote a photothermal chemotherapeutic action (Li et al., 2020). On the other hand, in gene-based treatments for repetitive gene transfection, the biodegradability of nanomedicine is still a crucial factor (Li et al., 2020). In order for nanocarriers to successfully unfold their gene payloads, such as pDNA and siRNA, via degradation, they must first leave intracellular compartments like endosomes and lysosomes after cell absorption (Islam et al., 2018). Severe molecular weight and non-degradable bonding nanocarriers can significantly accumulate in healthy cells, impairing normal cell transport and metabolism and ultimately leading to severe cytotoxicity, particularly after repeated injection (Zhou et al., 2017). Because they efficiently unpack the loaded therapeutic genes, decrease buildup, and lessen harmful effects on specific cells, nanocarriers with biodegradable characteristics therefore aid gene delivery procedures. Given their significant impact on biocompatibility and biosafety, the biodegradability of NMs is currently the most important characteristic that affects the clinical application of matching final biomedical products. The creation of biodegradable ocular nanoparticles in clinical trials is still extremely difficult, even when they show good biodegradability and biocompatibility (Zhan et al., 2018).

To sum up, a growing understanding of how different aspects impact the "nano-bio" interaction has led to substantial advancements in ocular nanomedicine. Enhancing endocytosis, penetration, cargo release, biodistribution, and removal in ocular settings is made possible by this information. When it comes to boosting cellular absorption and entry into target cells and tissues across ocular physiological barriers, one of the most important elements is the size of ocular nanomedicines. *In vivo*, surface charge is crucial because it affects the distribution of nanoparticles by electrostatically interacting with particular ocular tissues. Furthermore, transport and passage through the many biological interfaces within eye structures can be significantly impacted by hydrophilicity or hydrophobicity, whereas biodegradability is necessary for biosafety, regulated cargo release, and preservation in target ocular cells. Therefore, it is crucial to improve and modify these characteristics to improve therapeutic results in upcoming ocular nanomedicine applications.

6.4. Nanotechnology-Based Drug Delivery System (DDS)

Drug bioavailability, drug targeting, and the uptake of poorly soluble medications can all be enhanced by the use of nanoparticles in targeted drug delivery at the site of disease (Kipp, 2004; Ould-Ouali et al., 2005).

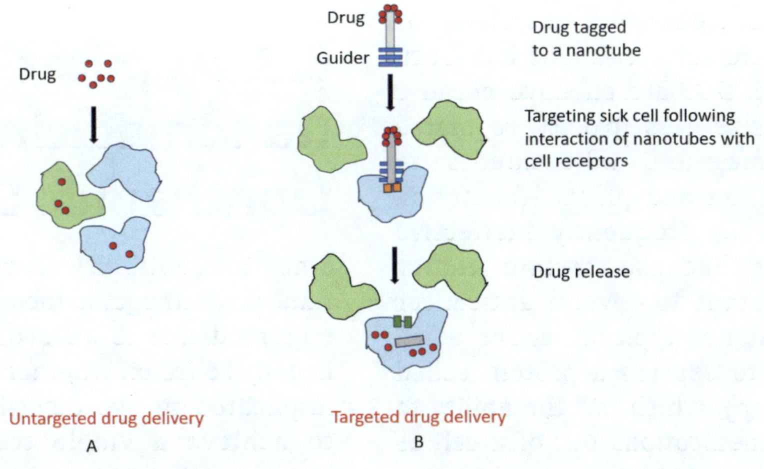

Figure 6.1. Comparison of targeted versus untargeted drug delivery. Nanomaterials (NMs) such as PLA and PLGA nanoparticles encapsulate dexamethasone for effective intracellular anti-inflammatory and anti-proliferative action.

Figure 6.1 depicts a schematic comparison of targeted and untargeted medication delivery systems. NMs have been successfully used in the formulation of several anti-cancer medications, such as doxorubicin (Yoo et al., 2000), 5-fluorouracil (Bhadra et al., 2003), dexamethasone (Panyam and Labhasetwar, 2004), and paclitaxel (Fonseca, Simoes, and Gaspar, 2002; Koziara et al., 2006).

Nanoparticles based on polylactic acid (PLA), and poly(lactic-co-glycolic acid) (PLGA) have been developed to encapsulate the glucocorticoid dexamethasone, which acts intracellularly. One chemotherapy drug with anti-inflammatory and anti-proliferative properties is dexamethasone. Following the drug's binding to the cytoplasmic receptors, the drug-receptor complex is carried to the nucleus, where it causes the production of specific genes that regulate cell division (Panyam and Labhasetwar, 2004). Vascular smooth muscle cell growth was totally suppressed by these drug-loaded nanoparticle formulations that release larger dosages of the medication over an extended period of time (Suri et al., 2007).

The application of colloidal drug delivery methods, such as liposomes, micelles, or nanoparticles, in cancer treatment has been thoroughly studied. DDS are effective because of their compact size, less toxicity, regulated drug release time, and adjustments to biological distribution and pharmacokinetics. Chemotherapy is too frequently ineffective in curing cancer because certain tumor cells become resistant to several anticancer medications. Resistance typically arises when cancer cells start to express a protein called p-glycoprotein (P-gp), which has the ability to pump anticancer medications out of a cell as fast as they pass through the outer membrane of the cell. According to recent studies, anticancer medications may be delivered into cells using nanoparticles without activating the P-gp pump (Koziara et al., 2004, 2006). The effectiveness of paclitaxel-loaded nanoparticles in paclitaxel-resistant human colorectal cancers was investigated *in vivo* by the researchers. In a human colon cancer cell line (HCT-15), paclitaxel encapsulated in emulsifying wax nanoparticles was demonstrated to overcome drug resistance. Paclitaxel's insolubility issues can be resolved by conjugating the medication with albumin. The injectable nano-suspension paclitaxel coupled to biocompatible proteins, such as albumin (Abraxane), is authorized for the treatment of breast cancer.

Acute hypersensitivity reactions are caused by the solvent Cremophor-EL, which was employed in earlier paclitaxel formulations. Patients must receive paclitaxel via modest infusions over a few hours and undergo pre-medication with steroids and antihistamines to lower the likelihood of adverse responses. Paclitaxel was delivered at a larger dose in a shorter amount of time when it bound to albumin. It also eliminates toxicities connected to solvents because it is solvent-free. Abraxane's response rate in a Phase III clinical trial was roughly double that of Taxol, a medication that contains solvents (Suri et al., 2007).

6.5. Applications of Nanomedicine in Ophthalmic Diseases

Since susceptibility frequently declines with time, the pathogenic-focused approach of ocular nanomedicine is an evolutionary notion that heavily relies on whether various pathogenesis implicated in eye disorders may be targeted to achieve a viable treatment window. In many ocular diseases, the most common pathological processes have been identified and are primarily divided into the following categories: inflammatory (such as uveitis, diabetic cataracts, and dry AMD), elevated intraocular pressure (such as glaucoma), bacterial infection (such as bacterial keratitis and endophthalmitis), neovascularization (such as corneal neovascularization and wet AMD), tumors (such as retinoblastoma and UM), and refractive error (such as myopia) (Figure 6.2).

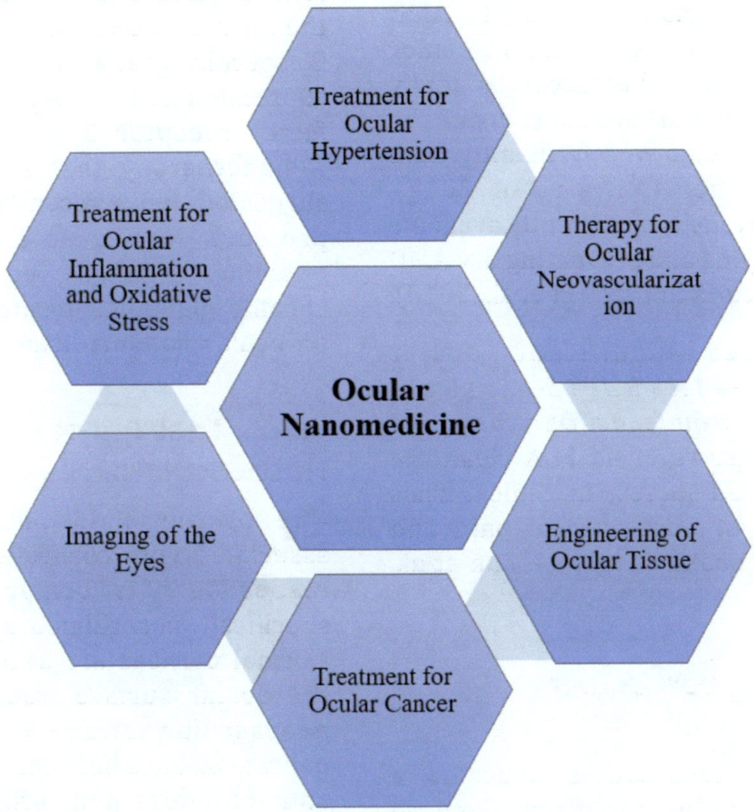

Figure 6.2. Diagrammatic representation of ophthalmic nanomedicine for various biomedical applications in ophthalmology.

6.5.1. Treatment for Ocular Inflammatory Reaction and Oxidative Damage

It is believed that the retina is a "immune-privileged" area and that human eyes are closed off from systemic circulation (Zhu et al., 2019). Therefore, by rupturing phospholipids in the cell membrane and causing an excessive release of inflammatory compounds like prostaglandins, inflammation in the eye plays a pathogenic role in a number of ocular illnesses, such as uveitis, diabetic cataracts, and dry AMD. Photophobia, opacification, discomfort, posterior capsule, vasodilatation, increased vascular permeability, and intraocular pressure are some of the common clinical signs of inflammatory ocular disease that these dangerous drugs may cause. Uveitis, for instance, is a common ocular inflammatory condition in the uvea that may be brought on by a bacterial or viral infection or an overreactive immune response brought on by particulate matter (Kamoi et al., 2021). In an experimental animal model of autoimmune uveitis, the controlled release of medications via biodegradable nanocarriers, namely PLGA-based nanoparticles, has been effectively accomplished the long-term release of medications that reduce inflammation, thereby controlling ocular inflammation without consequences (Luo et al., 2019).

Unquestionably, excessive ROS contributes to the pathogenic genesis of aberrant inflammatory responses during ocular inflammatory illnesses, particularly AMD and diabetic cataracts. AMD is the main reason for vision loss in senior people with progressive photoreceptor death, and diabetic cataract is an eye consequence in individuals with diabetes who frequently have reduced visual function (Mitra et al., 2017). However, the effectiveness of currently available medications in delaying and preventing dry AMD and diabetic cataracts is limited (Li et al., 2018).

Remarkably, three significant ocular nanomedicines—*INVELTYS* (Kala Pharmaceuticals), *bromfenac DuraSite*, and *DexaSite*—have either received FDA clearance or have demonstrated success in clinical trials for the treatment of post-surgical pain and inflammation after ocular surgery (Zhan et al., 2018).

6.5.2. Treatment for Ocular Hypertension

The injured optic nerve causes glaucoma, a form of optic neuropathy that affects about 60 million individuals globally (Stein, Khawaja, and Weizer, 2021). Elevated intraocular pressure, optic nerve ischemia, and activation linked to oxidative stress are among the pathogenic criteria that have been linked to the evolution of glaucoma (Wang et al., 2020). Decreasing the increased IOP directly provides efficient neuroprotection and is a main changeable goal for glaucoma control from a pathophysiological standpoint, even if it is not the only component linked to the development of glaucoma (Stein, Khawaja, and Weizer, 2021). The fabrication of various nanosystems, including layer-by-layer coated siRNA nano-sized particles hollow ceria nanoparticles, and lipid DNA nanoparticles, has been made possible by nanotechnology. According to reports, nanoparticles' strong intrinsic antioxidant and anti-inflammatory properties, as well as their controlled and prolonged release of anti-IOP medications or siRNA gene silencing, could provide long-term relief of glaucomatous damage without changing the form of the vesicles (Dillinger et al., 2018). By specifically attaching to Schlemm's canal cells' expression of the vascular endothelial growth factor receptor 3 (VEGFR3)/FLT4 receptor, A nanotherapy that softens cells has been suggested, more recently to lower intraocular pressure (Stack et al., 2020). Promising outcomes highlight the great potential of a chronic glaucoma treatment approach based on ocular nanomedicine.

6.5.3. Therapy for Ocular Neovascularization

One of the main pathogenic phenotypes associated with corneal and retinal disorders, respectively, is ocular neovascularization, specifically corneal neovascularization and CNV. Normal corneas are avascular, and injuries to the ocular surface frequently cause corneal neovascularization, which can upset the delicate balance between angiogenic stimulators and inhibitors and ultimately lead to vision impairment (Senturk et al., 2016). Initial CNV and altered central vision are caused by pathogenic vasculature that expand into the subretinal region after protruding through Bruch's membrane in wet AMD (Ling et al., 2021).

Clinically, one of the main treatment approaches for CNV is the monthly or biweekly intravitreal injection of big protein anti-VEGF medications, like bevacizumab (Ling et al., 2021). Furthermore, it has been possible to successfully engineer ocular nanomedicine-assisted possessing innate antiangiogenic qualities that come from a natural item. These procedures can be delivered intraocularly with minimal invasiveness via eye drops or conjunctival sac instillation, or through the focused and continuous release of siRNA-oriented intracellular therapeutic agents and anti-VEGF peptide/antibody to reduce dose intervals at medically effective concentrations (Jo et al., 2016; Senturk et al., 2016; Xin et al., 2020). All things considered, the ocular nanomedicine-assisted approach offers a different approach to effectively prevent ocular neovascularization without endangering wholesome tissues in a minimally invasive or non-invasive, while lowering the frequency of management needed to achieve curative control.

6.5.4. Engineering of Eye Tissue

If recovery after trauma, infection, or inflammation is not satisfactory, damaged cells, tissues, and organs may lose their structure and function. For instance, the death of RPE and/or photoreceptors has been regarded as a frequent etiology, and retinal degeneration is acknowledged as one of the main causes of irreversible visual impairment and even blindness globally (Schwartz et al., 2015). Therefore, to produce monolayer cells and restore the RPE-photoreceptor interface, RPE/photoreceptor-based transplantation into sick areas is required. Over the last 20 years, it has been demonstrated that engineering of eye tissue—which includes corneal, conjunctival, and retinal repair—is possible through the transplantation of implants produced from cells or tissues. They fall short, nonetheless, in terms of superior reconstruction of normal processes and particular reactions to biological signals (Dehghani et al., 2018). However, by triggering the signaling pathway through communication with the environment or acting as a sensor to track and monitor tissue healing and transplanted cell replacement, based on eye-related nanomedicine approaches could initiate and direct ocular tissue regeneration (Rizwan et al., 2017).

6.5.5. Treatment for Ocular Cancer

While UM, the most prevalent intraocular cancer in adults, usually affects the choroid, iris, and ciliary body, retinoblastoma is a harmful and rapidly growing tumor within the eye in infants and children (Everett and Copperman, 2019). The discovery of effective treatments is urgently needed due to the significantly high mortality rates of retinoblastoma and UM. Chemoreduction, chemotherapy, external beam/episcleral plaque radiation, and enucleation (eye removal) are the main medical therapies currently accessible (Liu et al., 2020). The only effective treatment for advanced retinoblastoma is enucleation; nevertheless, surgical lesions cause facial abnormalities. One of the many adverse consequences of radiation therapy is dry eye, which necessitates ongoing eye lubrication. Chemoreduction can cause serious side effects, such as transient pancytopenia, renal toxicity, and secondary malignancy, even if it addresses a number of issues with other methods (Gao et al., 2018).

6.5.6. Imaging of the Eyes

Early clinical diagnosis, treatment, and real-time monitoring of eye illnesses all depend on ocular imaging. For example, Preliminary diagnostic imaging is required to stop blindness and even mortality due to the fast growth of intraocular malignancies (Wang et al., 2020). The physiological state of ocular tissues could be ascertained by selectively using nanomedicine-based techniques that are rigorously screened in order to see the tissues of the eyes and precisely and quantitatively analyze changed levels of proteins, nucleic acids, or small molecules (Evans et al., 2014). Improved imaging techniques and improved predictive and diagnostic outcomes should be the main goals of efforts to improve theranostic NMs.

6.6. Obstacles in Clinical Nanomedicine Translation

A number of significant barriers pertaining to the design and development of nanotherapeutics make the process of transferring nanomedicine from the lab to the clinic intricate and difficult. First, the primary obstacles to bringing nanomedicine to the clinic are quality control (QC) testing for physicochemical characterization and large-scale manufacture of nanotherapeutics in compliance with good manufacturing practice (GMP) standards. Figure 6.3 depicts the essential elements of the product development process, ranging from pre-formulation (lab-scale) to commercialization (production scale) (Iqbal et al., 2024).

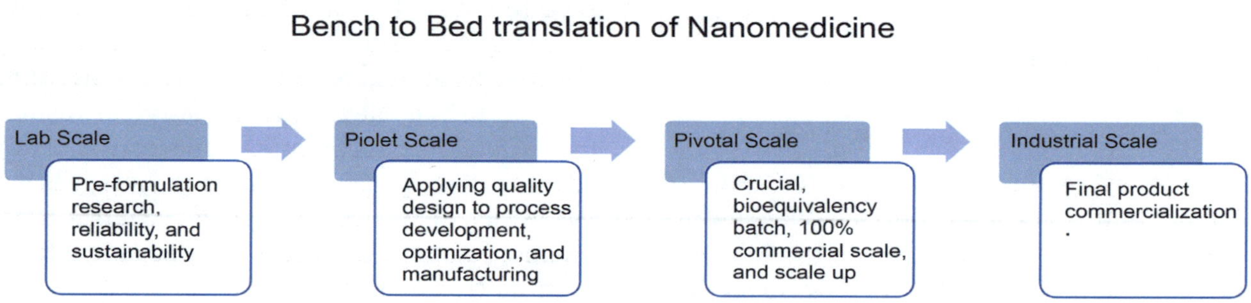

Figure 6.3. The essential elements of the procedure for developing a product, from laboratory-scale preliminary formulation to production-scale commercialization.

Second, the marketed product should meet established standards for safety, efficacy, stability, and patient acceptability. The formulation procedure must be repeatable and adhere to accepted standards. With less harmful side effects, the nanomedicine's therapeutic effectiveness is on par with or even better than that of conventional hypotensive eye drops (Kompella, Hartman, and Patil, 2021).

Thirdly, poor clinical translation results from inadequate information and comprehension of the intraocular bio-performance of nanopharmaceuticals. In contrast to extraocular or periocular nanomedicine, intraocular nanomedicine is difficult to remove from the eyes without the use of a non-invasive procedure. Before administering nanomedicine intraocularly, researchers may focus particularly on the biological effects and pharmacological reactions of the building blocks. The general physicochemical properties of nanosystems, like particle size, shape, and surface charge, are usually the focus of studies. However, little research has been done on how various intraocular conditions, such as prior intraocular surgery, repeated implantation, and vitreous liquefaction in elderly eyes, may impact the unique characteristics of nanomedicine. For instance, in vitrectomized and aphakic eyes, the movement and removal of particles following administration (Shen, Sun, and Sun, 2023).

Fourth, because the architecture of model eyes differs greatly from that of human eyes, the results of investigations using animal models may not transfer to identical results in human eyes (Lyu et al., 2021).

Fifth, large-scale industrial production, batch-to-batch stability, validation, reproducibility, and controllability of physical and chemical properties were all necessary for the real-time clinical translation of nanomedicines. Furthermore, clinical translation usually requires an optimized nanoformulation with a determined strategy, thus complex manufacturing processes might make reproducible nanomedicine production extremely challenging. Therefore, sufficient reproducibility and large-scale production with minimal batch-to-batch variations or changes must be resolved before gaining access to the real-time clinical application (Cabrera et al., 2019). Furthermore, the production of nanomedicines is often a multi-step procedure involving multiple components, which can be expensive and time-consuming (Lyu et al., 2021). Finally, there is a greater chance of severe adverse effects, such as entophthalmia or retinal detachment, due to the intrusive nature of intraocular nanomedicine administration. Standard operating procedures (SOPs) and procedural recommendations for each form of nanomedicine must be established and should be easy to follow in clinical practice, even with the current standards for intracameral and intravitreal injection (Shen, Sun, and Sun, 2023).

6.7. Future Perspectives and Innovations

The way we detect, track, and treat corneal illnesses could be completely changed by recent advancements in nanotechnology that allow for the creation and engineering of nanoparticles. It can make it unnecessary to apply the medication repeatedly in order to produce a long-lasting impact. Despite being extremely promising, there are still a lot of obstacles to be addressed. The quick clearance during systemic distribution is one of the biggest obstacles to the creation of the best therapeutic NPs (Chaurasia et al., 2015). Therefore, for the next generation of therapeutic nanoparticles, the aspects that affect physicochemical qualities, long-term stability, low toxicity, and targeted distribution should be taken into account. For the treatment of corneal diseases and vision restoration, the concept of "Theragonostics" (Sumer and Gao, 2008), in which nanoparticles administer treatment and offer disease monitoring, is highly appealing (Zarbin et al., 2010). High drug bioavailability at the anterior tissues, like the conjunctiva and cornea, can be achieved through controlled drug delivery using nanoformulations like nanomicelles, nanoparticles, liposomes, dendrimers, nanowafers, and microneedles. At the moment, all back of the eye conditions are treated with invasive procedures. Patients who receive intravitreal injections frequently may have pain, bleeding, and retinal detachment. It is difficult for ocular drug delivery experts to design a noninvasive sustained DDS for the posterior segment. Therefore, the creation of innovative noninvasive drug delivery methods that can get past ocular barriers, maintain drug release, and keep effective medication levels at the back of the eye is desperately needed (Tian et al., 2022).

6.8. Conclusion

Nanomedication delivery systems seem to have a lot of promise for removing some of the obstacles to effective cell and molecular targeting in cancer and inflammation. Additionally, there is an intriguing opportunity to help medications travel through barriers like those in the brain and to overcome issues with drug resistance in target cells. The exact characterization of molecular targets and ensuring that these molecules are expressed only in the targeted organs to avoid effects on healthy tissues continue to be challenges. Second, it is critical to comprehend what happens to the medications after they are delivered to the nucleus and other organelles of sensitive cells. Furthermore, doses may need to be recalibrated since nanosystems improve drug delivery efficiency. The future is still bright and exciting, though (Koziara et al., 2004).

KEY TERMS FROM THIS CHAPTER

- diabetic retinopathy
- glaucoma
- ocular neovascularization
- drug delivery
- nanotechnology
- ophthalmology

References

1. Apaolaza, P. S., et al. (2016). Structural recovery of the retina in a retinoschisin-deficient mouse after gene replacement therapy by solid lipid nanoparticles. *Biomaterials, 90*, 40–49.

2. Barar, J., et al. (2009). Ocular drug delivery; impact of *in vitro* cell culture models. *Journal of Ophthalmic & Vision Research, 4*(4), 238–252.

3. Begines, B., et al. (2020). Polymeric nanoparticles for drug delivery: Recent developments and future prospects. *Nanomaterials, 10*(7), 1403.

4. Bhadra, D., et al. (2003). A PEGylated dendritic nanoparticulate carrier of fluorouracil. *International Journal of Pharmaceutics, 257*(1, 2), 111–124.

5. Bochot, A., & Fattal, E. (2012). Liposomes for intravitreal drug delivery: A state of the art. *Journal of Controlled Release, 161*(2), 628–634.

6. Bourlais, C. L., et al. (1998). Ophthalmic drug delivery systems—recent advances. *Progress in Retinal and Eye Research, 17*(1), 33–58. https://doi.org/10.1016/s1350-9462(97)00002-5.

7. Brannon-Peppas, L., & Blanchette, J. O. (2004). Nanoparticle and targeted systems for cancer therapy. *Advanced Drug Delivery Reviews, 56*(11), 1649–1659. https://doi.org/10.1016/j.addr.2004.02.014.

8. Cabrera, F. J., et al. (2019). Challenges and opportunities for drug delivery to the posterior of the eye. *Drug Discovery Today, 24*(8), 1679–1684.

9. Chang, M. C., et al. (2020). Liposomal dexamethasone–moxifloxacin nanoparticle combinations with collagen/gelatin/alginate hydrogel for corneal infection treatment and wound healing. *Biomedical Materials, 15*(5), 055022.

10. Chaurasia, S. S., et al. (2015). Nanomedicine approaches for corneal diseases. *Journal of Functional Biomaterials, 6*(2), 277–298. https://doi.org/10.3390/jfb6020277.

11. Chaw, S. Y., et al. (2021). *In vivo* fate of liposomes after subconjunctival ocular delivery. *Journal of Controlled Release, 329*, 162–174.

12. Chen, X., et al. (2020). Toxicity and mechanism of mesoporous silica nanoparticles in eyes. *Nanoscale, 12*(25), 13637–13653.

13. Chun, Y. Y., et al. (2021). Positive-charge tuned gelatin hydrogel-siSPARC injectable for siRNA anti-scarring therapy in post-glaucoma filtration surgery. *Scientific Reports, 11*(1), 1470.

14. Dehghani, S., et al. (2018). 3D-Printed membrane as an alternative to amniotic membrane for ocular surface/conjunctival defect reconstruction: An *in vitro* & *in vivo* study. *Biomaterials, 174*, 95–112.

15. Deng, C. L., et al. (2021). Photoreceptor protection by mesenchymal stem cell transplantation identifies exosomal MiR-21 as a therapeutic for retinal degeneration. *Cell Death & Differentiation, 28*(3), 1041–1061.

16. Dillinger, A. E., et al. (2018). Intracameral delivery of layer-by-layer coated siRNA nanoparticles for glaucoma therapy. *Small, 14*(50), 1803239.

17. Evans, S. M., et al. (2014). Molecular probes for imaging of hypoxia in the retina. *Bioconjugate Chemistry, 25*(11), 2030–2037.

18. Everett, L., & Copperman, T. (2019). Metastatic uveal melanoma. *New England Journal of Medicine, 380*(19), 1853.

19. Fan, Z., et al. (2024). Rationalized landscape on protein-based cancer nanomedicine: Recent progress and challenges. *International Journal of Pharmaceutics: X, 7*, 100238. https://doi.org/10.1016/j.ijpx.2024.100238.

20. Fonseca, C., Simoes, S., & Gaspar, R. (2002). Paclitaxel-loaded PLGA nanoparticles: Preparation, physicochemical characterization and *in vitro* anti-tumoral activity. *Journal of Controlled Release, 83*(2), 273–286.

21. Freitas, R. A. Jr. (2005). What is nanomedicine? *Nanomedicine: Nanotechnology, Biology, and Medicine, 1*(1), 2–9. https://doi.org/10.1016/j.nano.2004.11.003.

22. Gao, R., et al. (2018). Developing nanoceria-based pH-dependent cancer-directed drug delivery system for retinoblastoma. *Advanced Functional Materials, 28*(52), 1806248.

23. Gómez-Ballesteros, M., et al. (2019). Osmo protectants in hybrid liposome/HPMC systems as potential glaucoma treatment. *Polymers, 11*(6), 929.

24. Gulsen, D., & Chauhan, A. (2004). Ophthalmic drug delivery through contact lenses. *Investigative Ophthalmology & Visual Science, 45*(7), 2342–2347. https://doi.org/10.1167/iovs.03-0959.

25. Hackett, S. F., et al. (2020). Sustained delivery of acriflavine from the suprachoroidal space provides long term suppression of choroidal neovascularization. *Biomaterials, 243*, 119935.

26. Han, H., et al. (2020). Biofilm microenvironment activated supramolecular nanoparticles for enhanced photodynamic therapy of bacterial keratitis. *Journal of Controlled Release, 327*, 676–687.

27. Heredero-Bermejo, I., et al. (2020). Ultrastructural study of *Acanthamoeba polyphaga* trophozoites and cysts treated *in vitro* with cationic carbonian dendrimers. *Pharmaceutics, 12*(6), 565.

28. Iqbal, H., et al. (2024). Nanomedicine in glaucoma treatment; Current challenges and future perspectives. *Materials Today Bio, 28*, 101229. https://doi.org/10.1016/j.mtbio.2024.101229.

29. Islam, M. A., et al. (2018). Restoration of tumor-growth suppression *in vivo* via systemic nanoparticle-mediated delivery of PTEN mRNA. *Nature Biomedical Engineering, 2*(11), 850–864.

30. Jo, D. H., et al. (2016). Nanoparticle–protein complexes mimicking corona formation in ocular environment. *Biomaterials, 109*, 23–31.

31. Jung, J. H., et al. (2018). Ocular drug delivery targeted by iontophoresis in the suprachoroidal space using a microneedle. *Journal of Controlled Release, 277*, 14–22. https://doi.org/10.1016/j.jconrel.2018.03.001.

32. Kamoi, K., et al. (2021). Horizontal transmission of HTLV-1 causing uveitis. *The Lancet Infectious Diseases, 21*(4), 578.

33. Kari, O. K., et al. (2020). Light-activated liposomes coated with hyaluronic acid as a potential drug delivery system. *Pharmaceutics, 12*(8), 763.

34. Kim, Y. C., et al. (2020). Gelling hypotonic polymer solution for extended topical drug delivery to the eye. *Nature Biomedical Engineering, 4*(11), 1053–1062.

35. Kipp, J. E. (2004). The role of solid nanoparticle technology in the parenteral delivery of poorly water-soluble drugs. *International Journal of Pharmaceutics, 284*(1, 2), 109–122.

36. Kompella, U. B., Hartman, R. R., & Patil, M. A. (2021). Extraocular, periocular, and intraocular routes for sustained drug delivery for glaucoma. *Progress in Retinal and Eye Research, 82*, 100901.

37. Koziara, J. M., et al. (2004). Paclitaxel nanoparticles for the potential treatment of brain tumors. *Journal of Controlled Release, 99*(2), 259–269.

38. Koziara, J. M., et al. (2006). *In-vivo* efficacy of novel paclitaxel nanoparticles in paclitaxel-resistant human colorectal tumors. *Journal of Controlled Release, 112*(3), 312–319.

39. Li, H., et al. (2024). Biomarker-driven molecular imaging probes in radiotherapy. *Theranostics, 14*(10), 4127–4146. https://doi.org/10.7150/thno.97768.

40. Li, J., et al. (2015). Positively charged micelles based on a triblock copolymer demonstrate enhanced corneal penetration. *International Journal of Nanomedicine, 10*, 6027–6037.

41. Li, L., et al. (2018). A broad-spectrum ROS-eliminating material for prevention of inflammation and drug-induced organ toxicity. *Advanced Science, 5*(10), 1800781.

42. Li, L., et al. (2018). Gelatin-based photocurable hydrogels for corneal wound repair. *ACS Applied Materials & Interfaces, 10*(16), 13283–13292.

43. Li, L., et al. (2020). Microenvironment-triggered degradable hydrogel for imaging diagnosis and combined treatment of intraocular choroidal melanoma. *ACS Nano, 14*(11), 15403–15416.

44. Li, T., et al. (2020). Co-delivery of brinzolamide and miRNA-124 by biodegradable nanoparticles as a strategy for glaucoma therapy. *Drug Delivery, 27*(1), 410–421.

45. Lin, S., et al. (2019). Overcoming the anatomical and physiological barriers in topical eye surface medication using a peptide-decorated polymeric micelle. *ACS Applied Materials & Interfaces, 11*(43), 39603–39612.

46. Ling, S., et al. (2021). Lentiviral delivery of co-packaged Cas9 mRNA and a Vegfa-targeting guide RNA prevents wet age-related macular degeneration in mice. *Nature Biomedical Engineering, 5*(2), 144–156.

47. Liu, C., et al. (2016). Facile noninvasive retinal gene delivery enabled by penetrating. *ACS Applied Materials & Interfaces, 8*(30), 19256–19267.

48. Liu, H., et al. (2020). Human embryonic stem cell-derived organoid retinoblastoma reveals a cancerous origin. *Proceedings of the National Academy of Sciences, 117*(52), 33628–33638.

49. Liu, S., et al. (2020). Incorporation of ion exchange functionalized-montmorillonite into solid lipid nanoparticles with low irritation enhances drug bioavailability for glaucoma treatment. *Drug Delivery, 27*(1), 652–661.

50. Luo, L., et al. (2019). Controlled release of corticosteroid with biodegradable nanoparticles for treating experimental autoimmune uveitis. *Journal of Controlled Release, 296*, 68–80.

51. Lyu, Q., et al. (2021). Smart nano-micro platforms for ophthalmological applications: The state-of-the-art and future perspectives. *Biomaterials, 270*, 120682.

52. Ma, Y., et al. (2019). Mammalian near-infrared image vision through injectable and self-powered retinal nanoantennae. *Cell, 177*(2), 243–255.e15. https://doi.org/10.1016/j.cell.2019.01.038.

53. Mahaling, B., et al. (2018). A non-invasive nanoparticle mediated delivery of triamcinolone acetonide ameliorates diabetic retinopathy in rats. *Nanoscale, 10*(35), 16485–16498.

54. Mandal, A., et al. (2017). Polymeric micelles for ocular drug delivery: From structural frameworks to recent preclinical studies. *Journal of Controlled Release, 248*, 96–116.
55. Mead, B., & Tomarev, S. T. (2017). Bone marrow-derived mesenchymal stem cells-derived exosomes promote survival of retinal ganglion cells through miRNA-dependent mechanisms. *Stem Cells Translational Medicine, 6*(4), 1273–1285.
56. Mitra, R. N., et al. (2017). Glycol chitosan engineered auto regenerative antioxidant significantly attenuates pathological damages in models of age-related macular degeneration. *ACS Nano, 11*(5), 4669–4685.
57. Morita, T., et al. (2021). Unveiling the interaction potential surface between drug-entrapped polymeric micelles clarifying the high drug nanocarrier efficiency. *Nano Letters, 21*(3), 1303–1310.
58. Morrow, K. J. Jr., Graham, R. D., & Ford, M. E. (2007). Recent advances in basic and clinical nanomedicine. *The Medical Clinics of North America, 91*(5), 805–843. https://doi.org/10.1016/j.mcna.2007.05.009.
59. Nguyen, D. D., Luo, L. J., & Lai, J. Y. (2020). Effects of shell thickness of hollow poly(lactic acid) nanoparticles on sustained drug delivery for pharmacological treatment of glaucoma. *Acta Biomaterial, 111*, 302–315.
60. Ogunjimi, A. T., et al. (2017). Hydrophilic polymeric nanoparticles prepared from Delonix galactomannan with low cytotoxicity for ocular drug delivery. *Carbohydrate Polymers, 157*, 1065–1075.
61. Ould-Ouali, L., et al. (2005). Self-assembling PEG-p(CL-co-TMC) copolymers for oral delivery of poorly water-soluble drugs: A case study with risperidone. *Journal of Controlled Release, 102*(3), 657–668.
62. Paek, J., et al. (2019). Micro physiological engineering of self-assembled and perusable microvascular beds for the production of vascularized three-dimensional human microtissues. *ACS Nano, 13*(7), 7627–7643.
63. Panyam, J., & Labhasetwar, V. (2004). Sustained cytoplasmic delivery of drugs with intracellular receptors using biodegradable nanoparticles. *Molecular Pharmaceutics, 1*(1), 77–84.
64. Patel, S., et al. (2019). Brief update on endocytosis of nanomedicines. *Advanced Drug Delivery Reviews, 144*, 90–111.
65. Pison, U., Poirier, J., & Ploquin, L. (2006). Nanomedicine for respiratory diseases. *European Journal of Pharmacology, 533*(1–3), 341–350. https://doi.org/10.1016/j.ejphar.2005.12.068.
66. Qin, C., et al. (2020). Are poly (amidoamine) dendrimers safe for ocular applications? Toxicological evaluation in ocular cells and tissues. *Journal of Ocular Pharmacology and Therapeutics, 36*(10), 715–724.
67. Rizwan, M., et al. (2017). Sequentially-crosslinked bioactive hydrogels as nano-patterned substrates with customizable stiffness and degradation for corneal tissue engineering applications. *Biomaterials, 120*, 139–154.
68. Robinson, R., et al. (2011). Nanospheres delivering the EGFR TKI AG1478 promote optic nerve regeneration: The role of size for intraocular drug delivery. *ACS Nano, 5*(6), 4392–4400.
69. Samaeekia, R., et al. (2018). Effect of human corneal mesenchymal stromal cell-derived exosomes on corneal epithelial wound healing. *Investigative Ophthalmology & Visual Science, 59*(12), 5194–5200.

70. Schätzlein, A. G. (2006). Delivering cancer stem cell therapies: A role for nanomedicines? *European Journal of Cancer, 42*(9), 1309–1315. https://doi.org/10.1016/j.ejca.2006.01.044.

71. Schnichels, S., et al. (2021). Improved treatment options for glaucoma with brimonidine-loaded lipid DNA nanoparticles. *ACS Applied Materials & Interfaces, 13*(8), 9445–9456.

72. Schnichels, S., Oellerich, T., & Kruse, F. E. (2020). Self-assembled DNA nanoparticles loaded with travoprost for glaucoma treatment. *Nanomedicine: Nanotechnology, Biology, and Medicine, 29*, 102260. https://doi.org/10.1016/j.nano.2020.102260.

73. Schwartz, S. D., et al. (2015). Human embryonic stem cell-derived retinal pigment epithelium in patients with age-related macular degeneration and Stargardt's macular dystrophy: Follow-up of two open-label phase 1/2 studies. *The Lancet, 385*(9967), 509–516.

74. Senturk, B., et al. (2016). Inhibition of VEGF mediated corneal neovascularization by anti-angiogenic peptide nanofibers. *Biomaterials, 107*, 124–132.

75. Sharma, A., et al. (2020). Dense hydroxyl polyethylene glycol dendrimer targets activated glia in multiple CNS disorders. *Science Advances, 6*(4), eaay8514. https://doi.org/10.1126/sciadv.aay8514.

76. Shen, Y., Sun, J., & Sun, X. (2023). Intraocular nano-microscale drug delivery systems for glaucoma treatment: Design strategies and recent progress. *Journal of Nanobiotechnology, 21*(1), 84.

77. Soiberman, U., et al. (2017). Subconjunctival injectable dendrimer-dexamethasone gel for the treatment of corneal inflammation. *Biomaterials, 125*, 38–53.

78. Stack, T., et al. (2020). Targeted delivery of cell softening micelles to Schlemm's canal endothelial cells for treatment of glaucoma. *Small, 16*(43), 2004205.

79. Stein, J. D., Khawaja, A. P., & Weizer, J. S. (2021). Glaucoma in adults—Screening, diagnosis, and management: A review. *JAMA, 325*(2), 164–174.

80. Stylios, G. K., McGetrick, P. D., & Stewart, R. A. (2005). Applications of nanotechnologies in medical practice. *Injury, 36*(Suppl 4), S6–S13. https://doi.org/10.1016/j.injury.2005.10.011.

81. Sumer, B., & Gao, J. (2008). Theragnostic nanomedicine for cancer. *Nanomedicine, 3*(2), 137–140.

82. Sun, K., & Hu, K. (2021). Preparation and characterization of tacrolimus-loaded SLNs *in situ* gel for ocular drug delivery for the treatment of immune conjunctivitis. *Drug Design, Development and Therapy, 15*, 141–150.

83. Suri, S. S., et al. (2007). Nanotechnology-based drug delivery systems. *Journal of Occupational Medicine and Toxicology, 2*, 16. https://doi.org/10.1186/1745-6673-2-16.

84. Taghe, S., et al. (2020). Polymeric inserts containing Eudragit® L100 nanoparticle for improved ocular delivery of azithromycin. *Biomedicines, 8*(11), 466.

85. Tan, Y. F., et al. (2018). Controlled-release nanotherapeutics: State of translation. *Journal of Controlled Release: Official Journal of the Controlled Release Society, 284*, 39–48. https://doi.org/10.1016/j.jconrel.2018.06.014.

86. Tang, Z., et al. (2022). Ocular nanomedicine. *Advanced Science (Weinheim, Baden-Wurttemberg, Germany), 9*(15), e2003699. https://doi.org/10.1002/advs.202003699.

87. Tavakoli, S., et al. (2020). Ocular barriers to retinal delivery of intravitreal liposomes: Impact of vitreoretinal interface. *Journal of Controlled Release, 328*, 952–961.

88. Than, A., et al. (2018). Self-implantable double-layered micro-drug-reservoirs for efficient and controlled ocular drug delivery. *Nature Communications, 9*(1), 4433.

89. Tian, B., et al. (2022). Ocular drug delivery: Advancements and innovations. *Pharmaceutics, 14*(9), 1931. https://doi.org/10.3390/pharmaceutics14091931.

90. Tighsazzadeh, M., & Boateng, J. (2024). Matrix hyaluronic acid and bilayer poly-hydroxyethyl methacrylate-hyaluronic acid films as potential ocular drug delivery platforms. *International Journal of Biological Macromolecules, 260*, 129496.

91. Valencia, P. M., et al. (2011). Effects of ligands with different water solubilities on self-assembly and properties of targeted nanoparticles. *Biomaterials, 32*(26), 6226–6233.

92. Van Hoorick, J., et al. (2020). Designer Descemet membranes containing PDLLA and functionalized gelatins as corneal endothelial scaffold. *Advanced Healthcare Materials, 9*(16), 2000760.

93. Vighi, E., et al. (2018). Combination of cGMP analogue and drug delivery system provides functional protection in hereditary retinal degeneration. *Proceedings of the National Academy of Sciences, 115*(13), E2997–E3006.

94. Wang, M., et al. (2020). Multifunctional nanoparticles for multimodal imaging-guided low-intensity focused ultrasound/immunosynergistic retinoblastoma therapy. *ACS Applied Materials & Interfaces, 12*(5), 5642–5657.

95. Wang, X., et al. (2020). An ocular glymphatic clearance system removes β-amyloid from the rodent eye. *Science Translational Medicine, 12*(536), eaaw3210.

96. Wang, Y., et al. (2020). A pH-responsive silica–metal–organic framework hybrid nanoparticle for the delivery of hydrophilic drugs, nucleic acids, and CRISPR-Cas9 genome-editing machineries. *Journal of Controlled Release, 324*, 194–203.

97. Weng, Y. H., et al. (2018). Nano micelle-assisted targeted ocular delivery with enhanced anti-inflammatory efficacy *in vivo*. *Advanced Science, 5*(1), 1700455.

98. Willoughby, C. E., et al. (2010). Anatomy and physiology of the human eye: Effects of mucopolysaccharidoses disease on structure and function—A review. *Clinical & Experimental Ophthalmology, 38*, 2–11.

99. Wong, C. W., et al. (2022). Liposomal drug delivery system for anti-inflammatory treatment after cataract surgery: A phase I/II clinical trial. *Drug Delivery and Translational Research*, 1–8.

100. Xie, G., Zhang, Z., & Wu, Y. (2023). Nanomaterial-based ophthalmic drug delivery. *Advanced Drug Delivery Reviews, 200*, 115004. https://doi.org/10.1016/j.addr.2023.115004.

101. Xin, G., et al. (2020). Ophthalmic drops with nanoparticles derived from a natural product for treating age-related macular degeneration. *ACS Applied Materials & Interfaces, 12*(52), 57710–57720.

102. Yokoyama, M. (2005). Drug targeting with nano-sized carrier systems. *Journal of Artificial Organs: The Official Journal of the Japanese Society for Artificial Organs, 8*(2), 77–84. https://doi.org/10.1007/s10047-005-0285-0.

103. Yoo, H. S., et al. (2000). *In vitro* and *in vivo* anti-tumor activities of nanoparticles based on doxorubicin–PLGA conjugates. *Journal of Controlled Release, 68*(3), 419–431.

104. Zarbin, M. A., et al. (2010). Nanomedicine in ophthalmology: The new frontier. *American Journal of Ophthalmology, 150*(2), 144–162.

105. Zhan, C., et al. (2018). Long-acting liposomal corneal anesthetics. *Biomaterials, 181*, 372–377.

106. Zhang, X., et al. (2018). Effects of mesenchymal stem cells and their exosomes on the healing of large and refractory macular holes. *Graefe's Archive for Clinical and Experimental Ophthalmology, 256*(11), 2041–2052. https://doi.org/10.1007/s00417-018-4097-3.

107. Zhou, Z., et al. (2017). Nonviral cancer gene therapy: Delivery cascade and vector nano property integration. *Advanced Drug Delivery Reviews, 115*, 115–154.

108. Zhu, S., et al. (2019). Safety assessment of nanomaterials to eyes: An important but neglected issue. *Advanced Science, 6*(16), 1802289.

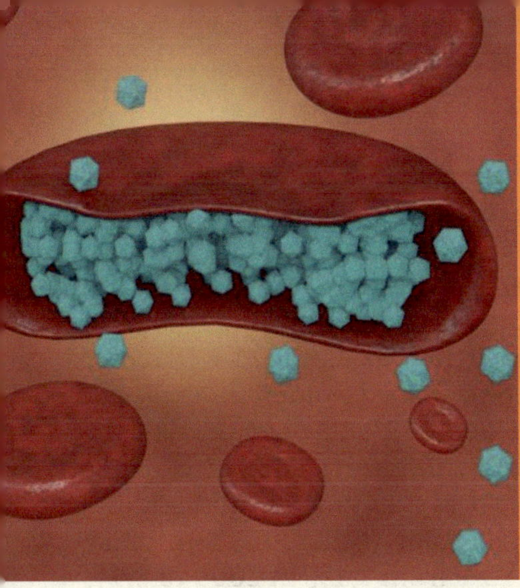

Chapter 7

NANOMEDICINE IN DIABETES

Contents

Kusum Rani,[1] Shyam Tripathi,[1] Nikita Malik,[2] V. Samuel Raj,[1,2] and Pratibha Gaur[1,2,]*

[1]Center for Drug Design Discovery and Development, SRM University Delhi-NCR, Rajiv Gandhi Education City, Sonepat, Haryana, India

[2]Department of Biotechnology and Microbiology, School of Science and Humanities, SRM University Delhi-NCR, Sonepat, Haryana, India

**Corresponding author.*

Abstract

Diabetes is one of the major health problems on a global scale, with the burden raising at a really fast pace. The population burdened by diabetes has increased manifold over time. It is projected that, by the year 2019, 537 million people would be ailing from diabetes. Type 1 diabetes, accounting for less than 10% of the cases, is prevalent in adolescence and teenage years and is characterized by little production of insulin as the immune system fights it. On the other hand, 85–90% of type 2 diabetes cases occur in adults and older populations and living habits such as obesity are contributory factors. Enthusiasm for the "open loop" method of classic insulin replacement requires subcutaneous injections, which can be a challenge for some patients. Nanomedicine is oriented to improve treatment in diabetes by allowing more precise glucose monitoring, optimum medication administration, and establishing a basis for personalized treatments in specific diseases. NPs are being developed with potential to revolutionize the treatment of diabetes and the care of patients suffering from these diseases, notably by way of early detection, precise monitoring, and better ways of drug administration.

7.1. Introduction

The number of diabetics has risen substantially, from 108 million in 1980 to 422 million by 2014. In 2019, an estimated 537 million persons were living with diabetes globally (Deshpande, Harris-Hayes, and Schootman, 2008). There are age groupings, sexes, and ethnic groups where diabetes is more prevalent. Type 1 diabetes (T1D) primarily affects young people and adolescents, while it can affect anyone at any age. Type 2 diabetes affects 85–90% of cases, and it is more common in adults and older persons (Wild et al., 2004). In the United States, 38.4 million adults (11.6% of the population) had diabetes in 2021. The prevalence is higher among certain racial/ethnic groups, affecting 13.6% of American Indians/Alaskan Natives, 12.1% of non-Hispanic Blacks, and 11.7% of Hispanics compared to 6.9% of non-Hispanic Whites (Haw et al., 2021). Diabetes disproportionately impacts older adults, with 29.2% of those aged 65 and older having the condition. Globally, the prevalence of diabetes is increasing most rapidly in low- and middle-income countries (Lam et al., 2021). In India, the prevalence rose from 7.1% in 2009 to 8.9% in 2019, with an estimated 77 million adults affected (Pradeepa and Mohan, 2021). A major concern is the high percentage of undiagnosed cases, which exceeds 50% in many developing nations like Bangladesh, Vietnam, and Ghana. Diabetes is a leading cause of mortality, contributing to over 1.5 million deaths directly in 2019 and an additional 4,60,000 deaths from kidney disease (Groop et al., 2009). It is also a major risk factor for cardiovascular disease, vision loss, and limb amputations. The economic burden is substantial, with the total cost of diagnosed diabetes in the United States reaching $412.9 billion in 2022 (Butt, Khalid, Ahmad, and Khan, 2024).

T1D, also known as young-onset diabetes, accounts for approximately 10% of all cases of diabetes mellitus globally (Dabelea, 2009). It has resulted from a deficiency of insulin hormone which is derived from 51 amino acid peptide produced by the pancreatic islets of Langerhans' β-cells. Insulin is responsible for the absorption of glucose within the blood by the liver cells and muscle cells; hence, it regulates the levels of glucose in blood. This deficit is brought on by an autoimmune response in the afflicted patients whereby T-cells cause the death of β cells, hence lowering insulin levels and raising blood sugar. On the other hand, type 2 diabetes is often linked to lifestyle factors such as obesity and lack of physical activity. In patients with a diagnosis of type 2 diabetes, insulin resistance occurs, in which the sensitivity of the body to insulin secreted by β-cells is reduced enough to result in high blood sugar levels (Veiseh et al., 2015).

Insulin and other diabetic therapies that are macromolecular in nature, like glucagon-like peptide-1 (GLP-1), are normally administered subcutaneously due to the unpleasant gastrointestinal environment, and such painful and rather inconvenient injections result in low compliance by patients. This traditional method of insulin replacement, termed 'open loop,' relies on past information in determining insulin doses if the blood glucose response of the patient to his meals and treatments is known (Pickup, 2024). Various technologies, such as insulin pumps and continuous glucose monitors, aim to dynamically control insulin levels in real-time, reducing the burden on patients. For instance, the dual hormone bionic pancreas system, combining insulin and glucagon, has shown significant improvements in glucose control and fewer hypoglycemic episodes in patients with T1D. Despite these advancements, maintaining optimal glucose levels remains challenging for many patients, with around 50% not achieving target glucose levels throughout the day. To achieve these objectives, researchers are looking into different ways to administer insulin, improving insulin pharmacokinetics, and developing novel treatment approaches (Owens, 2002). Advances in sensor technology are now opening up the opportunity for nanomedicine in the creation of more accurate and frequent methods of glucose monitoring. The potentials of NPs would raise the performance of glucose biosensors tremendously and thus help diabetics in better controlling their blood sugar levels (Odularu and Ajibade, 2021). Trends in the unprecedented use of nanotechnology in medicine are nanoparticle-based glucose biosensors. This technology diagnoses, treats, and understands a growing number of complicated pathways of disease processes by using nanoparticles. These nanoscale devices aim to enhance the solubility of drugs, their bioavailability, and enhance targeted specificity, which improves the quality of life. The category of nanomedicines includes both biological and non-biological products, the former which are obtained from biological sources and the latter known as non-biological complex pharmaceuticals (Soares et al., 2018).

In addition, nanotechnology is facilitating novel means of insulin delivery. Advancements in nanotechnology could serve to revolutionize the management of diabetes, either by increasing effectiveness or making treatments more friendly to the patient. Indeed, the International Diabetes Federation projects that by 2030 there will be 439 million people worldwide living with diabetes, making-healthcare costs of $490 billion, thus placing a critical need for creative new approaches to the treatment of this disease (Lemmerman et al., 2020).

In the case of insulin or other antidiabetic drugs, nanomedicine does give quite an edge over traditional therapy. Several nanoparticle-based pathways for the delivery of drugs, like lipid NPs, liposomes, and polymeric NPs, enhance the bioavailability of a drug and reduce side effects by targeted delivery (Sajeesh, Sharma, and Vauthier, 2012). Extensive research on mucoadhesive NPs for oral insulin delivery holds out the potential for increased patient compliance. Nanomedicine has also been proposed for enhancement of transplantation of islet cells into T1D patients by preventing or minimizing immunological rejection, thus promoting survival and functionality. Nanomedicine plays a part in the treatment of diabetic diseases like neuropathy, nephropathy, and retinopathy, either by targeted drug delivery into the tissues or due to the attenuation of inflammation and oxidative stress (Odularu and Ajibade, 2021). NPs are being created as contrast agents to help identify type 1 diabetes early on. Implantable CGMS devices are being equipped with glucose nanosensors to enhance the precision and practicality of real-time blood glucose monitoring (Lemmerman et al.,

2020; Veiseh et al., 2015). These developments have shown that nanomedicine could be the breakthrough that will revolutionize diabetes care by delivering accurate and non-invasive monitoring tools, therefore improving the standard of care in patients with diabetes (Luo, Yan, and Feng, 2021). Nanomedicine is revolutionizing the management of diabetes in the areas of glucose monitoring, drug delivery, and targeted therapy of complications. Further improvements in the quality of life and diabetes management will be witnessed in the near future. Even with all the benefits that nanomedicine gives, safety is always the priority. Therefore, it is very important and gated to study in detail the potential toxicity of NPs. Ongoing research aims to improve the biocompatibility of nanomedicines through strategies like surface modification and immunomodulation (Kujawa and Winnik, 2013).

Development of nanomedicines involves a number of challenges, including evaluating physicochemical qualities, biocompatibility, nanotoxicity, pharmacokinetics, and pharmacodynamics. Nanomedicines have shown promise in clinical applications, ranging from medical devices to nano-pharmaceuticals, but the regulation of these innovative products remains a work in progress, especially in defining harmonized standards and protocols for their characterization and evaluation (Astruc, 2016).

7.2. Diabetes Management with Nanomedicine

Diabetes mellitus is a serious global health burden, impacting millions of individuals globally. Traditional treatment options often fall short in providing optimal glycemic control, leading to the exploration of innovative solutions like nanomedicine. Nanotechnology offers a range of benefits in diabetes care, revolutionizing diagnostics, monitoring, and therapeutics.

7.2.1. Diagnostics and Monitoring

Recent advances in nanotechnology make diabetes management a realistic option for enhancing people's quality of life. Traditional diabetes treatment options, such as continuous glucose monitoring and insulin injections, may be costly and uncomfortable. To solve these issues, novel ways are being studied using nanotechnology. Implantable nanosensors are being developed for continuous glucose monitoring, and innovative nanoparticle-based imaging approaches are being researched for early detection by detecting minute changes in beta cell mass. Nanoparticle contrast agents are being developed for non-invasive imaging modalities, such as magnetic resonance imaging (MRI), to measure β-cell mass and monitor pancreatic inflammation. For example, a pilot investigation utilizing a clinically authorized superparamagnetic iron oxide nanoparticles (SPIONs)-based MRI contrast agent revealed a twofold difference in pancreatic T2 relaxation time between healthy volunteers and recently diagnosed diabetes patients owing to islet inflammation (Sim and Wong, 2021; Veiseh et al., 2015). Ferrimagnetic iron oxide nanocubes with high MRI relaxivity allow visualization of single pancreatic islet cells using clinical MRI, enabling monitoring of endogenous and transplanted islet cells. Nanomedicine approaches are also being explored for regenerative therapies to treat diabetic tissues and organs. Nanostructures provide an appropriate scaffold for regeneration of islet β cells, retinal tissue, nerves, and wounds (Li, Liu, and Wu, 2022; Veiseh et al., 2015). In the near future, nanotechnology might be highly useful in developing improved glucose sensors that would provide equity users with more user-friendly interfaces, quicker readings, and more accurate results than those of current technologies. Glucose oxidase, glucose-binding proteins, and tiny glucose-binding molecules are the three main kinds of glucose-sensing compounds that have been employed to create glucose sensors based on nanoparticles (Soares et al., 2018; Veiseh et al., 2015). Glucose oxidase-based nanosensors have been built onto metallic NPs and carbon nanotubes (CNTs) but have limitations such as batch-to-batch variability, diminishing activity over time, and the need for constant oxygen, pH, and temperature. Non-enzymatic nanosensors have been developed to improve reliability by eliminating drift and inconsistent enzyme activity. These include oxidation-based sensors using metal oxide catalysts like copper oxide or gold NPs, and binding-based sensors using fluorescent or voltametric readouts with glucose-binding moieties like lectins, phenylboronic acid, or molecularly imprinted polymers (Soares et al., 2018). As a result, NPs such as CNTs and quantum dots (QDs) have been developed. When designed properly, these NPs can emit fluorescence and have shown to have a respectable lifespan. To lessen reliance on a single sensor, several nanosensors that measure blood glucose in parallel can be implanted throughout the body. The field of glucose nanosensor development is young; thus far, *in vivo* experiments have only been documented in animals. The next generation of continuous glucose monitoring sensors, which will show less variability than the current glucose oxidase-based sensors, can more easily be developed using nonenzymatic technology. Non-invasive nanosensors are significantly more likely to replace manual glucose detection techniques that rely on finger pricking since they can provide ultrafast readouts and do not require batteries or an enzyme-based catalyst (Safarkhani et al., 2023).

7.2.2. Drug Delivery

Nanoparticle mediated drug delivery systems (DDS) are being used to boost the efficacy of anti-diabetic treatments (Figure 7.1) (Saini and Sharma, 2023). The goal of producing glucose-responsive nanoparticles is to more closely mimic the physiological needs of the human body for insulin (Veiseh et al., 2015). Nano-biotechnology is revolutionizing insulin delivery methods to improve efficacy, safety, and patient convenience. Key advancements include:

- Development of nanoparticulate insulin formulations for extended action, hence less frequent injections. These minimize the need for frequent subcutaneous injections, which can be painful and inconvenient for patients (Kesharwani et al., 2018).
- Glucose-responsive insulin formulations that modulate insulin release based on real-time glucose levels, enabling tighter glycemic control while minimizing hypoglycemia risk. This mimics the body's natural insulin response more accurately (Hunt et al., 2024; Kesharwani et al., 2018).
- Novel delivery routes like oral, transdermal, and inhaled insulin to provide less invasive options. Oral insulin delivery is a particularly active research area, with nanocarriers designed to protect insulin from degradation and enhance absorption (Bahman, Greish, and Taurin, 2019; Kesharwani et al., 2018).
- Multifunctional nanoparticle formulations that combine various strategies to overcome delivery challenges. For example, using pH-sensitive polymers, enzyme-triggered release, and liver targeting to improve oral insulin bioavailability (Bahman, Greish, and Taurin, 2019; Kesharwani et al., 2018).

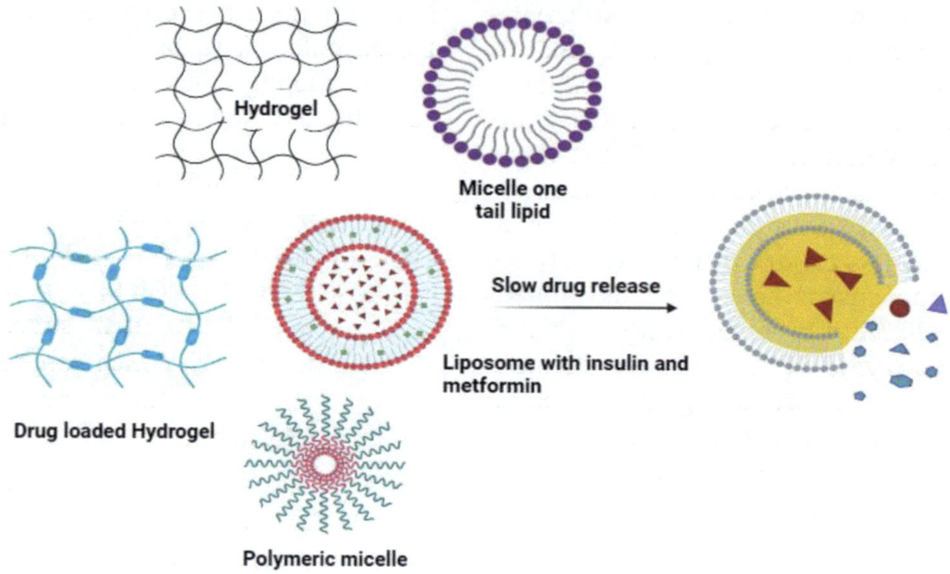

Figure 7.1. Insulin and antidiabetic drugs such as metformin are being explored for delivery using various types of liposomes, nanoparticles, and micelles for targeted, slow, and sustained release. For the diabetic wound healing process, hydrogel-based drug delivery systems (DDS) can efficiently be used to carry various substances such as antimicrobial agents, hemostatic agents, growth factors, and nutrients to the wound site.

Source: Figure created with BioRender.

These nanotechnology-enabled insulin delivery systems are rapidly advancing, with some early-generation carriers already in clinical trials. They have the capability to significantly enhance patient quality of life and diabetes treatment by optimizing insulin delivery. Nanomedicines based on trace elements like zinc, selenium, and magnesium can help lower blood glucose, promote insulin secretion, and alleviate diabetic complications (Ruan et al., 2023). Nanoparticle delivery systems can enhance the solubility, stability, and bioavailability of antidiabetic drugs, improving their therapeutic efficacy (Ruan et al., 2023). Functionalized NPs loaded with antidiabetic drugs, plant extracts, or other bioactive molecules have demonstrated therapeutic potential in managing diabetes (Sharma et al., 2023).

For diabetic wound healing, nano-based DDS can efficiently carry various substances like antimicrobial agents, hemostatic agents, growth factors, and nutrients to the wound site (Liu et al., 2023). The poor healing and high susceptibility to infection resulting from hyperglycemia in the wound bed make diabetic wounds difficult to treat. In these wounds, bacteria that have formed biofilms become very resistant to medications. Smart hydrogels refer to stimuli-responsive hydrogels that have recently drawn interest as a potentially effective treatment for diabetic wound healing (Chen et al., 2023). Under a variety of stimuli, such as temperature, pH, enzymes, and biological factors, smart hydrogels can alter their mechanical characteristics, expanding capacity, hydrophilicity, and the permeability of biologically active molecules (Zhang et al., 2023). pH-responsive antibiotics loaded hydrogels (Figure 7.1) can break down bacterial cell membranes and speed up drug release in acidic conditions, greatly lowering the inhibitory dosage of antibiotics on bacteria that are resistant to several drugs (Wang and Zhang, 2024). Some examples of nano-based therapies for diabetic wounds include silver NPs with antimicrobial properties combined with calcium alginate NPs for hemostasis and chitosan (CH) hydrogel, Ferulic acid nano-formulations to enhance wound healing, Quercetin-loaded silver NPs in hydrogel matrices, Nano-insulin formulations that modulate cytokines and promote wound remodeling (Liu et al., 2023).

Insulin oral bioavailability has been reported to be enhanced by polymeric nanoparticles and micelles in preclinical animal models (Alai, Lin, and Pingale, 2015). Metformin hydrochloride, a popular oral antidiabetic drug, was encapsulated for long-term treatment using porcine casein micelles. Additionally, *sambiloto*, a natural anti-diabetic drug, was encapsulated using casein micelles, which rapidly degraded in artificial stomach juice to release the active ingredients (Mazhar, Shrivastava, and Tomar, 2021). Insulin and calcitonin can be better absorbed by the lungs with the help of polyamidoamine dendrimers (Table 7.1). Nonionic surfactant vesicles known as niosomes have the ability to carry active pharmaceutical ingredients (APIs) with a wide range of solubility. They have demonstrated to be effective drug transporters for amphiphilic, lipophilic, and hydrophilic compounds. Because they are nonionic, they are considered safe drug delivery methods (Fouad et al., 2023). A new formulation including gliclazide and metformin was employed to create anti-diabetic niosomes (Kumar and Jeyabalan, 2017). Bile salt-based liposomes increase both oral bioavailability and intestinal insulin absorption. As a result, liposomes can be an excellent option for delivering insulin and other medications that reduce blood sugar, such as metformin, enabling improved management of the hyperglycemic stage through several administration methods (Kumar and Jeyabalan, 2017). In an effort to combat diabetes, dual CH/albumin-coated alginate/dextran sulfate nanoparticles have been researched for better oral insulin administration (Lopes et al., 2016).

Table 7.1. Nanomedicines Used for Diabetes Management

Nanomedicine	Nanoparticles Used as Carriers	References
Insulin	Alginate NPs, Chitosan NPs, Dextran NPs	Veiseh et al. (2015)
Metformin, Calcein, Insulin	Liposome NPs	Wang et al. (2021)
Gliclazide, Metformin	Niosome NPs	Olatunde et al. (2022)
Calcitonin	Dendrimer NPs	Olatunde et al. (2022)
Porcine insulin	Micelle NPs	He, Al-Mureish, and Wu (2021)

7.2.3. Immunotherapy

In an effort to find a cure, nanotechnology is being employed to create T1D vaccines, which could be more effective (Veiseh et al., 2015). NPs are being explored for immunomodulation in cell-based therapies for diabetes. While nanomedicine holds great promise, challenges remain in ensuring long-term safety and efficacy. Rigorous evaluation of these novel therapies is needed before they can be widely adopted in clinical practice (Saini and Sharma, 2023). Nanoparticle-based immunotherapy seems to be a very promising means of treatment against diabetes, especially T1D, which is an autoimmune disorder (Nigam et al., 2022). Some key reasons why NPs are important for use in immunotherapy against diabetes are explained in subsections.

7.2.3.1. Nanoparticle-Mediated T Cell Therapy

In diabetes treatment, nanoparticle-mediated T cell therapy involves using NPs targeting and modulating T cells for therapeutic purposes. These will allow the delivery of siRNA/miRNA into T cells, which are involved in modulating effector arms of the immune response and lead to immunosuppression and a decrease in beta cell loss (Nigam et al., 2022). It aims at re-establishing immune tolerance and preventing further autoimmune obliteration of insulin-producing beta cells. Research in this field is aimed at enhancing treatment effectiveness and patient outcomes for patients with diabetes and, more specifically, T1D. This is accomplished by testing the ability of NPs to deliver insulin, immunomodulators, or modified vaccinations to immune cells in order to raise insulin levels and decrease beta cell death in response to hyperglycemia. Evidence has established that nanoparticle-based DDS allow for targeting of T cells, offering a number of advantages in controlled drug release, improved pharmacokinetics, and cell-specific targeting (Cevaal et al., 2021). In addition, the encapsulation of multiple recombinant pancreatic T cell proteins within tolerogenic immune-modifying NPs has been potent in preventing both onset and progression in preclinical T1D models. This novel approach underlines the potential of nanoparticle-mediated T cell therapy as a novel strategy for the treatment of diabetes (Podojil et al., 2022).

As in any other organ-specific autoimmune disease, in T1D, autoreactive T cells mount an immune response against insulin-producing beta cells. These pathogenic T cells are normally held in a balance by the Tregs, and an imbalance or dysfunction of this control mechanism may subsequently lead to T1D. Current and developing immunotherapies either prevent activation of the autoimmune response or reestablish regulatory control over autoreactive T cells. Strategies include abatacept-based co-stimulation blockade based on alteration in the levels of $CD4^+$ memory T cells and Tregs in the population, inhibition of autoimmune T cells, delaying T1D through teplizumab through enhancement of inhibitory molecules and reduction of $CD4^+$ and $CD8^+$ T cells, and the identification of markers to correct dysfunctional Tregs and restore tolerance. Engineering Tregs with chimeric antigen receptors against insulin for redirecting their specificity toward autoimmune T cells in T1D has also been tried. Indeed, autoimmune T cells, notably $CD4^+$ and $CD8^+$ T cells, play a central role in the destruction of insulin-producing beta cells in individuals with T1D. These pathogenic T cells are normally kept in check by regulatory T cells (Tregs), but an imbalance or dysfunction in this control mechanism can lead to the onset of T1D.

Nanomedicine has introduced novel techniques to precisely control immunomodulation using NPs. Methods include using dextran particles to deliver autoantigen and immunosuppressant, which acts selectively on effector T cells; co-encapsulating autoantigen and vitamin D3 into liposomes to induce antigen-specific Tregs; and creating NPs loaded with a hybrid peptide of insulin-chromogranin A, which impairs $CD4^+$ T cell function and increases the ratio of Tregs over effector T cells to prevent diabetes (Nigam et al., 2022). In order to restore immunological tolerance and regulatory functions, these designed nanomaterials (NMs) can conjugate immunomodulators and target particular areas of the innate and adaptive immune responses in T1D.

7.2.3.2. B Cell Depletion via NPs

SiRNA/miRNA-conjugated monoclonal antibodies and NPs have been utilized to induce the apoptosis event and the depletion of autoreactive B cells (Nigam et al., 2022). This treatment has aimed to halt disease progression by eliminating the generally one B cells causative agents for driving the autoimmune response. Nanoparticle-based immunotherapies are of high potential in the treatment of T1D by targeting autoreactive B cells specifically (Huang et al., 2023). It is known that B cells are centrally involved in the pathogenesis of T1D, and their depletion halts disease at a pre-insulitis stage. However, current B cell-targeted treatments, including rituximab, have Gordon crossover and fast re-emergence of autoreactive B cells, and have been shown to deplete regulatory cells (Zhang et al., 2022). Nanomedicine provides a more targeted approach where NPs are conjugated with siRNA to silence antiapoptotic factors in autoreactive B cells. Also, polymeric NPs have been designed to release their payload of insulin, proinsulin DNA, and siRNAs according to changes in glucose level. In other words, controlled releases can be adjusted to react appropriately to changing environmental factors and situations (Kopan et al., 2018; Zhang et al., 2022).

Administration of nanoparticles to certain places on autoreactive B cells is becoming more and more popular as an alternative to monoclonal antibodies that target surface antigens. Therapeutic genetic expression can be provided via CRISPR-encased NPs in the B cell milieu, which can lower expression and cause autoreactive B cells to be eliminated. This approach aims to break the detrimental loop between autoreactive B and T cells that leads to beta cell destruction in T1D. While limited studies have directly investigated nanoparticle-based immunotherapies targeting B cells in T1D, successful depletion of B cells using this approach has been demonstrated in other autoimmune diseases (Deshpande, Harris-Hayes, and Schootman, 2008; Lam et al., 2021; Pradeepa and Mohan, 2021). Nanomedicine offers a promising strategy for the actual reversal of Type 1 Diabetes by addressing both individual genetic predispositions and environmental factors that promote the condition (Bresson and Von Herrath, 2009).

7.2.3.3. Immune Checkpoint Modulation with Liposome

NPs and liposome can be engineered to deliver siRNA/miRNA that upregulates the production of immune checkpoint proteins like PD-L1 and CTLA4 (Nigam et al., 2022). This leads to the abrogation of T-cell activation and suppression of the autoimmune response. Immune checkpoint proteins are essential for regulating the immune system and maintaining self-tolerance. They function as co-stimulatory and co-inhibitory receptors that precisely control T cell activation and proliferation (Paluch et al., 2018). Co-stimulatory checkpoints, such as CD28 expressed on $CD4^{+}$ T cells, bind to B7.1 and B7.2 ligands to promote T cell proliferation and migration. $CD8^{+}$ T cell activation relies more on CD70, CD137, and CD134 interactions. On the other hand, immune response suppression is achieved by inhibitory checkpoints such as PD-1 and its ligands PD-L1/PD-L2, which induce apoptosis and reduce the proliferation of T cells (Deshpande, Harris-Hayes, and Schootman, 2008; Lam et al., 2021; Pradeepa and Mohan, 2021). Furthermore, B7.1/2 is bound by the CD28 homolog CTLA-4 and inhibits T cell activation through inhibitory signaling pathways (Huang et al., 2019). The most current strategy to treating cancer is the use of epigenetic therapies, such as immune checkpoint inhibitors (ICIs), which reconstitute immune-mediated tumor targeting and killing. By inhibiting T cell inhibitory receptors including CTLA-4 and PD-1, ICIs stimulate the body's natural anticancer immune responses (Zhang et al., 2020). However, such a powerful drug comes with a distinct set of side effects called immune-related adverse events (irAEs), some of which impact the endocrine system. T1DM, which develops when ICIs trigger an autoimmune attack on the insulin-producing beta cells in the pancreas, is one of the most serious irAEs. ICIs trigger T cell responses generally, including autoreactive T cells that attack pancreatic beta cells, by suppressing CTLA-4 or PD-1 (Liao et al., 2023; Zhang et al., 2020). Liposome conjugated with specific microRNAs (miRNAs) show promise as a potential therapeutic approach to increase the expression of co-inhibitory immune checkpoint proteins like PD-L1 and CTLA-4 in beta cells of the pancreas (Figure 7.2).

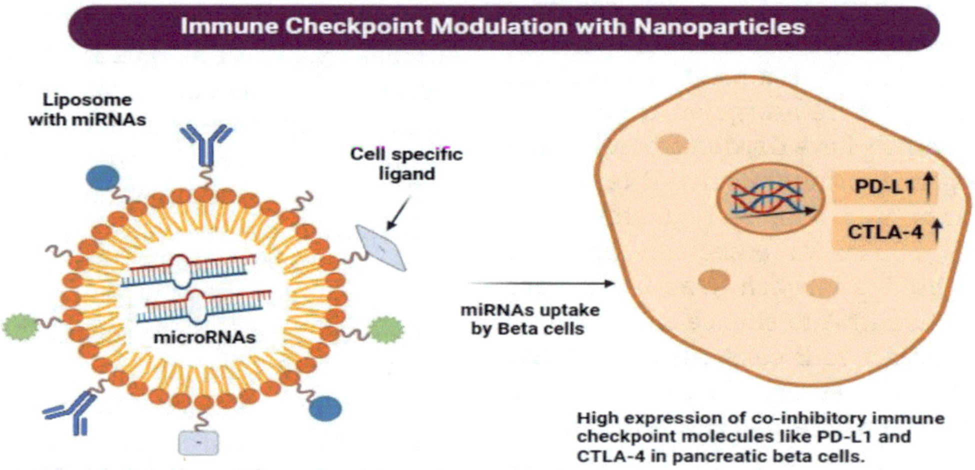

Figure 7.2. Pictorial representation of a liposome coupled to specific microRNAs (miRNAs), which have emerged as a promising therapeutic approach for increasing the expression of co-inhibitory checkpoint immune molecules, including PD-L1 and CTLA-4, in pancreatic beta cells. Conjugation of several miRNAs with Fe-oxide nanoparticles and liposomes enhances their expression and promotes protection of endogenous beta cells, potentially aiding in the treatment of type 1 diabetes (T1D).

Source: Figure created with BioRender.

This could help protect beta cells from autoimmune destruction in type 1 diabetes (T1D). Approaches include using dextran particles in the delivery of autoantigen and immunosuppressant to selectively affect effector T cells, co-encapsulating autoantigen and vitamin D_3 in liposomes to induce antigen-specific Tregs, and fabricating NPs loaded with insulin–chromogranin A hybrid peptide to prevent diabetes by impairing $CD4^+$ T cell function and increasing the proportion of Tregs to effector T cells (Zhang et al., 2020). Some studies have reported that NPs conjugated with miR-200c exhibit higher potency in the inhibition of PD-L1 expression compared to naked miR-200c. Other miRNAs, such as miR-138-5p, miR-513, miR-200a, and miR-34a, also modulate the expression of PD-L1 and CTLA-4. In sum, NPs are an effective delivery vehicle for miRNA-based therapeutics. Conversely, NPs can be used to deliver antisense oligonucleotides (ASO) that will up-modulate the expression of PD-L1 and CTLA-4 in pancreatic islets (Marin-Acevedo, Kimbrough, and Lou, 2021).

7.2.3.4. Stem Cell Therapy Enhanced by NPs

Stem cell treatment is now recognized as a viable approach for treating T1D by transplanting insulin-producing beta cells derived from stem cells. This regenerative medicine therapy aims to provide a long-term solution by replacing the destroyed beta cells and reducing the patient's reliance on insulin injections (Wan et al., 2022).

Several clinical studies have explored different stem cell-based approaches for T1D treatment:

i. **Autologous Nonmyeloablative Hematopoietic Stem Cell Transplantation (AHST):** In one study, 14 out of 15 patients were able to continue being insulin independent for at least six months after AHST, and they also showed lower levels of anti-GAD antibodies and higher C-peptide levels (Voltarelli et al., 2007).

ii. **Autologous Mesenchymal Stromal Cells (MSCs) Derived from Umbilical Cord Tissue:** Transplantation of these cells led to improved C-peptide levels and reduced insulin dependence in all treated patients (Jayasinghe et al., 2022).

These studies demonstrate the prospective of stem cell therapy to improve patient outcomes and reduce the burden of T1D management. However, challenges remain, such as the need for immunosuppression to prevent graft rejection and the potential risks associated with stem cell transplantation. MRI, also known as magnetic particle imaging, is the main technique used for molecular imaging of stem cells and stem cell transplantation. SPIONs are used to target extracellular and intracellular markers throughout the imaging process. These NPs are specifically designed to track stem cells, islet cells, and immune cells.

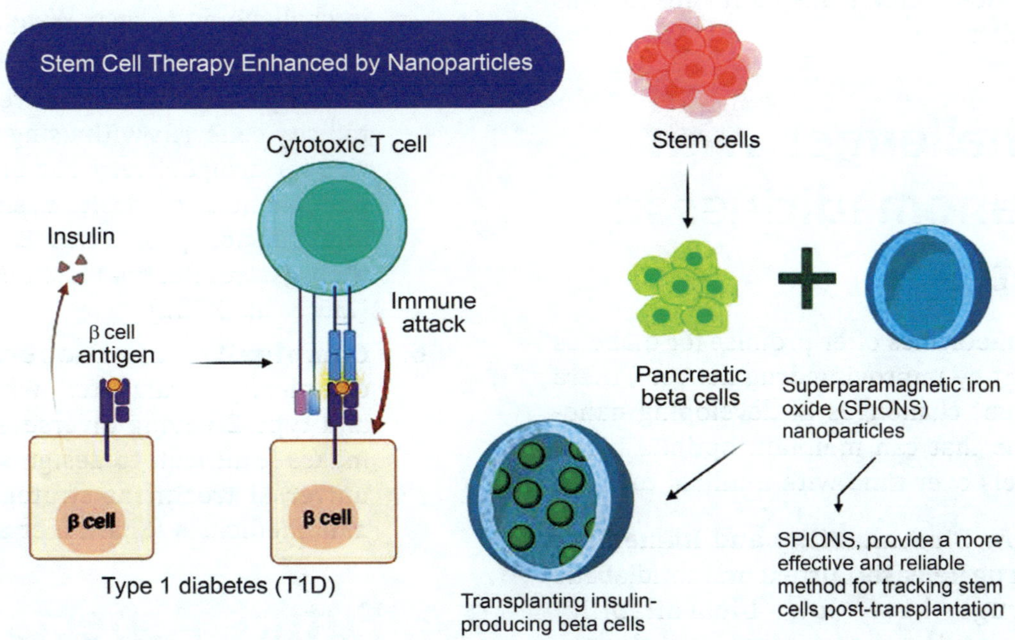

Figure 7.3. Stem cell therapy may help regenerate pancreatic beta cells and improve insulin production in diabetes. Nanomedicine techniques, such as encapsulating stem cells in nanoparticles (NPs), can enhance targeted delivery and improve the survival of these cells.

Source: Figure created with BioRender.

As such, they provide an invaluable longitudinal monitoring tool for cell transplantation, particularly in the treatment of autoimmune illnesses such as T1D (Ernst, Wang, Ma, and Ma, 2019). NPs, particularly SPIONs, provide a more effective and reliable method for tracking stem cells post-transplantation (Figure 7.3) compared to traditional methods like organic dyes or fluorescent probes due to their optimal magnetic and optical properties. SPIONs have proven to be a useful tool for tracking and photographing stem cells in both human and animal research, indicating their potential for therapeutic and precision medicine applications. These NPs enable targeted therapy and imaging, offering a platform for specific cell targeting and combined therapy approaches (Ernst, Wang, Ma, and Ma, 2019). While MPI has emerged as a promising imaging modality for tracking labeled cells, its limitations include challenges in distinguishing viable from non-viable cell transplants over time, especially as dead cells and their NPs degrade, potentially leading to false positive signals. Despite these limitations, NPs, particularly SPIONs, continue to be a focus of research for enhancing the monitoring and efficacy of stem cell transplants in various clinical applications.

7.3. Challenges with the Nanomedicines in Diabetes

While nanomedicines offer promise for diabetes management by improving drug delivery, there are significant challenges in developing nano-formulations that can maintain optimal blood glucose levels over time with minimal toxicity:

1. **Low Bioavailability and Immediate Drug Release:** Current oral antidiabetic drugs have low bioavailability and release the drug immediately, requiring higher dosing frequencies which can lead to adverse side effects and reduce patient compliance (Simos et al., 2021).
2. **Difficulty Maintaining Optimal Blood Glucose Levels:** Nano-drug formulations face the challenge of maintaining stable blood glucose levels over long periods of time. It is not ideal to have sharp declines followed by similar increases. The ideal nano-drug should gradually release the drug to maintain progressively low glucose levels over time (Simos et al., 2021).
3. **Clearing the Drug from Circulation:** Maintaining low blood glucose levels requires long-term blood circulation of nano-drug formulations, however this can be challenging because the body gradually eliminates the medication from circulation (Simos et al., 2021).
4. **Lack of Smart Glucose-Responsive Release:** It is ideal for nano-carriers to react to blood glucose levels and adjust their delivery of drugs accordingly, but creating such intelligent nano-carriers is challenging (Ernst, Wang, Ma, and Ma, 2019; Simos et al., 2021).
5. **Toxicity Concerns:** There are potential toxicity concerns with using inorganic NPs for drug delivery. Factors like the nanoparticle composition, size, shape, and surface properties can impact their gastrointestinal fate and toxicity (Liu et al., 2022).
6. **Complexity of Diabetes:** The complexity of diabetes, with type 1 and type 2 having diverse etiologies, makes it difficult to design successful universal treatment strategies using nanomedicines (Sharma et al., 2023).

7.4. Future Aspects of Nanomedicines in Diabetes Management

Future aspects of nanomedicines in diabetes management involve promising advancements in the treatment and care of diabetes through the utilization of nanotechnology. Nanomedicines offer a potential solution to the challenges faced in diabetes therapy, such as the need for more effective treatment options with fewer side effects. The integration of nanotechnology in diabetes management aims to enhance the precision, bioavailability, absorption, and biocompatibility of therapeutic interventions. Key areas of focus comprise the synthesis of potent glucose-sensitive NPs, nanosensors for monitoring blood glucose levels, and integrated glucose-sensing and insulin-delivering nanoformulations (Table 7.1). These advancements are crucial for achieving tighter glucose control, reducing lag times in response to glucose levels, and enhancing the way diabetes is managed generally throughout the next 10 years.

7.5. Conclusion

In conclusion, nanomedicine is transforming diabetes care by offering novel methods for diagnostics, monitoring, and treatments. NPs have been used in non-invasive imaging to quantify β-cell mass and monitor inflammation, implantable nano-sensors for continuous glucose monitoring, DDS to improve insulin and antidiabetic drug availability, regenerative therapies using nanomedicine scaffolds, immunotherapies to restore immune tolerance in T1D and stem cell therapy enhanced by NPs for longitudinal tracking and treatment monitoring. Nanoformulations are critical in delivering medications to specific areas in a regulated way, minimizing toxicity while increasing stability, solubility, absorption, penetration, and bioavailability. Lipid-based nanoformulations show potential for delivering therapeutic components to the intestinal lymphatic system without first-pass digestion. Nanocarriers can target organs and tissues associated with diabetes, enhancing medicine delivery to particular cells. Advanced nanomedicines, such as liposomes, niosomes, nanocarriers, and other NPs, have therapeutic promise for diabetes therapy, providing better control and fewer problems. However, there are still certain areas in the field of nanomedicine that require development, such as biocompatibility, physico-chemical characterization, nanotoxicology, pharmacokinetics, and pharmacodynamics. Nanomedicine is promising in diabetes management, potentially significantly improving patient care and treatment results.

KEY TERMS FROM THIS CHAPTER

bioavailability
drug delivery
nanomedicine
nanosensors
diabetes
immunotherapy
nanoparticles
nanotechnology

References

1. Alai, M. S., Lin, W. J., & Pingale, S. S. (2015). Application of polymeric nanoparticles and micelles in insulin oral delivery. *Journal of Food and Drug Analysis, 23*(3), 351–358. https://doi.org/10.1016/j.jfda.2015.01.007.
2. Astruc, D. (2016). Introduction to nanomedicine. *Molecules, 21*(1), 4. https://doi.org/10.3390/molecules21010004.
3. Bahman, F., Greish, K., & Taurin, S. (2019). Nanotechnology in insulin delivery for management of diabetes. *Pharmaceutical Nanotechnology, 7*(2), 113–128. https://doi.org/10.2174/2211738507666190321110721.
4. Bresson, D., & Von Herrath, M. (2009). Immunotherapy for the prevention and treatment of type 1 diabetes: Optimizing the path from bench to bedside. *Diabetes Care, 32*(10), 1753–1768. https://doi.org/10.2337/dc09-0373.
5. Butt, M. D., Khalid, S., Ahmad, R., & Khan, S. (2024). A systematic review of the economic burden of diabetes mellitus: Contrasting perspectives from high and low middle-income countries. *Journal of Pharmaceutical Policy and Practice, 17*(1). https://doi.org/10.1080/20523211.2024.2322107.
6. Cevaal, P. M., Cockrell, A. S., Thorp, E. B., Karp, J. M., & Boehm, T. (2021). *In vivo* T cell-targeting nanoparticle drug delivery systems: Considerations for rational design. *ACS Nano, 15*(3), 3736–3753. https://doi.org/10.1021/acsnano.0c09514.
7. Chen, Y., et al. (2023). Research advances in smart responsive-hydrogel dressings with potential clinical diabetic wound healing properties. *Military Medical Research, 10*(1), 37. https://doi.org/10.1186/s40779-023-00473-9.
8. Dabelea, D. (2009). The accelerating epidemic of childhood diabetes. *The Lancet, 373*(9680), 1999–2000. https://doi.org/10.1016/S0140-6736(09)60874-6.
9. Deshpande, A. D., Harris-Hayes, M., & Schootman, M. (2008). Epidemiology of diabetes and diabetes-related complications. *Physical Therapy, 88*(11), 1254–1264. https://doi.org/10.2522/ptj.20080020.
10. Ernst, A. U., Wang, L., Ma, M., & Ma, M. (2019). Nanotechnology in cell replacement therapies for type 1 diabetes. *Advanced Drug Delivery Reviews, 139*, 116–138. https://doi.org/10.1016/j.addr.2019.01.013.
11. Fouad, S. A., Teaima, M. H., Gebril, M. I., Abd Allah, F. I., El-Nabarawi, M. A., & Elhabal, S. F. (2023). Formulation of novel niosomal repaglinide chewable tablets using coprocessed excipients: *In vitro* characterization, optimization and enhanced hypoglycemic activity in rats. *Drug Delivery, 30*(1), 2181747. https://doi.org/10.1080/10717544.2023.2181747.
12. Groop, P. H., Thomas, M. C., Moran, J. L., Wadèn, J., Thorn, L. M., Mäkinen, V. P., & FinnDiane Study Group. (2009). The presence and severity of chronic kidney disease predicts all-cause mortality in type 1 diabetes. *Diabetes, 58*(7), 1651–1658. https://doi.org/10.2337/db08-1543.
13. Haw, J. S., Shah, M., Turbow, S., Egeolu, M., & Umpierrez, G. (2021). Diabetes complications in racial and ethnic minority populations in the USA. *Current Diabetes Reports, 21*(1). https://doi.org/10.1007/s11892-020-01369-x.

14. He, Y., Al-Mureish, A., & Wu, N. (2021). Nanotechnology in the treatment of diabetic complications: A comprehensive narrative review. *Journal of Diabetes Research, 2021*, 6612063. https://doi.org/10.1155/2021/6612063.
15. Huang, C., Zhang, Q., Feng, W., & Chen, W. (2019). Immune checkpoint molecules: Possible future therapeutic implications in autoimmune diseases. *Journal of Autoimmunity, 104*, 102333. https://doi.org/10.1016/j.jaut.2019.102333.
16. Huang, M., Wang, H., Lin, J., Yang, X., Wu, Y., & Gu, Y. (2023). Advanced delivery strategies for immunotherapy in type I diabetes mellitus. *Bio Drugs, 37*(3), 331–352. https://doi.org/10.1007/s40259-023-00594-6.
17. Hunt, N. J., et al. (2024). Oral nanotherapeutic formulation of insulin with reduced episodes of hypoglycemia. *Nature Nanotechnology, 19*(4), 534–544. https://doi.org/10.1038/s41565-023-01565-2.
18. Jayasinghe, M., de Silva, T., Fernando, R., & Jayasinghe, C. D. (2022). The role of mesenchymal stem cells in the treatment of type 1 diabetes. *Cureus, 14*(7), e27337. https://doi.org/10.7759/cureus.27337.
19. Kesharwani, P., et al. (2018). Nanotechnology-based approaches for anti-diabetic drugs delivery. *Diabetes Research and Clinical Practice, 136*, 52–77. https://doi.org/10.1016/j.diabres.2017.11.018.
20. Kopan, C., Tucker, T., Alexander, M., Mohammadi, M. R., Pone, E., & Lakey, J. R. T. (2018). Approaches in immunotherapy, regenerative medicine, and bioengineering for type 1 diabetes. *Frontiers in Immunology, 9*, 1354. https://doi.org/10.3389/fimmu.2018.01354.
21. Kujawa, P., & Winnik, F. M. (2013). Innovation in nanomedicine through materials nano architectonics. *Langmuir, 29*(24), 7354–7361. https://doi.org/10.1021/la4014619.
22. Kumar, B., & Jeyabalan, G. (2017). Development of anti-diabetic niosomes formulation containing metformin and gliclazide. *International Journal of Pharmaceutical and Biological Research.* http://www.ijpbr.in (accessed on 8 May 2025).
23. Lam, A. A., Lepe, A., Wild, S. H., & Jackson, C. (2021). Diabetes comorbidities in low-and middle-income countries: An umbrella review. *Journal of Global Health, 11*, 04040. https://doi.org/10.7189/jogh.11.04040.
24. Lemmerman, L. R., Das, D., Higuita-Castro, N., Mirmira, R. G., & Gallego-Perez, D. (2020). Nanomedicine-based strategies for diabetes: Diagnostics, monitoring, and treatment. *Trends in Endocrinology & Metabolism, 31*(6), 448–458. https://doi.org/10.1016/j.tem.2020.02.001.
25. Li, D., Liu, Y., & Wu, N. (2022). Application progress of nanotechnology in regenerative medicine of diabetes mellitus. *Diabetes Research and Clinical Practice, 190*, 109966. https://doi.org/10.1016/j.diabres.2022.109966.
26. Liao, D., Li, X., Guo, Y., Zheng, H., Liu, Q., & Sun, L. (2023). Recent advances in immune checkpoint inhibitor-induced type 1 diabetes mellitus. *International Immunopharmacology, 122*, 110414. https://doi.org/10.1016/j.intimp.2023.110414.
27. Liu, M., et al. (2023). Recent advances in nano-drug delivery systems for the treatment of diabetic wound healing. *International Journal of Nanomedicine, 18*, 1537–1560. https://doi.org/10.2147/IJN.S395438.

28. Liu, Y., et al. (2022). Emerging theragnostic nanomaterials in diabetes and its complications. *Advanced Science, 9*(3). https://doi.org/10.1002/advs.202102466.

29. Lopes, M., Andrade, F., Egea, M. A., Garcia, M. L., Fernandes, C., & Sarmento, B. (2016). Dual chitosan/albumin-coated alginate/dextran sulfate nanoparticles for enhanced oral delivery of insulin. *Journal of Controlled Release, 232*, 29–41. https://doi.org/10.1016/j.jconrel.2016.04.012.

30. Luo, X. M., Yan, C., & Feng, Y. M. (2021). Nanomedicine for the treatment of diabetes-associated cardiovascular diseases and fibrosis. *Advanced Drug Delivery Reviews, 172*, 234–248. https://doi.org/10.1016/j.addr.2021.01.004.

31. Marin-Acevedo, J. A., Kimbrough, E. O., & Lou, Y. (2021). Next generation of immune checkpoint inhibitors and beyond. *Journal of Hematology & Oncology, 14*(1), 45. https://doi.org/10.1186/s13045-021-01056-8.

32. Mazhar, T., Shrivastava, V., & Tomar, R. S. (2021). Biogenic synthesis of bi-metallic (Zn-Cu) nanoparticles by leaf extract of *Citrus limon* and evaluation of its antibiofilm activity against *E. coli*. *Biomedical and Pharmacology Journal, 14*, 2017+. https://link.gale.com/apps/doc/A690838433/HRCA?u=anon~3330ba3d&sid=googleScholar&xid=70a65562 (accessed on 8 May 2025).

33. Nigam, S., Bishop, J. O., Hayat, H., Quadri, T., Hayat, H., & Wang, P. (2022). Nanotechnology in immunotherapy for type 1 diabetes: Promising innovations and future advances. *Pharmaceutics, 14*(3), 644. https://doi.org/10.3390/pharmaceutics14030644.

34. Odularu, A. T., & Ajibade, P. A. (2021). Challenge of diabetes mellitus and researchers' contributions to its control. *Open Chemistry, 19*(1), 614–634. https://doi.org/10.1515/chem-2020-0153.

35. Olatunde, A., et al. (2022). Nanomedicine for diabetes mellitus management. In C. Egbuna, M. A. Găman, & J. Jeevanandam (Eds.), *Applications of Nanotechnology in Drug Discovery and Delivery* (pp. 179–203). Elsevier. https://doi.org/10.1016/B978-0-12-824408-1.00009-0.

36. Owens, D. R. (2002). New horizons—Alternative routes for insulin therapy. *Nature Reviews Drug Discovery, 1*(7), 529–540. https://doi.org/10.1038/nrd836.

37. Paluch, C., Santos, A. M., Anzilotti, C., Cornall, R. J., & Davis, S. J. (2018). Immune checkpoints as therapeutic targets in autoimmunity. *Frontiers in Immunology, 9*, 2306. https://doi.org/10.3389/fimmu.2018.02306.

38. Pickup, J. C. (2024). Insulin-pump therapy for type 1 diabetes mellitus. *New England Journal of Medicine, 366*(17), 1616–1624. https://doi.org/10.1056/NEJMct1113948.

39. Podojil, J. R., Glaser, A. P., Scott, D. W., & Miller, S. D. (2022). Tolerogenic immune-modifying nanoparticles encapsulating multiple recombinant pancreatic β cell proteins prevent onset and progression of type 1 diabetes in nonobese diabetic mice. *The Journal of Immunology, 209*(3), 465–475. https://doi.org/10.4049/jimmunol.2200208.

40. Pradeepa, R., & Mohan, V. (2021). Epidemiology of type 2 diabetes in India. *Indian Journal of Ophthalmology, 69*(11), 2932–2938. https://doi.org/10.4103/ijo.IJO_1627_21.

41. Ruan, S., Guo, X., Ren, Y., Cao, G., Xing, H., & Zhang, X. (2023). Nanomedicines based on trace elements for intervention of diabetes mellitus. *Biomedicine & Pharmacotherapy, 168*, 115684. https://doi.org/10.1016/j.biopha.2023.115684.

42. Safarkhani, M., et al. (2023). Nanomaterial-assisted wearable glucose biosensors for noninvasive real-time monitoring: Pioneering point-of-care and beyond. *Nano Materials Science.* https://doi.org/10.1016/j.nanoms.2023.11.009.

43. Saini, K., & Sharma, S. (2023). Nanomedicine's transformative impact on anti-diabetic drug discovery: An appraisal. *Journal of Nanoparticle Research, 25*(11), 227. https://doi.org/10.1007/s11051-023-05870-8.

44. Sajeesh, S., Sharma, C. P., & Vauthier, C. (2012). Mucoadhesive nanoparticles for oral delivery of insulin. In *Nanotechnology and Nanomedicine in Diabetes* (pp. 9780429087134). https://doi.org/10.1201/b11775-13.

45. Sharma, R., et al. (2023). Emerging trends in nano-based antidiabetic therapeutics: A path to effective diabetes management. *Materials Advances, 4*(15), 3091–3113. https://doi.org/10.1039/d3ma00159h.

46. Sim, S., & Wong, N. K. (2021). Nanotechnology and its use in imaging and drug delivery (Review). *Biomedical Reports, 14*(5). https://doi.org/10.3892/br.2021.1418.

47. Simos, Y. V., et al. (2021). Trends of nanotechnology in type 2 diabetes mellitus treatment. *Asian Journal of Pharmaceutical Sciences, 16*(1), 62–76. https://doi.org/10.1016/j.ajps.2020.05.001.

48. Soares, S., Sousa, J., Pais, A., & Vitorino, C. (2018). Nanomedicine: Principles, properties, and regulatory issues. *Frontiers in Chemistry, 6*, Article 360. https://doi.org/10.3389/fchem.2018.00360.

49. Veiseh, O., Tang, B. C., Whitehead, K. A., Anderson, D. G., & Langer, R. (2015). Managing diabetes with nanomedicine: Challenges and opportunities. *Nature Reviews Drug Discovery, 14*(1), 45–57. https://doi.org/10.1038/nrd4477.

50. Voltarelli, J. C., Couri, C. E. B., Stracieri, A. B. P. L., Oliveira, M. C., Moraes, D. A., Pieroni, F., ... & Burt, R. K. (2007). Autologous nonmyeloablative hematopoietic stem cell transplantation in newly diagnosed type 1 diabetes mellitus. *JAMA, 297*(14), 1568–1576. https://doi.org/10.1001/jama.297.14.1568.

51. Wan, X. X., Zhang, X. Q., Wang, H., Chen, H. J., Zhang, Q., & Li, D. X. (2022). Stem cell transplantation in the treatment of type 1 diabetes mellitus: From insulin replacement to beta-cell replacement. *Frontiers in Endocrinology, 13*, 859638. https://doi.org/10.3389/fendo.2022.859638.

52. Wang, H., & Zhang, L. M. (2024). Intelligent biobased hydrogels for diabetic wound healing: A review. *Chemical Engineering Journal, 484*, 149493. https://doi.org/10.1016/j.cej.2024.149493.

53. Wang, Y., et al. (2021). Recent advances of nanomedicine-based strategies in diabetes and complications management: Diagnostics, monitoring, and therapeutics. *Journal of Controlled Release, 330*, 618–640. https://doi.org/10.1016/j.jconrel.2021.01.002.

54. Wild, S., Roglic, G., Green, A., Sicree, R., & King, H. (2004). Global prevalence of diabetes: Estimates for the year 2000 and projections for 2030. *Diabetes Care, 27*(5), 1047–1053. https://doi.org/10.2337/diacare.27.5.1047.

55. Zhang, R., Cai, X. L., Liu, L., Han, X. Y., & Ji, L. N. (2020). Type 1 diabetes induced by immune checkpoint inhibitors. *Chinese Medical Journal, 133*(21), 2595–2598. https://journals.lww.com/cmj/fulltext/2020/11050/type_1_diabetes_induced_by_immune_checkpoint.9.aspx (accessed on 8 May 2025).

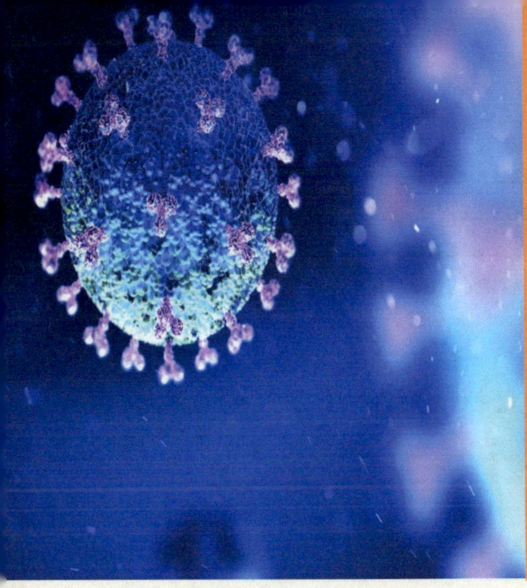

Chapter 8

NANOMEDICINE'S CRUCIAL ROLE IN ADVANCING COVID-19 DIAGNOSTICS AND THERAPEUTICS

Contents

Arpana Vibhuti,[1,*] Sandeep Kumar Shukla,[2,*] and Rishav Kumar[1,2]

[1]Department of Biotechnology, SRM University, Rajiv Gandhi Education City, Sonepat, Haryana, India

[2]Institute of Nuclear Medicine and Allied Sciences (INMAS), Defense Research and Development Organization (DRDO), Brig S.K. Mazumdar Marg, Timarpur, Delhi, India

**Corresponding author.*

Abstract

The COVID-19 pandemic has highlighted the urgent need for novel approaches to evaluate and treat patients in the virus's combat. Since there is not an approved drug that targets the Coronavirus family well at the moment, finding new therapeutic targets is necessary. The use of nanosensors in different diseases and medication delivery in nanomedicine has already demonstrated its worth. Research on COVID-19 diagnosis and therapy can greatly benefit from the application of nanomedicine and its constituent parts at different phases. The ability of nanoparticles to alter their surfaces with polymers, antibodies, or aptamers extends their half-lives and reduces their potential toxicity, even if their unique optical, magnetic, and size-dependent properties make them desirable candidates for disease diagnostics. These nanoparticles are conjugated with aptamers to create sensors that provide label-free, highly selective, reusable, fluorescent, optical, and electrochemical detection signals. Nanostructures have improved medical diagnosis by providing low-cost, reproducible, sensitive, and highly specific methods for illness diagnosis, either as imaging agents or as sensors. The current chapter covers the cutting-edge materials being utilized in nanomedicine to diagnose diseases. Moving beyond diagnostics, the explores the application of nanomedicine in COVID-19 therapeutics. Drug delivery technologies based on nanoparticles have shown great promise in improving the effectiveness of antiviral medications and vaccine formulations. These nanocarriers enhance overall safety and curative impact by reducing off-target effects and allowing focused administration of drugs to sick cells. Furthermore, the development of nano-formulations for vaccine delivery has accelerated global vaccination efforts, offering innovative approaches to generating robust and long-lasting immune responses. The application of nanomedicine in the prognosis and treatment of COVID-19-related illnesses is covered in this book. The creation of highly sensitive diagnostic tests and innovative therapy tactics made possible by the extensive toolbox of materials and processes that nanotechnology offers.

8.1. An Overview of Nanotechnology in Healthcare

The manipulation of matter at sizes between 1 and 100 nanometers, or nanotechnology, reveals special chemical, biological, and physical qualities that lead to the development of innovative materials and medical procedures (Gommersall et al., 2007) (Figure 8.1).

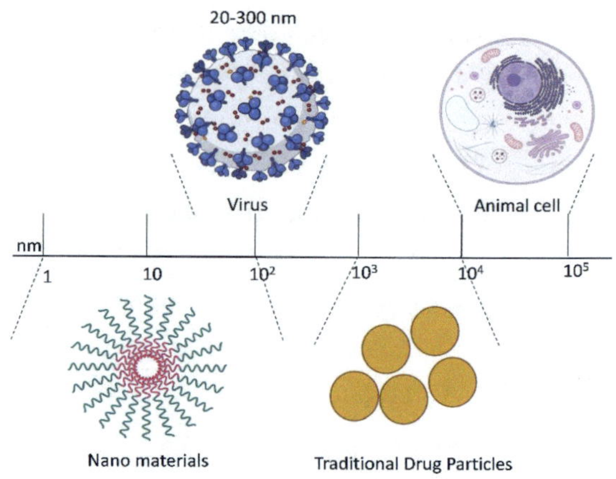

Figure 8.1. Scale comparison of nanoparticles.

Nanomaterials (NMs) have unique properties that improve their use in medical applications. For targeted therapeutics, the enhanced surface area of nanoparticles resulting from a larger surface area-to-volume ratio enhances drug loading capacity and bioavailability (Alekhin et al., 2010; Rizvi and Saleh, 2018). Their customizable characteristics make them versatile for a range of medical uses by enabling exact control over size, shape, and surface chemistry

(Mele and Pisignano, 2009). Some NMs also exhibit enhanced biocompatibility, which lowers immunological responses and possible toxicity.

There are several uses for nanomedicine in the medical field. Targeted drug delivery makes use of the size and surface properties of nanoparticles to improve medication uptake by cells and guarantee accurate delivery to particular organs (Rani et al., 2022; Singh and Lillard, 2009). Additionally, the larger surface area promotes quicker drug release. Effective drug loading maximizes therapeutic efficacy using the fewest carrier materials possible (Jia et al., 2021). This is accomplished by incorporation and adsorption techniques. Different systems based on nanoparticles, such as polymers and liposomes, enhance drug transport and make it possible to pass across biological barriers like the blood–brain barrier (BBB) (Lockman et al., 2002). Diagnostic imaging is greatly advanced by nanotechnology. By increasing sensitivity, resolution, and specificity, NMs such as nanoparticles, nanotubes, and quantum dots (QDs) improve modalities like MRI, CT, PET, and optical imaging (Avgoustakis et al., 2002; Power, Slattery, and Lee, 2011; Rosen et al., 2011). Research is still primarily focused on developing biocompatible and biodegradable NMs to integrate multimodal imaging with theranostic nanoplatforms. This would enable accurate disease detection and customized treatment plans, revolutionizing healthcare.

8.2. Diagnostics at the Point-of-Care (POC) and Nano-Biosensors

To diagnose COVID-19, doctors currently mostly use conventional diagnostic techniques including RT-PCR, ELISA, and chest X-ray radiography (Carter et al., 2020). When it comes to high specificity and sensitivity in viral nucleic acid amplification, RT-PCR is still the gold standard. Through distinctive consolidation lesions, complementary radiological exams—especially CT imaging—help identify COVID-19 (Song et al., 2020; Younes et al., 2020; Zu et al., 2020). However, the need for highly trained staff and complex laboratory facilities limits the applicability of these procedures for mass screening, particularly in distant or resource-poor environments (Ravi et al., 2020; Zainol et al., 2020). Moreover, diminishing viral loads cause molecular diagnostic test reliability to decline with illness progression, requiring creative solutions for effective large-scale screening. Point-of-care (POC) diagnostic devices have several benefits, including low sample processing requirements, portability, and affordability. These tools use readily collectible samples, such as saliva or nasal swabs, and do away with the need to transfer samples to laboratories for analysis. They also shorten processing times. As a result, POC diagnostics allow for the quick identification of the virus, antigens, or antibodies, which helps with timely clinical judgments and quarantine procedures. Immunoassay platforms used in POC diagnostics have attracted a lot of interest due to their rapid on-site detection capabilities, which reduce false-positive rates and improve disease management (Morales-Narváez and Dincer, 2020; Ravi et al., 2020; Wen et al., 2020). In order to better integrate these platforms into epidemiological investigations and outbreak control, research is actively focused on their refinement.

8.2.1. Utilizing Nanomaterials (NMs) to Improve POC Diagnostics

POC diagnostics are revolutionized by NMs, which dramatically increase assay sensitivity and specificity. Their special qualities, like high surface area, tunability, and biocompatibility, make it possible to create sophisticated diagnostic tests (Barbosa et al., 2021; Nasirzadeh, Golbabaei, and Omari, 2022; Sui et al., 2021).

Because of their adaptability and capacity to interact with biomolecules such as antibodies and antigens, nanoparticles, nanotubes, and nanowires are frequently employed in POC diagnostics (Erathodiyil and Ying, 2011; Li et al., 2020; Wan et al., 2011). These interactions increase the sensitivity of the assay, making it possible to identify minuscule amounts of analytes. Nanotubes and nanowires offer special electrical and optical properties for sensitive biosensor applications, while nanoparticles can be functionalized with certain antibodies for targeted detection (Li et al., 2020; Sui et al., 2021).

8.2.2. Nano-Biosensor Technologies: Applications for Point-of-Care (POC)

A viable platform for quick and portable POC diagnostics is lateral flow immunoassay (LFIA) with colloidal gold nanoparticles (AuNPs). Through the conjugation of particular SARS-CoV-2 antigens to AuNPs fixed on a nitrocellulose membrane, LFIA demonstrates remarkable sensitivity and specificity in facilitating the detection of COVID-19 antibodies in blood samples in as little as 15 to 20 minutes (Li et al., 2020; Pan et al., 2020). Even with the potential, there are still issues with cost-effectiveness, manufacturing simplicity, regulatory barriers, and analytical specificity. Ongoing research aims to improve the usability and accessibility of nanobiosensors for efficient POC diagnostics by developing low-cost NMs, integrating microfluidic technologies, and incorporating artificial intelligence (AI).

8.3. Diagnostic Imaging Technologies Based on Nanoparticles

Radiation exposure and ambiguous results are two major limitations of conventional procedures like CT scans and X-rays (Pal et al., 2021). To overcome these obstacles, scientists are utilizing nanoparticle-based technologies, taking advantage of their special characteristics to improve imaging accuracy and security.

Improved contrast capabilities and the ability to target certain disease biomarkers with nanoparticles lead to improved diagnostic accuracy (Chouhan, Verma, and Singh, 2024). Nanoparticles such as QDs and AuNPs are especially attractive for COVID-19 because of their biocompatibility and capacity to improve imaging modalities including CT and fluorescence-based techniques (Cao et al., 2020; Oliveira et al., 2023). These nanoparticles reduce radiation exposure concerns in addition to improving imaging clarity of lung abnormalities linked to COVID-19 (Sodickson et al., 2009).

To improve diagnostic capacities even further, research is currently being conducted to produce sophisticated nanoparticle probes and investigate multimodal imaging techniques (Trivedi et al., 2022). Nanoparticle-based imaging has the potential to transform COVID-19 diagnosis by utilizing these developments, allowing for early detection, accurate disease monitoring, and individualized treatment plans (Skjøt-Arkil et al., 2021; World Health Organization [WHO], 2020). In addition to improving patient care, this revolutionary technology is expected to increase readiness for potential infectious disease epidemics in the future (Duan et al., 2021; Wang, Liu, and Pang, 2021).

8.4. PCR and Quick Testing Enhanced by Nanotechnology

The ongoing COVID-19 pandemic has brought attention to how urgently accessible, quick, and accurate diagnostic methods are needed. Modern techniques including LFIAs and polymerase chain reaction (PCR) have proven essential in detecting SARS-CoV-2 infections (Meumann and Robson, 2023). The gold standard, PCR, has a high sensitivity for detecting viral RNA but is expensive, time-consuming, and needs skilled workers and specialized equipment (Kashif, Acharya, and Khalil, 2024; To et al., 2020). Though they produce answers quickly, rapid antigen tests are less sensitive, especially when it comes to identifying low viral loads, which can result in false negative results (Cavalera et al., 2021; Smithgall et al., 2021). There are promising opportunities to improve these diagnostic techniques through nanotechnology. Similar to AuNPs, nanoparticle probes can lower cycle thresholds, increase amplification through better temperature uniformity, and improve local concentration effects, all of which can increase PCR efficiency (Li et al., 2005). Moreover, real-time monitoring is made possible by nanobiosensors combined with PCR, which expedites processing and shortens test times (Pradhan et al., 2021). Antibody-conjugated nanoparticles improve sensitivity in fast antigen tests by making it simpler to capture and identify viral antigens, which is essential for increasing accuracy, particularly in situations with low viral loads (Chen et al., 2022; Muttaqien et al., 2023). These developments in nanotechnology have the potential to completely transform COVID-19 diagnosis, providing quicker, more accurate, and more affordable testing options—all of which are critical for managing the disease and implementing global public health initiatives.

8.5. Antiviral Drug Delivery Using Nanocarriers

Viral infections are the primary cause of many global health issues, from minor colds to serious illnesses like HIV/AIDS. The cornerstone of treatment techniques is antiviral medicines, which target different stages of the viral life cycle (Kausar et al., 2021). However, classical delivery methods have several drawbacks, including low bioavailability, drug resistance brought on by viral alterations, and non-specific targeting that can have negative effects (Chen et al., 2021; Yao et al., 2020).

The COVID-19 pandemic has highlighted how urgently improved antiviral therapies are needed. Even with the introduction of vaccines, the creation of effective and safe antiviral drugs is still essential. A potential remedy is provided by nanotechnology, more especially using nanocarriers, which are microscopic particles that can transport medications precisely (Maus, Strait, and Zhu, 2021; Milovanovic et al., 2017). By removing biological barriers, increasing medication absorption, and facilitating targeted therapy to sick cells, these nanocarriers can improve drug delivery and perhaps lower side effects while increasing therapeutic efficacy.

Regarding COVID-19, researchers are investigating the potential of several nanocarriers, such as polymeric nanoparticles, liposomes, dendrimers, and carbon nanotubes (CNTs)/graphene, to encapsulate vaccines and antiviral medications (Charelli et al., 2022; Loutsch, Ong, and Hill, 2003; Muzata, Gebrekrstos, and Ray, 2021; Orecchioni et al., 2014; Ramana et al., 2015; Zhou et al., 2023). Through the precise delivery of therapeutic payloads, these systems aim to improve treatment outcomes by utilizing both active targeting through particular ligands and passive targeting through the lung's inflammatory milieu (Attia et al., 2019; Bandopadhyay et al., 2019). To fully realize the potential of nanocarriers in the fight against viral diseases such as COVID-19, further research should concentrate on improving their design and targeting tactics. This could pave the way for the development of more potent antiviral treatments (Figures 8.2 and 8.3).

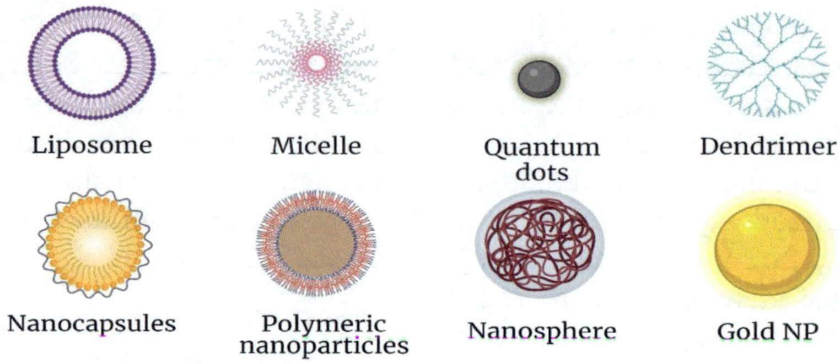

Figure 8.2. Types of nanocarriers.

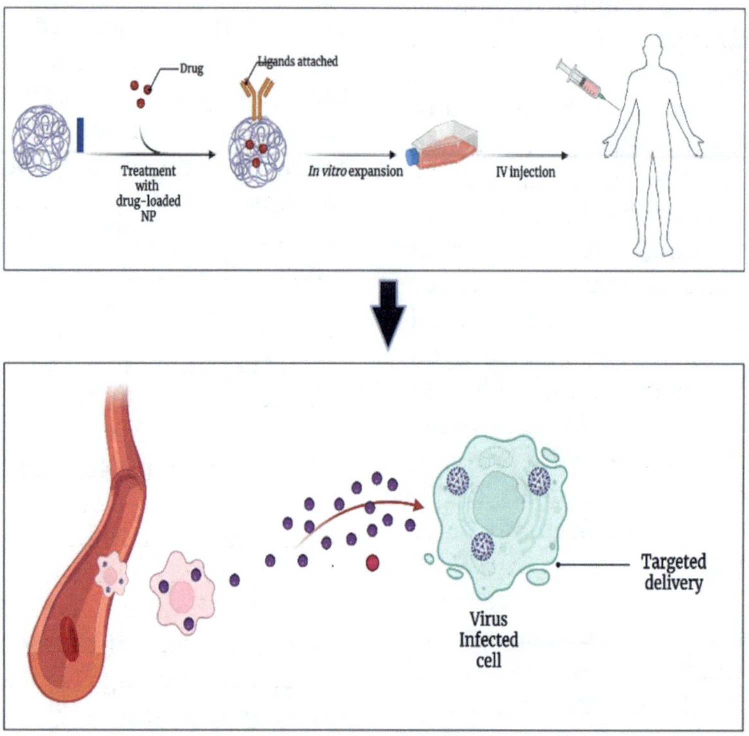

Figure 8.3. Targeted drug delivery through nanocarriers.

8.6. Design and Development of Nanovaccines

The COVID-19 pandemic, which was sparked by SARS-CoV-2, has presented significant challenges to international healthcare systems, underscoring the urgent need for efficacious vaccinations. Conventional vaccine development encounters many challenges, including long manufacturing lead times and scaling constraints (Allebeck, 2021; Ellebedy and Ahmed, 2016). Through the use of materials at the nanoscale to improve stability, precise antigen delivery, and immune system activation, nanotechnology offers a viable answer in the form of nanovaccines (Gurunathan et al., 2024; Shahbazi and Santos, 2015).

Vaccine design is being revolutionized by nanovaccines, which address issues like as genetic diversity and antigenic drift observed in viruses such as SARS-CoV-2 (Kennedy et al., 2023; Yewdell, 2021). These vaccines enhance immune responses by improving antigen stability, extending antibody release, and facilitating targeted delivery of antigens to immune cells by the encapsulation of antigens in nanoparticles (Bhardwaj et al., 2020; Gheibi Hayat, and Darroudi, 2019). A variety of platforms, each with specific benefits in antigen presentation and immune activation, are available for the delivery of vaccines, including liposomes, polymeric nanoparticles, and dendrimers (Ben-Akiva et al., 2019; Peng et al., 2009; Tretiakova and Vodovozova, 2022).

The potential of nanovaccines to transform preventive healthcare by inducing strong and long-lasting immune responses is highlighted by our growing understanding of their underlying mechanisms (Celis-Giraldo et al., 2021; Kim, Kye, and Yun, 2019). Nanovaccines have the potential to address not only COVID-19 but also future viral threats by utilizing sophisticated vaccination technologies and overcoming the limits of regular vaccines (Hasanzadeh et al., 2021; Smith, Simon, and Baker, 2013).

8.7. Repurposing Drugs Enabled by Nanotechnology

The urgent need for efficient medicines to stop the virus's spread and severity has been highlighted by the COVID-19 pandemic. Despite major advancements in vaccines, there is still a pressing need for easily available therapies for individuals who have already contracted the disease. By utilizing pharmaceuticals with proven safety profiles and pharmacokinetics, repurposing authorized medications offers a quick solution to address this demand and speed up clinical testing procedures (Cha et al., 2018; Govender and Chuturgoon, 2022). Nevertheless, there are issues with conventional repurposing methods, like low bioavailability and potential for toxicity and off-target effects (Dey, 2021; Pushpakom et al., 2018), which call for creative ways to increase their efficacy.

To precisely manage medication distribution, nanotechnology leverages the unique qualities of nanoparticles, such as size and surface characteristics (Singh and Lillard, 2009). This presents a disruptive answer to these problems. Medication stability and bioavailability can be greatly increased by encasing it in nanoparticles, which maximizes therapeutic effects (Kumari et al., 2014). Additionally, targeted distribution to diseased cells or tissues is made possible by nanotechnology, which minimizes systemic side effects and maximizes treatment efficacy (Elumalai, Srinivasan, and Shanmugam, 2024; Mishra and Singh, 2020). By lowering dosage frequency and sustaining therapeutic levels for longer periods, controlled release mechanisms further improve therapy efficacy (Cheng, Xie, and Sun, 2023; Kumar et al., 2023).

This novel strategy not only makes repurposed drugs more effective against COVID-19, but it also creates opportunities for combination therapies and targeted immunomodulatory treatments—both of which are essential for treating severe cases (El-Saber Batiha, Al-Gareeb, Saad, and Al-Kuraishy, 2022; Gurunathan et al., 2018). Ongoing developments promise to speed the transfer of nanotechnology-driven treatments from the lab to clinical practice, providing optimism for better outcomes in the worldwide fight against COVID-19 (De Ribeiro and Fonseca, 2020; Petkar et al., 2021), despite obstacles in nanocarrier optimization and regulatory approval.

8.8. Nanotherapeutics: COVID-19-Targeted Methods

The COVID-19 epidemic has presented challenges to the international healthcare community, emphasizing the need for novel ways to therapy. With the development of innovative techniques for targeted drug delivery through nanotherapeutics, nanotechnology has emerged as a viable remedy (Prasad et al., 2018). Through the utilization of distinct characteristics of NMs such as liposomes, polymeric nanoparticles, and micelles, these systems improve the stability, solubility, and efficacy of medicinal medications in the context of COVID-19 (Kumari et al., 2014). By using functionalized nanocarriers with ligands or antibodies, nanotherapeutics enable precise targeting of virus-infected cells or tissues, minimizing off-target effects, and optimizing treatment outcomes (Rizvi and Saleh, 2018; Singh and Lillard, 2009). These systems' built-in controlled release mechanisms guarantee continuous drug delivery, enhancing patient compliance and preserving therapeutic concentrations at the infection site (Calvo et al., 1997; Sofia, 2015).

A paradigm shift has occurred with the use of nanotechnology into COVID-19 therapy, especially in addressing the virus's range of clinical symptoms, from asymptomatic patients to severe respiratory illness (National Institutes of Health [NIH], 2020). While supportive care and symptom control are the main focuses of current treatment approaches, nanotherapeutics provide a special platform for targeted therapy that minimizes systemic exposure and maximizes therapeutic effects (Mishra and Singh, 2020). Micelles, liposomes, and polymeric nanoparticles are examples of nanocarrier-based drug delivery systems (DDS) that are specifically made to encapsulate and transport therapeutic chemicals. By increasing the solubility, stability, and bioavailability of the drug, these systems maximize therapeutic efficacy while minimizing systemic side effects (Charelli et al., 2022; Elumalai, Srinivasan, and Shanmugam, 2024; Gurunathan et al., 2018; Kumar et al., 2023; Milovanovic et al., 2017). Both active and passive targeting techniques improve the accuracy of drug administration; active targeting attaches ligands to overexpressed receptors on infected cells, while passive targeting takes advantage of the pathological characteristics of infected tissues (Attia et al., 2019; Ben-Akiva et al., 2019; Khatun et al., 2023; Milovanovic et al., 2017). Antiviral or immunomodulatory drugs can be delivered precisely by using nanocarriers that are aimed towards SARS-CoV-2 spike proteins or ACE2 receptors, which are essential for viral entry (Kim et al., 2022; Rak, Isakova-Sivak, and Rudenko, 2023). Through the maintenance of ideal drug concentrations at the infection site, the reduction of dosage frequency, and the improvement of patient compliance, controlled release mechanisms further improve treatment outcomes (Chen et al., 2021; Moghimi, Hunter, and Murray, 2001; Vandervoort and Ludwig, 2007). Furthermore, combined therapy strategies utilizing nanotherapeutics exhibit potential in tackling the complex nature of COVID-19, providing synergistic outcomes by focusing on distinct phases of the virus' lifecycle (Gurunathan et al., 2018). In general, nanotherapeutics provide a fresh and practical approach to getting beyond the drawbacks of traditional medication delivery systems, improving treatment outcomes and possibly revolutionizing the way that global health crises are handled (Jeon et al., 2023; Kausar et al., 2021).

8.8.1. Personal Protective Equipment (PPE) and Nanomaterials (NMs) for COVID-19

The COVID-19 epidemic has highlighted the vital role that personal protective equipment (PPE) plays in protecting the public and frontline workers (Hoernke et al., 2021). Although face masks, gloves, eye protection, and gowns are examples of traditional PPE, they have drawbacks, including discomfort, waste generation, and shortages of supplies (Atta et al., 2023; Çiriş et al., 2022; Kolb et al., 2023; Li et al., 2020; Manookian et al., 2022). PPE can be significantly improved with nanotechnology thanks to the introduction of materials that increase durability, comfort, and protection. NMs, such as self-cleaning surfaces and antibacterial nanoparticles, lower the risk of contamination and increase the longevity of PPE (Phuna et al., 2023). Furthermore, hydrophobic coatings improve breathability and lessen fogging, while nanoporous membranes boost filtration effectiveness (Mahapatra et al., 2020; Palmieri et al., 2021). PPE with smart sensor integration can monitor in real time, improving safety (Nanjunda et al., 2022).

The use of nanotechnology in PPE offers notable improvements. Superior filtration is provided by nanofiber masks, and the risk of viral transmission is decreased by gowns coated with antimicrobial nanoparticles (Essa et al., 2021). NMs enable PPE that is durable and reusable, which addresses supply chain and waste issues (Phuna et al., 2023). By using this novel strategy, PPE becomes more sustainable and effective while offering users increased comfort and protection. In order to overcome present obstacles and realize the full potential of nanotechnology in PPE, ongoing research and development are essential. In the end, this will help the public and frontline workers combat COVID-19 and other pandemics.

8.8.2. Air Filtration and Purification Using Nanotechnology for COVID-19

In order to stop the spread of SARS-CoV-2, modern air filtration and purification technologies are necessary, as the COVID-19 pandemic has highlighted. The need for creative solutions is highlighted by the fact that while conventional techniques like HEPA and mechanical filters have offered basic protection, they are limited in their ability to capture virus particles and bioaerosols (Oberg and Brosseau, 2008; Roy et al., 2018; Yit, Chew, and Yau, 2020). Nanotechnology provides a revolutionary potential for air filtration systems with materials like nanoporous membranes, electrostatic nanofibers, photocatalytic NMs, and antimicrobial nanoparticles, improving filtration efficiency and viral inactivation (Damokhi et al., 2022; Le et al., 2024; Mousavi et al., 2024).

High-efficiency (HE) nanofilters, for example, are nanotechnology-enabled air filters that are more effective than traditional HEPA filters at capturing smaller airborne particles (Leung and Sun, 2020). Novelties such as self-cleaning filters that employ photocatalytic or antimicrobial NMs consistently eliminate ensnared viruses, diminishing the possibility of contamination and prolonging the lifespan of the filter (Aghababai Beni, and Jabbari, 2022). By utilizing these technologies, portable air purifiers can effectively and conveniently clean the air in high-risk situations, hence reducing the spread of viruses (Guo et al., 2021; Zhai et al., 2021). Nonetheless, there are still issues with guaranteeing the safety, affordability, and scalability of air filters based on NMs (Zhai et al., 2021). Optimizing the application of nanotechnology in air purification will improve public health protection by addressing these problems through ongoing research and development (Singh, Ali, and Kale, 2023).

8.8.3. Cold Chain Management for Vaccines and Nanotechnology

The delivery of COVID-19 vaccinations, which is supported by the difficult effort of preserving the cold chain to guarantee vaccine efficacy, represents a critical turning point in the pandemic's fight (Wouters et al., 2021). Because vaccines are sensitive biological products, they must be kept at a precise temperature throughout the production and administration processes to avoid deterioration (Dumpa et al., 2019). The COVID-19 pandemic has brought to light issues with the cold chain, including susceptibility to temperature, limitations in infrastructure, and the requirement for ongoing maintenance and monitoring (Hanson et al., 2017; Hatchett, 2017). These challenges highlight the need for creative ways to improve vaccine stability and simplify distribution.

Nanotechnology offers viable solutions to these cold chain problems. Improved lyophilization methods, desiccant NMs, and thermostabilizing nanocarriers can all increase vaccine stability and possibly enable greater storage and transportation temperatures (Abdelwahed et al., 2006; Ghaemmaghamian et al., 2022; Pati, Shevtsov, and Sonawane, 2018). Particularly in environments with limited resources, these developments can lower expenses, loosen temperature restrictions, and increase vaccination accessibility (Ghaemmaghamian et al., 2022; Pati, Shevtsov, and Sonawane, 2018). Strict testing, regulatory clearance, public acceptability, and environmental monitoring are necessary to fully achieve these benefits (Ensar and Topaloglu, 2023; Jia et al., 2021; Pati, Shevtsov, and Sonawane, 2018). In order to fully utilize nanotechnology's revolutionary potential in vaccine cold chain management and eventually improve international vaccination campaigns against COVID-19 and other infectious illnesses, more research and cooperation are required.

8.9. Regulatory Aspects of Nanomedicine for COVID-19

Global efforts to create new treatments have been sparked by the emergence of COVID-19, with nanomedicine emerging as a particularly promising approach. This quickly developing discipline has the potential to completely change how diseases, like COVID-19, are identified, treated, and prevented. But there are several obstacles to overcome to guarantee the safe and efficient application of nanomedicines when negotiating the intricate regulatory environment (Vahedifard and Chakravarthy, 2021). This subtopic looks at the complexities of the regulations, emphasizing how to balance innovation with efficacy and safety—especially in light of the pandemic's pressing demands.

Traditional pharmaceutical regulatory frameworks, such as those overseen by the EMA and FDA, involve rigorous preclinical and clinical trials to ensure drug safety, efficacy, and quality (Marchetti and Schellens, 2007). However, these frameworks are often insufficient for nanomedicines due to their unique properties and potential risks (Ali, Neha, and Parveen, 2023). Specific considerations for nanomedicines in COVID-19 include thorough nanocarrier characterization, understanding biodistribution and pharmacokinetics, and assessing immunotoxicity and environmental impacts (Hofer et al., 2022; Hoshyar et al., 2016; Joseph et al., 2023; Manaia et al., 2017; Ray et al., 2021). Addressing these factors within regulatory frameworks is crucial for advancing nanomedicines from concept to clinical application.

In response to the pandemic, regulatory agencies have implemented expedited pathways, such as fast-track designations, rolling submissions, and guidance documents to hasten the approval of promising COVID-19 treatments, including nanomedicines (Bauer et al., 2022; Marinus et al., 2022; Michaeli et al., 2023). These measures aim to balance speed and safety, ensuring that potentially life-saving treatments reach patients quickly while maintaining rigorous safety standards (Cole et al., 2022). Ongoing challenges include harmonizing global regulatory frameworks and conducting comprehensive post-market surveillance to monitor long-term safety and efficacy (Scheppler et al., 2021).

These initiatives are essential for the global advancement of nanomedicine treatments for COVID-19, ultimately enhancing public health outcomes.

8.10. Ethical Concerns and Public View of COVID-19 Responses

The COVID-19 pandemic has posed not only scientific and medical challenges but also fundamental ethical dilemmas, sparking debates on the values guiding public health initiatives and resource allocation (Aliyu, 2021). These ethical concerns influence public opinion and legislative actions, shaping responses to the pandemic. Key ethical considerations include balancing public health measures with individual liberties, ensuring equitable access to vaccines and treatments, upholding research ethics amid accelerated vaccine development, and addressing misinformation that undermines public trust in scientific institutions (Bolcato et al., 2021; Coors et al., 2017; Foo et al., 2022; Grady, 2004; Purnat et al., 2021).

Public perception of COVID-19 responses varies, influenced by factors such as the perceived effectiveness of lockdowns and mask mandates, economic impacts, and concerns about personal freedoms (Mehta et al., 2020; Oberman, 2022). Vaccine hesitancy, fueled by misinformation and skepticism about vaccine safety and efficacy, remains a significant barrier to achieving widespread immunization (Rodrigues et al., 2023; Troiano and Nardi, 2021). The pandemic's economic and social impacts, including unemployment, business closures, and mental health issues, further affect public perceptions and trust in response efforts (Kamble et al., 2022; Levy and Filippini, 2021).

Addressing these ethical concerns and building public trust requires transparent, scientifically grounded communication from public health authorities (Kerr et al., 2022; Payne, 2007). Community engagement, equitable resource distribution, and maintaining scientific integrity are essential for fostering trust and promoting responsible decision-making (Maccaro et al., 2023). Combating misinformation through media literacy and factual information dissemination is also crucial. By understanding public attitudes and employing effective communication strategies, stakeholders can navigate ethical complexities and enhance pandemic preparedness for future crises (Dame Adjin-Tettey, 2022).

8.11. Beyond Nanomedicine: Future Directions in ARS-CoV-2 Therapeutics

In their quest to combat SARS-CoV-2, scientists have explored cutting-edge therapeutic approaches, leading to a paradigm shift toward innovative treatments. This sub-topic, "Beyond Nanomedicine: Future Directions in SARS-CoV-2 Therapeutics," delves into the evolving landscape of therapeutics, highlighting the urgent need for diverse strategies beyond conventional medicine. Gene editing, especially using CRISPR/Cas9 technology, offers a promising path for targeting viral replication and enhancing host immune responses. However, challenges such as delivery systems and off-target effects must be addressed to fully harness its potential (Alamgir and Haider, 2023; Machkovech et al., 2024) (Figure 8.4).

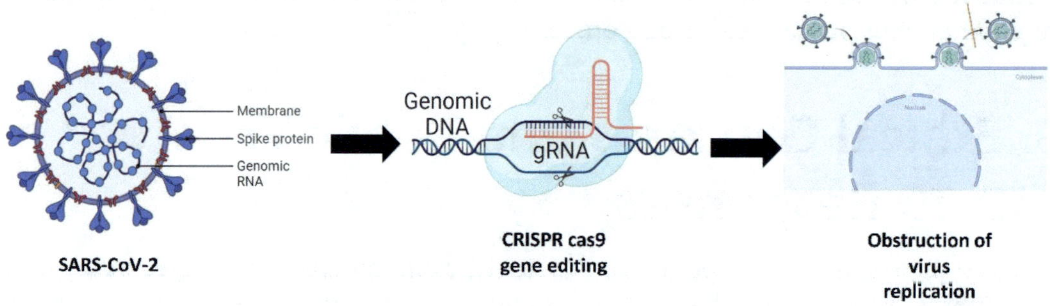

Figure 8.4. Gene-editing technologies for SARS-CoV-2.

Immunotherapy emerges as a key strategy, utilizing monoclonal antibodies, passive vaccination, and cell-based therapies like natural killer cells and mesenchymal stem cells (MSCs) to boost the body's defenses against COVID-19 (Bonam et al., 2020; Pashaei and Rezaei, 2020; Shanmugaraj et al., 2020; Shanmugaraj, Malla, and Phoolcharoen, 2020; Xu et al., 2020). Additionally, AI accelerates drug repurposing and vaccine development by analyzing molecular interactions and identifying potential therapeutic candidates (Beck et al., 2020; Kaushal et al., 2022; Wang et al., 2020). Personalized medicine further refines these approaches, tailoring treatments to patient subgroups based on genetic and clinical factors, thereby improving therapeutic efficacy and minimizing side effects (Su et al., 2024).

Phage display technology, antibody cocktails, and vaccines targeting proteins beyond the viral spike protein present further avenues for targeted viral neutralization and broader defense against new strains (Chakraborty, Bhattacharya, and Dhama, 2023; Du et al., 2009; Kuhn et al., 2016; Li et al., 2022). The integration of AI, immunotherapy, and personalized medicine represents a formidable arsenal against COVID-19, offering a path to more effective and tailored treatments. This sub-topic underscores the necessity of exploring these innovative therapeutic approaches to address the ongoing challenges posed by SARS-CoV-2 and enhance patient outcomes.

8.12. Research on Nanomedicine: Obstacles and Prospects

Nanomedicine is a cutting-edge field that offers customized and focused therapeutic treatments for the prevention and treatment of sickness. The difficulties and prospects in nanomedicine research are examined in this topic, along with the obstacles related to biocompatibility and regulations. These include the creation of DDS, diagnostic instruments, and therapeutic agents at the nanoscale. Notwithstanding these obstacles, nanomedicine offers the potential to enhance drug efficacy, minimize adverse effects, and facilitate tailored disease management. Offering a research roadmap, it also emphasizes promising opportunities such as tailored medication administration, drug resistance tactics, novel imaging techniques, and theranostics.

8.12.1. Overcoming Obstacles and Future Prospects

Although there is much potential for nanomedicine to revolutionize healthcare, there are still many obstacles to overcome. Size, surface properties, and drug loading capacity must all be carefully considered when designing nanocarriers for targeted drug delivery in order to effectively transport therapeutic payloads across physiological barriers (Tavares et al., 2021; Zhang et al., 2017). Clinical translation requires an understanding of *in vivo* behavior and biodistribution, which necessitates careful evaluation to guarantee safety and effectiveness (Kumar et al., 2010). Addressing scalability, cost-effectiveness, and regulatory compliance concerns is necessary to close the gap between preclinical success and clinical use (Han e al., 2019; Wolfram et al., 2015). To guarantee therapeutic efficacy and safety, standardizing characterization procedures and putting in place strong quality control (QC) methods are essential (Rani et al., 2022).

To address these obstacles, researchers use cutting-edge techniques like computational modeling, biocompatible NMs, and stakeholder engagement (Gimondi et al., 2023; Khan et al., 2022; Kyriakides et al., 2021; Lama, Merlin-Zhang, and Yang, 2020; Peltonen, 2018; Shamsi et al., 2019). The potential of nanomedicine includes fighting drug resistance, theranostics, and precise medication administration. By using nanocarriers to deliver medications straight to illness locations, systemic exposure and off-target effects are decreased, improving therapeutic efficacy (Patra et al., 2018; Rhaman et al., 2022). Real-time illness monitoring and individualized treatment are made possible by theranostic platforms, which integrate therapeutic and diagnostic capabilities (Prabhu and Patravale, 2012). By specifically targeting resistant cells and altering cellular absorption pathways, nanomedicines also treat drug resistance (Charelli et al., 2022; Hetta et al., 2023; Wang, Zhang, and Chen, 2019).

In conclusion, precise, customized therapies are the key to unlocking the revolutionary potential of nanomedicine. By utilizing creative solutions to address design, regulatory, and translational obstacles, nanomedicine can reach its full potential and usher in a new era of effective and customized healthcare delivery.

KEY TERMS FROM THIS CHAPTER

- artificial intelligence
- COVID-19
- nanomedicine
- point-of-care
- biosensor
- healthcare
- personal protective equipment
- polymerase chain reaction

References

1. Abdelwahed, W., Degobert, G., Stainmesse, S., & Fessi, H. (2006). Freeze-drying of nanoparticles: Formulation, process and storage considerations. *Advanced Drug Delivery Reviews, 58*(15). https://doi.org/10.1016/j.addr.2006.09.017.

2. Aghababai Beni, A., & Jabbari, H. (2022). Nanomaterials for environmental applications. *Results in Engineering, 15*. https://doi.org/10.1016/j.rineng.2022.100467.

3. Alamgir, W., & Haider, A. (2023). The nanomedicine revolution. *Life Sciences, 4*(2). https://doi.org/10.37185/lns.1.1.389.

4. Alekhin, A. P., Boleiko, G. M., Gudkova, S. A., et al. (2010). Synthesis of biocompatible surfaces by nanotechnology methods. *Nanotechnologies in Russia, 5*(9, 10). https://doi.org/10.1134/S1995078010090144.

5. Ali, F., Neha, K., & Parveen, S. (2023). Current regulatory landscape of nanomaterials and nanomedicines: A global perspective. *Journal of Drug Delivery Science and Technology, 80*. https://doi.org/10.1016/j.jddst.2022.104118.

6. Aliyu, A. A. (2021). Public health ethics and the COVID-19 pandemic. *Annals of African Medicine, 20*(3). https://doi.org/10.4103/aam.aam_80_20.

7. Allebeck, P. (2021). Richard Horton. The COVID-19 catastrophe: What's gone wrong and how to stop it happening again? *European Journal of Public Health, 31*(1). https://doi.org/10.1093/eurpub/ckaa216.

8. Atta, A. B., Imoro, A. Z., Agyemang, R. O., & Acheampong, N. A. (2023). The assessment of personal protective equipment waste management in a developing neighborhood: Examples of Tamale metropolis. *Clean Waste Systems, 6*. https://doi.org/10.1016/j.clwas.2023.100115.

9. Attia, M. F., Anton, N., Wallyn, J., Omran, Z., & Vandamme, T. F. (2019). An overview of active and passive targeting strategies to improve the nanocarriers efficiency to tumor sites. *Journal of Pharmacy and Pharmacology, 71*(8). https://doi.org/10.1111/jphp.13098.

10. Avgoustakis, K., Beletsi, A., Panagi, Z., Klepetsanis, P., Karydas, A. G., & Ithakissios, D. S. (2002). PLGA-mPEG nanoparticles of cisplatin: *In vitro* nanoparticle degradation, *in vitro* drug release, and *in vivo* drug residence in blood properties. *Journal of Controlled Release, 79*(1–3). https://doi.org/10.1016/S0168-3659(01)00530-2.

11. Bandopadhyay, S., Manchanda, S., Chandra, A., Ali, J., & Deb, P. K. (2019). Overview of different carrier systems for advanced drug delivery. In *Drug Delivery Systems*. https://doi.org/10.1016/B978-0-12-814487-9.00005-3.

12. Barbosa, A. I., Rebelo, R., Reis, R. L., Bhattacharya, M., & Correlo, V. M. (2021). Current nanotechnology advances in diagnostic biosensors. *Medical Devices & Sensors, 4*(1). https://doi.org/10.1002/mds3.10156.

13. Bauer, A., Eskat, A., Ntekim, A., et al. (2022). How COVID-19 changed clinical research strategies: A global survey. *Journal of International Medical Research, 50*(4). https://doi.org/10.1177/03000605221093179.

14. Beck, B. R., Shin, B., Choi, Y., Park, S., & Kang, K. (2020). Predicting commercially available antiviral drugs that may act on the novel coronavirus (SARS-CoV-2) through a drug-target interaction deep learning model. *Computational and Structural Biotechnology Journal, 18*.

https://doi.org/10.1016/j.csbj.2020.03.025.

15. Ben-Akiva, E., Est Witte, S., Meyer, R. A., Rhodes, K. R., & Green, J. J. (2019). Polymeric micro- and nanoparticles for immune modulation. *Biomaterials Science, 7*(1). https://doi.org/10.1039/c8bm01285g.
16. Bhardwaj, P., Bhatia, E., Sharma, S., Ahamad, N., & Banerjee, R. (2020). Advancements in prophylactic and therapeutic nano vaccines. *Acta Biomaterial, 108*. https://doi.org/10.1016/j.actbio.2020.03.020.
17. Bolcato, M., Rodriguez, D., Feola, A., et al. (2021). COVID-19 pandemic and equal access to vaccines. *Vaccines, 9*(6). https://doi.org/10.3390/vaccines9060538.
18. Bonam, S. R., Kaveri, S. V., Sakuntabhai, A., Gilardin, L., & Bayry, J. (2020). Adjunct immunotherapies for the management of severely ill COVID-19 patients. *Cell Reports Medicine, 1*(2). https://doi.org/10.1016/j.xcrm.2020.100016.
19. Calvo, P., Remuñan-López, C., Vila-Jato, J. L., & Alonso, M. J. (1997). Chitosan and chitosan/ethylene oxide-propylene oxide block copolymer nanoparticles as novel carriers for proteins and vaccines. *Pharmaceutical Research, 14*(10). https://doi.org/10.1023/A:1012128907225.
20. Cao, Z., Shu, Y., Qin, H., Su, B., & Peng, X. (2020). Quantum dots with highly efficient, stable, and multicolor electrochemiluminescence. *ACS Central Science, 6*(7). https://doi.org/10.1021/acscentsci.0c00484.
21. Carter, L. J., Garner, L. V., Smoot, J. W., et al. (2020). Assay techniques and test development for COVID-19 diagnosis. *ACS Central Science, 6*(5). https://doi.org/10.1021/acscentsci.0c00501.
22. Cavalera, S., Colitti, B., Rosati, S., et al. (2021). A multi-target lateral flow immunoassay enabling the specific and sensitive detection of total antibodies to SARS-CoV-2. *Talanta, 223*. https://doi.org/10.1016/j.talanta.2020.121737.
23. Celis-Giraldo, C. T., López-Abán, J., Muro, A., Patarroyo, M. A., & Manzano-Román, R. (2021). Nano vaccines against animal pathogens: The latest findings. *Vaccines, 9*(9). https://doi.org/10.3390/vaccines9090988.
24. Cha, Y., Erez, T., Reynolds, I. J., et al. (2018). Drug repurposing from the perspective of pharmaceutical companies. *British Journal of Pharmacology, 175*(2). https://doi.org/10.1111/bph.13798.
25. Chakraborty, C., Bhattacharya, M., & Dhama, K. (2023). SARS-CoV-2 vaccines, vaccine development technologies, and significant efforts in vaccine development during the pandemic: The lessons learned might help to fight against the next pandemic. *Vaccines, 11*(3). https://doi.org/10.3390/vaccines11030682.
26. Charelli, L. E., de Mattos, G. C., de Jesus Sousa-Batista, A., Pinto, J. C., & Balbino, T. A. (2022). Polymeric nanoparticles as therapeutic agents against coronavirus disease. *Journal of Nanoparticle Research, 24*(1). https://doi.org/10.1007/s11051-022-05396-5.
27. Chen, C., Hu, H., Li, X., et al. (2022). Rapid detection of anti-SARS-CoV-2 antibody using a selenium nanoparticle-based lateral flow immunoassay. *IEEE Transactions on Nano Bioscience, 21*(1). https://doi.org/10.1109/TNB.2021.3105662.
28. Chen, R., Wang, T., Song, J., et al. (2021). Antiviral drug delivery system for enhanced bioactivity, better metabolism and pharmacokinetic characteristics. *International Journal of Nanomedicine, 16*. https://doi.org/10.2147/IJN.S315705.

29. Cheng, X., Xie, Q., & Sun, Y. (2023). Advances in nanomaterial-based targeted drug delivery systems. *Frontiers in Bioengineering and Biotechnology, 11*. https://doi.org/10.3389/fbioe.2023.1177151.

30. Chouhan, A. P. S., Verma, A., & Singh, V. (2024). The significance of nanomaterials in medical imaging and diagnostics. In *Advancements in Nanomedicine* (Chap. 12). https://doi.org/10.4018/979-8-3693-0448-8.ch012.

31. Çiriş Yildiz, C., Ulaşli Kaban, H., & Tanriverdi, F. Ş. (2022). COVID-19 pandemic and personal protective equipment: Evaluation of equipment comfort and user attitude. *Archives of Environmental & Occupational Health, 77*(1). https://doi.org/10.1080/19338244.2020.1828247.

32. Cole, A., Webster, P., Van Liew, D., Salas, M., Aimer, O., & Malikova, M. A. (2022). Safety surveillance and challenges in accelerated COVID-19 vaccine development. *Therapeutic Advances in Drug Safety, 13*. https://doi.org/10.1177/20420986221116452.

33. Coors, M., Bauer, L., Edwards, K., et al. (2017). Ethical issues related to clinical research and rare diseases. *Translational Science of Rare Diseases, 2*(3, 4). https://doi.org/10.3233/trd-170013.

34. Dame Adjin-Tettey, T. (2022). Combating fake news, disinformation, and misinformation: Experimental evidence for media literacy education. *Cogent Arts & Humanities, 9*(1). https://doi.org/10.1080/23311983.2022.2037229.

35. Damokhi, A., Yousefinejad, S., Fakherpour, A., & Jahangiri, M. (2022). Improvement of performance and function in respiratory protection equipment using nanomaterials. *Journal of Nanoparticle Research, 24*(4). https://doi.org/10.1007/s11051-022-05460-0.

36. De M Ribeiro, L. N., & Fonseca, B. B. (2020). The role of pharmaceutical nanotechnology in the time of COVID-19 pandemic. *Future Microbiology, 15*(16). https://doi.org/10.2217/fmb-2020-0118.

37. Dey, P. (2021). Low bioavailability hinders drug discovery against COVID-19, guided by *in silico* docking. *British Journal of Pharmacology, 178*(3). https://doi.org/10.1111/bph.15325.

38. Du, L., He, Y., Zhou, Y., Liu, S., Zheng, B. J., & Jiang, S. (2009). The spike protein of SARS-CoV–A target for vaccine and therapeutic development. *Nature Reviews Microbiology, 7*(3). https://doi.org/10.1038/nrmicro2090.

39. Duan, Y., Wang, S., Zhang, Q., Gao, W., & Zhang, L. (2021). Nanoparticle approaches against SARS-CoV-2 infection. *Current Opinion in Solid State and Materials Science, 25*(6). https://doi.org/10.1016/j.cossms.2021.100964.

40. Dumpa, N., Goel, K., Guo, Y., et al. (2019). Stability of vaccines. *AAPS Pharm SciTech, 20*(2). https://doi.org/10.1208/s12249-018-1254-2.

41. Ellebedy, A. H., & Ahmed, R. (2016). Antiviral vaccines: Challenges and advances. In *The Vaccine Book (2nd ed.)*. https://doi.org/10.1016/B978-0-12-802174-3.00015-1.

42. El-Saber Batiha, G., Al-Gareeb, A. I., Saad, H. M., & Al-Kuraishy, H. M. (2022). COVID-19 and corticosteroids: A narrative review. *Inflammopharmacology, 30*(4). https://doi.org/10.1007/s10787-022-00987-z.

43. Elumalai, K., Srinivasan, S., & Shanmugam, A. (2024). Review of the efficacy of nanoparticle-based drug delivery systems for cancer treatment. *Biomedical Technology, 5*. https://doi.org/10.1016/j.bmt.2023.09.001.

44. Ensar Işık, E., & Topaloglu Yildiz, S. (2023). Optimizing the COVID-19 cold chain vaccine distribution network with medical waste management: A robust optimization approach. *Expert Systems with Applications, 229*. https://doi.org/10.1016/j.eswa.2023.120510.

45. Erathodiyil, N., & Ying, J. Y. (2011). Functionalization of inorganic nanoparticles for bioimaging applications. *Accounts of Chemical Research, 44*(10). https://doi.org/10.1021/ar2000327.

46. Essa, W. K., Yasin, S. A., Saeed, I. A., & Ali, G. A. M. (2021). Nanofiber-based face masks and respirators as COVID-19 protection: A review. *Membranes, 11*(4). https://doi.org/10.3390/membranes11040250.

47. Foo, C. D., Verma, M., Tan, S. M., et al. (2022). COVID-19 public health and social measures: A comprehensive picture of six Asian countries. *BMJ Global Health, 7*(11). https://doi.org/10.1136/bmjgh-2022-009863.

48. Ghaemmaghamian, Z., Zarghami, R., Walker, G., O'Reilly, E., & Ziaee, A. (2022). Stabilizing vaccines via drying: Quality by design considerations. *Advanced Drug Delivery Reviews, 187*. https://doi.org/10.1016/j.addr.2022.114313.

49. Gheibi Hayat, S. M., & Darroudi, M. (2019). Nano vaccine: A novel approach in immunization. *Journal of Cellular Physiology, 234*(8). https://doi.org/10.1002/jcp.28120.

50. Gimondi, S., Ferreira, H., Reis, R. L., & Neves, N. M. (2023). Microfluidic devices: A tool for nanoparticle synthesis and performance evaluation. *ACS Nano, 17*(15). https://doi.org/10.1021/acsnano.3c01117.

51. Gommersall, L., Shergill, I. S., Ahmed, H. U., et al. (2007). Nanotechnology and its relevance to the urologist. *European Urology, 52*(2). https://doi.org/10.1016/j.eururo.2007.04.065.

52. Govender, K., & Chuturgoon, A. (2022). An overview of repurposed drugs for potential COVID-19 treatment. *Antibiotics, 11*(12). https://doi.org/10.3390/antibiotics11121678.

53. Grady, C. (2004). Ethics of vaccine research. *Nature Immunology, 5*(5). https://doi.org/10.1038/ni0504-465.

54. Guo, L., Torii, R., Epstein, R., et al. (2021). Using portable air purifiers to reduce airborne transmission of infectious respiratory viruses–A computational fluid dynamics study. *medRxiv*. https://doi.org/10.1101/2021.02.03.21251057.

55. Gurunathan, S., Kang, M. H., Qasim, M., & Kim, J. H. (2018). Nanoparticle-mediated combination therapy: Two-in-one approach for cancer. *International Journal of Molecular Sciences, 19*(10). https://doi.org/10.3390/ijms19103264.

56. Gurunathan, S., Thangaraj, P., Wang, L., Cao, Q., & Kim, J. H. (2024). Nano vaccines: An effective therapeutic approach for cancer therapy. *Biomedicine & Pharmacotherapy, 170*. https://doi.org/10.1016/j.biopha.2023.115992.

57. Han, X., Xu, K., Taratula, O., & Farsad, K. (2019). Applications of nanoparticles in biomedical imaging. *Nanoscale, 11*(3). https://doi.org/10.1039/c8nr07769j.

58. Hanson, C. M., George, A. M., Sawadogo, A., & Schreiber, B. (2017). Is freezing in the vaccine cold chain an ongoing issue? A literature review. *Vaccine, 35*(17). https://doi.org/10.1016/j.vaccine.2016.09.070.

59. Hasanzadeh, A., Alamdaran, M., Ahmadi, S., et al. (2021). Nanotechnology against COVID-19: Immunization, diagnostic and therapeutic studies. *Journal of Controlled Release, 336*. https://doi.org/10.1016/j.jconrel.2021.06.036.

60. Hatchett, R. (2017). The medicines refrigerator and the importance of the cold chain in the safe storage of medicines. *Nursing Standard, 32*(6). https://doi.org/10.7748/ns.2017.e10960.

61. Hetta, H. F., Ramadan, Y. N., Al-Harbi, A. I., et al. (2023). Nanotechnology as a promising approach to combat multidrug resistant bacteria: A comprehensive review and future perspectives. *Biomedicines, 11*(2). https://doi.org/10.3390/biomedicines11020413.

62. Hoernke, K., Djellouli, N., Andrews, L., et al. (2021). Frontline healthcare workers' experiences with personal protective equipment during the COVID-19 pandemic in the UK: A rapid qualitative appraisal. *BMJ Open, 11*(1). https://doi.org/10.1136/bmjopen-2020-046199.

63. Hofer, S., Hofstätter, N., Punz, B., Hasenkopf, I., Johnson, L., & Himly, M. (2022). Immunotoxicity of nanomaterials in health and disease: Current challenges and emerging approaches for identifying immune modifiers in susceptible populations. *Wiley Interdisciplinary Reviews: Nanomedicine and Nanobiotechnology, 14*(6). https://doi.org/10.1002/wnan.1804.

64. Hoshyar, N., Gray, S., Han, H., & Bao, G. (2016). The effect of nanoparticle size on *in vivo* pharmacokinetics and cellular interaction. *Nanomedicine, 11*(6). https://doi.org/10.2217/nnm.16.5.

65. Jeon, W. J., Lee, H. K., Na, Y. G., et al. (2023). Antiviral lipid nanocarrier loaded with remdesivir effective against SARS-CoV-2 *in vitro* model. *International Journal of Nanomedicine, 18*. https://doi.org/10.2147/IJN.S391462.

66. Jia, L., Zhang, P., Sun, H., et al. (2021). Optimization of nanoparticles for smart drug delivery: A review. *Nanomaterials, 11*(11). https://doi.org/10.3390/nano11112790.

67. Joseph, T. M., Kar Mahapatra, D., Esmaeili, A., et al. (2023). Nanoparticles: Taking a unique position in medicine. *Nanomaterials, 13*(3). https://doi.org/10.3390/nano13030574.

68. Kamble, S., Joshi, A., Kamble, R., & Kumari, S. (2022). Influence of COVID-19 pandemic on psychological status: An elaborate review. *Cureus, 14*(10), e29820. https://doi.org/10.7759/cureus.29820.

69. Kashif, M., Acharya, S., & Khalil, A. (2024). Molecular interactions leading to advancements in the techniques for COVID-19 detection: A review. *Journal of AOAC International*. https://doi.org/10.1093/jaoacint/qsae010.

70. Kausar, S., Said Khan, F., Ishaq Mujeeb Ur Rehman, M., et al. (2021). A review: Mechanism of action of antiviral drugs. *International Journal of Immunopathology and Pharmacology, 35*. https://doi.org/10.1177/20587384211002621.

71. Kaushal, K., Sarma, P., Rana, S. V., Medhi, B., & Naithani, M. (2022). Emerging role of artificial intelligence in therapeutics for COVID-19: A systematic review. *Journal of Biomolecular Structure and Dynamics, 40*(10). https://doi.org/10.1080/07391102.2020.1855250.

72. Kennedy, N. A., Janjua, M., Chanchlani, N., et al. (2023). Vaccine escape, increased breakthrough and reinfection in infliximab-treated patients with IBD during the Omicron wave of the SARS-CoV-2 pandemic. *Gut, 72*(2). https://doi.org/10.1136/gutjnl-2022-327570.

73. Kerr, J. R., Schneider, C. R., Freeman, A. L. J., Marteau, T., & Van der Linden, S. (2022). Transparent communication of evidence does not undermine public trust in evidence. *PNAS Nexus, 1*(5). https://doi.org/10.1093/pnasnexus/pgac280.

74. Khan, I. S., Kauppila, O., Fatima, N., & Majava, J. (2022). Stakeholder interdependencies in a collaborative innovation project. *Journal of Innovation and Entrepreneurship, 11*(1). https://doi.org/10.1186/s13731-022-00229-0.

75. Khatun, S., Putta, C. L., Hak, A., & Rengan, A. K. (2023). Immunomodulatory nano systems: An emerging strategy to combat viral infections. *Biomaterials and Biosystems, 9*. https://doi.org/10.1016/j.bbiosy.2023.100073.

76. Kim, C. G., Kye, Y. C., & Yun, C. H. (2019). The role of nano vaccine in cross-presentation of antigen-presenting cells for the activation of CD8+ T cell responses. *Pharmaceutics, 11*(11). https://doi.org/10.3390/pharmaceutics11110612.

77. Kim, J., Jozic, A., Mukherjee, A., et al. (2022). Rapid generation of circulating and mucosal decoy human ACE2 using mRNA nanotherapeutics for the potential treatment of SARS-CoV-2. *Advanced Science, 9*(35). https://doi.org/10.1002/advs.202202556.

78. Kolb, J. P., Hättich, A., Strahl, A., et al. (2023). Does the COVID-19 personal protective equipment impair the surgeon's performance? *Archives of Orthopedic and Trauma Surgery, 143*(4). https://doi.org/10.1007/s00402-022-04416-2.

79. Kuhn, P., Fühner, V., Unkauf, T., et al. (2016). Recombinant antibodies for diagnostics and therapy against pathogens and toxins generated by phage display. *Proteomics–Clinical Applications, 10*(9, 10). https://doi.org/10.1002/prca.201600002.

80. Kumar, M., Hilles, A. R., Almurisi, S. H., Bhatia, A., & Mahmood, S. (2023). Micro and nano-carriers-based pulmonary drug delivery system: Their current updates, challenges, and limitations–A review. *JCIS Open, 12*. https://doi.org/10.1016/j.jciso.2023.100095.

81. Kumar, R., Roy, I., Ohulchanskky, T. Y., et al. (2010). *In vivo* biodistribution and clearance studies using multimodal organically modified silica nanoparticles. *ACS Nano, 4*. https://doi.org/10.1021/nn901146y.

82. Kumari, A., Singla, R., Guliani, A., & Yadav, S. K. (2014). Nanoencapsulation for drug delivery. *EXCLI Journal, 13*.

83. Kyriakides, T. R., Raj, A., Tseng, T. H., et al. (2021). Biocompatibility of nanomaterials and their immunological properties. *Biomedical Materials, 16*(4). https://doi.org/10.1088/1748-605X/abe5fa.

84. Lama, S., Merlin-Zhang, O., & Yang, C. (2020). *In vitro* and *in vivo* models for evaluating the oral toxicity of nanomedicines. *Nanomaterials, 10*(11). https://doi.org/10.3390/nano10112177.

85. Le, B., Omran, N., Elnabawy, E., et al. (2024). Exploring advances in nanofiber-based face masks: A comprehensive review of mechanical, electrostatic, and antimicrobial functionality filtration for the removal of airborne particulate matter and pathogens. *Emergent Materials*. https://doi.org/10.1007/s42247-023-00622-9.

86. Leung, W. W. F., & Sun, Q. (2020). Charged PVDF multilayer nanofiber filter in filtering simulated airborne novel coronavirus (COVID-19) using ambient nano-aerosols. *Separation and Purification Technology, 245*. https://doi.org/10.1016/j.seppur.2020.116887.

87. Levy, E., & Filippini, F. (2021). Social and economic impact of COVID-19. *Global Economics and Development*.

88. Li, K. K. W., Joussen, A. M., Kwan, J. K. C., & Steel, D. H. W. (2020). FFP3, FFP2, N95, surgical masks and respirators: What should we be wearing for ophthalmic surgery in the COVID-19 pandemic? *Graefe's Archive for Clinical and Experimental Ophthalmology, 258*(8). https://doi.org/10.1007/s00417-020-04751-3.

89. Li, L., Wei, Y., Yang, H., et al. (2022). Advances in next-generation coronavirus vaccines in response to future virus evolution. *Vaccines, 10*(12). https://doi.org/10.3390/vaccines10122035.

90. Li, M., Lin, Y. C., Wu, C. C., & Liu, H. S. (2005). Enhancing the efficiency of a PCR using gold nanoparticles. *Nucleic Acids Research, 33*(21). https://doi.org/10.1093/nar/gni183.

91. Li, X., Mo, J., Fang, J., et al. (2020). Vertical nanowire array-based biosensors: Device design strategies and biomedical applications. *Journal of Materials Chemistry B, 8*(34). https://doi.org/10.1039/d0tb00990c.

92. Lockman, P. R., Mumper, R. J., Khan, M. A., & Allen, D. D. (2002). Nanoparticle technology for drug delivery across the blood-brain barrier. *Drug Development and Industrial Pharmacy, 28*(1). https://doi.org/10.1081/DDC-120001481.

93. Loutsch, J. M., Ong, D., & Hill, J. M. (2003). Dendrimers: An innovative and enhanced ocular drug delivery system. In *Ophthalmic Drug Delivery Systems (2nd ed.)*. https://doi.org/10.4324/9781003113423-19.

94. Maccaro, A., Audia, C., Stokes, K., et al. (2023). Pandemic preparedness: A scoping review of best and worst practices from COVID-19. *Healthcare, 11*(18). https://doi.org/10.3390/healthcare11182572.

95. Machkovech, H. M., Hahn, A. M., Garonzik Wang, J., et al. (2024). Persistent SARS-CoV-2 infection: Significance and implications. *The Lancet Infectious Diseases*. https://doi.org/10.1016/S1473-3099(23)00815-0.

96. Mahapatra, P. S., Chatterjee, S., Tiwari, M. K., Ganguly, R., & Megaridis, C. M. (2020). Surface treatments to enhance the functionality of PPEs. *Transactions of the Indian National Academy of Engineering, 5*(2). https://doi.org/10.1007/s41403-020-00110-0.

97. Manaia, E. B., Abuçafy, M. P., Chiari-Andréo, B. G., Silva, B. L., Oshiro Junior, J. A., & Chiavacci, L. A. (2017). Physicochemical characterization of drug nanocarriers. *International Journal of Nanomedicine, 12*. https://doi.org/10.2147/IJN.S133832.

98. Manookian, A., Dehghan Nayeri, N., & Shahmari, M. (2022). Physical problems of prolonged use of personal protective equipment during the COVID-19 pandemic: A scoping review. *Nursing Forum, 57*(5). https://doi.org/10.1111/nuf.12735.

99. Marchetti, S., & Schellens, J. H. M. (2007). The impact of FDA and EMEA guidelines on drug development in relation to Phase 0 trials. *British Journal of Cancer, 97*(5). https://doi.org/10.1038/sj.bjc.6603925.

100. Marinus, R., Mofid, S., Mpandzou, M., & Kühler, T. C. (2022). Rolling reviews during COVID-19: The European Union experience in a global context. *Clinical Therapeutics, 44*(3). https://doi.org/10.1016/j.clinthera.2022.01.001.

101. Maus, A., Strait, L., & Zhu, D. (2021). Nanoparticles as delivery vehicles for antiviral therapeutic drugs. *Engineering Regeneration, 2*. https://doi.org/10.1016/j.engreg.2021.03.001.

102. Mehta, R., Mehta, R., Balaji, A., & Mehta, H. (2020). Perceptions on COVID-19: A ground-level analysis to guide public policy. *Lung India, 37*(3). https://doi.org/10.4103/lungindia.lungindia_190_20.

103. Mele, E., & Pisignano, D. (2009). Nanobiotechnology: Soft lithography. *Progress in Molecular and Subcellular Biology, 47*. https://doi.org/10.1007/978-3-540-88552-8_15.

104. Meumann, E. M., & Robson, J. M. B. (2023). Testing for COVID-19: A 2023 update. *Australian Prescriber, 46*(1). https://doi.org/10.18773/austprescr.2023.007.

105. Michaeli, D. T., Michaeli, T., Albers, S., Boch, T., & Michaeli, J. C. (2023). Special FDA designations for drug development: Orphan, fast track, accelerated approval, priority review, and breakthrough therapy. *European Journal of Health Economics*. https://doi.org/10.1007/s10198-023-01639-x.

106. Milovanovic, M., Arsenijevic, A., Milovanovic, J., Kanjevac, T., & Arsenijevic, N. (2017). Nanoparticles in antiviral therapy. In *Antimicrobial Nano Architectonics: From Synthesis to Applications*. https://doi.org/10.1016/B978-0-323-52733-0.00014-8.

107. Mishra, B., & Singh, J. (2020). Novel drug delivery systems and significance in respiratory diseases. In *Targeting Chronic Inflammatory Lung Diseases Using Advanced Drug Delivery Systems*. https://doi.org/10.1016/B978-0-12-820658-4.00004-2.

108. Moghimi, S. M., Hunter, A. C., & Murray, J. C. (2001). Long-circulating and target-specific nanoparticles: Theory to practice. *Pharmacological Reviews, 53*(2).

109. Morales-Narváez, E., & Dincer, C. (2020). The impact of biosensing in a pandemic outbreak: COVID-19. *Biosensors and Bioelectronics, 163*. https://doi.org/10.1016/j.bios.2020.112274.

110. Mousavi, S. M., Pouramini, Z., Babapoor, A., et al. (2024). Photocatalysis air purification systems for coronavirus removal: Current technologies and future trends. *Chemosphere, 353*. https://doi.org/10.1016/j.chemosphere.2024.141525.

111. Muttaqien, S. El, Khoris, I. M., Pambudi, S., & Park, E. Y. (2023). Nanosphere structures using various materials: A strategy for signal amplification for virus sensing. *Sensors, 23*(1). https://doi.org/10.3390/s23010160.

112. Muzata, T. S., Gebrekrstos, A., & Ray, S. S. (2021). Recent progress in modified polymer-based PPE in fight against COVID-19 and beyond. *ACS Omega, 6*(43). https://doi.org/10.1021/acsomega.1c04754.

113. Nanjunda, S. B., Seshadri, V. N., Krishnan, C., et al. (2022). Emerging nanophotonic biosensor technologies for virus detection. *Nanophotonic, 11*(22). https://doi.org/10.1515/nanoph-2022-0571.

114. Nasirzadeh, N., Golbabaei, F., & Omari Shekaftik, S. (2022). Laboratory activities involving nanomaterials: Risk assessment and investigating researchers' symptoms. *Nanoscale, 15*(6). https://doi.org/10.1039/d2nr06118j.

115. National Institutes of Health. (2020). Clinical spectrum of SARS-CoV-2 infection. *Radiology: Cardiothoracic Imaging, 2*(2).

116. Oberg, T., & Brosseau, L. M. (2008). Surgical mask filter and fit performance. *American Journal of Infection Control, 36*(4). https://doi.org/10.1016/j.ajic.2007.07.008.

117. Oberman, K. (2022). Freedom and viruses. *Ethics, 132*(4). https://doi.org/10.1086/719516.

118. Oliveira, B. B., Ferreira, D., Fernandes, A. R., & Baptista, P. V. (2023). Engineering gold nanoparticles for molecular diagnostics and biosensing. *Wiley Interdisciplinary Reviews: Nanomedicine and Nanobiotechnology, 15*(1). https://doi.org/10.1002/wnan.1836.

119. Orecchioni, M., Bedognetti, D., Sgarrella, F., Marincola, F. M., Bianco, A., & Delogu, L. G. (2014). Impact of carbon nanotubes and graphene on immune cells. *Journal of Translational Medicine, 12*(1). https://doi.org/10.1186/1479-5876-12-138.

120. Pal, A., Ali, A., Young, T. R., et al. (2021). Comprehensive literature review on the radiographic findings, imaging modalities, and the role of radiology in the COVID-19 pandemic. *World Journal of Radiology, 13*(9). https://doi.org/10.4329/wjr.v13.i9.258.

121. Palmieri, V., De Maio, F., De Spirito, M., & Papi, M. (2021). Face masks and nanotechnology: Keep the blue side up. *Nano Today, 37*. https://doi.org/10.1016/j.nantod.2021.101077.

122. Pan, Y., Li, X., Yang, G., et al. (2020). Serological immunochromatographic approach in diagnosis with SARS-CoV-2 infected COVID-19 patients. *Journal of Infection, 81*(1). https://doi.org/10.1016/j.jinf.2020.03.051.

123. Pashaei, M., & Rezaei, N. (2020). Immunotherapy for SARS-CoV-2: Potential opportunities. *Expert Opinion on Biological Therapy, 20*(10). https://doi.org/10.1080/14712598.2020.1807933.

124. Pati, R., Shevtsov, M., & Sonawane, A. (2018). Nanoparticle vaccines against infectious diseases. *Frontiers in Immunology, 9*. https://doi.org/10.3389/fimmu.2018.02224.

125. Patra, J. K., Das, G., Fraceto, L. F., et al. (2018). Nano based drug delivery systems: Recent developments and future prospects. *Journal of Nanobiotechnology, 16*(1). https://doi.org/10.1186/s12951-018-0392-8.

126. Payne, K. (2007). Ethical issues related to pandemic flu planning and response. *AACN Advanced Critical Care, 18*(4). https://doi.org/10.1097/01.AACN.0000298627.07535.76.

127. Peltonen, L. (2018). Practical guidelines for the characterization and quality control of pure drug nanoparticles and nano-cocrystals in the pharmaceutical industry. *Advanced Drug Delivery Reviews, 131*. https://doi.org/10.1016/j.addr.2018.06.009.

128. Peng, X. C., Peng, X. H., Liu, S. M., & Zhao, J. Q. (2009). Synthesis and properties of new amphoteric poly(amidoamine) dendrimers. *Express Polymer Letters, 3*(8). https://doi.org/10.3144/expresspolymlett.2009.63.

129. Petkar, K. C., Patil, S. M., Chavhan, S. S., et al. (2021). An overview of nanocarrier-based adjuvants for vaccine delivery. *Pharmaceutics, 13*(4). https://doi.org/10.3390/pharmaceutics13040455.

130. Phuna, Z. X., Panda, B. P., Hawala Shivashekaregowda, N. K., & Madhavan, P. (2023). Nano protection from SARS-COV-2: Would nanotechnology help in personal protection equipment (PPE) to control the transmission of COVID-19? *International Journal of Environmental Health Research, 33*(7). https://doi.org/10.1080/09603123.2022.2046710.

131. Power, S., Slattery, M. M., & Lee, M. J. (2011). Nanotechnology and its relationship to interventional radiology. Part I: Imaging. *Cardiovascular and Interventional Radiology, 34*(2). https://doi.org/10.1007/s00270-010-9961-4.

132. Prabhu, P., & Patravale, V. (2012). The upcoming field of theragnostic nanomedicine: An overview. *Journal of Biomedical Nanotechnology, 8*(6). https://doi.org/10.1166/jbn.2012.1459.

133. Pradhan, A., Lahare, P., Sinha, P., et al. (2021). Biosensors as nano-analytical tools for COVID-19 detection. *Sensors, 21*(23). https://doi.org/10.3390/s21237823.

134. Prasad, M., Lambe, U. P., Brar, B., et al. (2018). Nanotherapeutics: An insight into healthcare and multi-dimensional applications in medical sector of the modern world. *Biomedicine & Pharmacotherapy, 97*. https://doi.org/10.1016/j.biopha.2017.11.026.

135. Purnat, T. D., Vacca, P., Czerniak, C., et al. (2021). Infodemic signal detection during the COVID-19 pandemic: Development of a methodology for identifying potential information voids in online conversations. *JMIR Infodemiology, 1*(1). https://doi.org/10.2196/30971.

136. Pushpakom, S., Iorio, F., Eyers, P. A., et al. (2018). Drug repurposing: Progress, challenges and recommendations. *Nature Reviews Drug Discovery, 18*(1). https://doi.org/10.1038/nrd.2018.168.

137. Rak, A., Isakova-Sivak, I., & Rudenko, L. (2023). Overview of nucleocapsid-targeting vaccines against COVID-19. *Vaccines, 11*(12). https://doi.org/10.3390/vaccines11121810.

138. Ramana, L. N., Sharma, S., Sethuraman, S., Ranga, U., & Krishnan, U. M. (2015). Stealth anti-CD4 conjugated immunoliposomes with dual antiretroviral drugs–Modern Trojan horses to combat HIV. *European Journal of Pharmaceutics and Biopharmaceutics, 89*. https://doi.org/10.1016/j.ejpb.2014.11.021.

139. Rani, N. N. I. M., Chen, X. Y., Al-Zubaidi, Z. M., et al. (2022). Surface-engineered liposomes for dual-drug delivery targeting strategy against methicillin-resistant *Staphylococcus aureus* (MRSA). *Asian Journal of Pharmaceutical Sciences, 17*(1). https://doi.org/10.1016/j.ajps.2021.11.004.

140. Ravi, N., Cortade, D. L., Ng, E., & Wang, S. X. (2020). Diagnostics for SARS-CoV-2 detection: A comprehensive review of the FDA-EUA COVID-19 testing landscape. *Biosensors and Bioelectronics, 165*. https://doi.org/10.1016/j.bios.2020.112454.

141. Ray, P., Haideri, N., Haque, I., et al. (2021). The impact of nanoparticles on the immune system: A gray zone of nanomedicine. *Journal of Immunology and Immunotherapy, 5*(1). https://doi.org/10.29245/2578-3009/2021/1.1206.

142. Rhaman, M. M., Islam, M. R., Akash, S., et al. (2022). Exploring the role of nanomedicines for the therapeutic approach of central nervous system dysfunction: At a glance. *Frontiers in Cell and Developmental Biology, 10*. https://doi.org/10.3389/fcell.2022.989471.

143. Rizvi, S. A. A., & Saleh, A. M. (2018). Applications of nanoparticle systems in drug delivery technology. *Saudi Pharmaceutical Journal, 26*(1). https://doi.org/10.1016/j.jsps.2017.10.012.

144. Rodrigues, F., Ziade, N., Jatuworapruk, K., Caballero-Uribe, C. V., Khursheed, T., & Gupta, L. (2023). The impact of social media on vaccination: A narrative review. *Journal of Korean Medical Science, 38*(40). https://doi.org/10.3346/jkms.2023.38.e326.

145. Rosen, J. E., Yoffe, S., Meerasa, A., Verma, M., & Gu, F. X. (2011). Nanotechnology and diagnostic imaging: New advances in contrast agent technology. *Journal of Nanomedicine and Nanotechnology, 2*(5). https://doi.org/10.4172/2157-7439.1000115.

146. Roy, A., Mishra, C., Jain, S., & Solanki, N. (2018). A review of general and modern methods of air purification. *Journal of Thermal Engineering, 5*(2). https://doi.org/10.18186/THERMAL.529054.

147. Scheppler, L., De Clercq, N., McGoldrick, M., & Dias, J. (2021). Regulatory harmonization and streamlining of clinical trial applications globally should lead to faster clinical development and earlier access to life-saving vaccines. *Vaccine, 39*(5). https://doi.org/10.1016/j.vaccine.2020.11.077.

148. Shahbazi, M. A., & Santos, H. A. (2015). Revolutionary impact of nano vaccines on immunotherapy. *New Horizons in Translational Medicine, 2*(2). https://doi.org/10.1016/j.nhtm.2014.11.058.

149. Shamsi, M., Mohammadi, A., Manshadi, M. K. D., & Sanati-Nezhad, A. (2019). Mathematical and computational modeling of nano-engineered drug delivery systems. *Journal of Controlled Release, 307*. https://doi.org/10.1016/j.jconrel.2019.06.014.

150. Shanmugaraj, B., Malla, A., & Phoolcharoen, W. (2020). Emergence of novel coronavirus 2019-nCoV: Need for rapid vaccine and biologics development. *Pathogens, 9*(2). https://doi.org/10.3390/pathogens9020148.

151. Shanmugaraj, B., Siriwattananon, K., Wangkanont, K., & Phoolcharoen, W. (2020). Perspectives on monoclonal antibody therapy as potential therapeutic intervention for Coronavirus disease-19 (COVID-19). *Asian Pacific Journal of Allergy and Immunology, 38*(1). https://doi.org/10.12932/AP-200220-0773.

152. Singh, P., Ali, S. W., & Kale, R. D. (2023). Antimicrobial nanomaterials as advanced coatings for self-sanitizing of textile clothing and personal protective equipment. *ACS Omega, 8*(9). https://doi.org/10.1021/acsomega.2c06343.

153. Singh, R., & Lillard, J. W. (2009). Nanoparticle-based targeted drug delivery. *Experimental and Molecular Pathology, 86*(3). https://doi.org/10.1016/j.yexmp.2008.12.004.

154. Skjøt-Arkil, H., Heltborg, A., Lorentzen, M. H., et al. (2021). Improved diagnostics of infectious diseases in emergency departments: A protocol of a multifaceted multicenter diagnostic study. *BMJ Open, 11*(9). https://doi.org/10.1136/bmjopen-2021-049606.

155. Smith, D. M., Simon, J. K., & Baker, J. R. (2013). Applications of nanotechnology for immunology. *Nature Reviews Immunology, 13*(8). https://doi.org/10.1038/nri3488.

156. Smithgall, M. C., Dowlatshahi, M., Spitalnik, S. L., Hod, E. A., & Rai, A. J. (2021). Types of assays for SARS-CoV-2 testing: A review. *Laboratory Medicine, 51*(5). https://doi.org/10.1093/labmed/lmaa039.

157. Sodickson, A., Baeyens, P. F., Andriole, K. P., et al. (2009). Recurrent CT, cumulative radiation exposure, and associated radiation-induced cancer risks from CT of adults. *Radiology, 251*(1). https://doi.org/10.1148/radiol.2511081296.

158. Sofia, A. P. (2015). *Review on Various Approaches on Preparation, Characterization and Applications of Polymeric Nanoparticles* (Vol. 4).

159. Song, F., Shi, N., Shan, F., et al. (2020). Emerging 2019 novel coronavirus (2019-NCoV) pneumonia. *Radiology, 295*(1). https://doi.org/10.1148/radiol.2020200274.

160. Su, J., Yang, L., Sun, Z., & Zhan, X. (2024). Personalized drug therapy: Innovative concept guided with proteoformics. *Molecular & Cellular Proteomics, 23*(3). https://doi.org/10.1016/j.mcpro.2024.100737.

161. Sui, X., Downing, J. R., Hersam, M. C., & Chen, J. (2021). Additive manufacturing and applications of nanomaterial-based sensors. *Materials Today, 48*. https://doi.org/10.1016/j.mattod.2021.02.001.

162. Tavares Luiz, M., Santos Rosa Viegas, J., Palma Abriata, J., et al. (2021). Design of experiments (DoE) to develop and to optimize nanoparticles as drug delivery systems. *European Journal of Pharmaceutics and Biopharmaceutics, 165*. https://doi.org/10.1016/j.ejpb.2021.05.011.

163. To, K. K. W., Tsang, O. T. Y., Yip, C. C. Y., et al. (2020). Consistent detection of 2019 novel coronavirus in saliva. *Clinical Infectious Diseases, 71*(15). https://doi.org/10.1093/cid/ciaa149.

164. Tretiakova, D. S., & Vodovozova, E. L. (2022). Liposomes as adjuvants and vaccine delivery systems. *Biochemistry (Moscow) Supplement Series A: Membrane and Cell Biology, 16*(1). https://doi.org/10.1134/S1990747822020076.

165. Trivedi, R., Upadhyay, T. K., Mujahid, M. H., et al. (2022). Recent advancements in plant-derived nanomaterials research for biomedical applications. *Processes, 10*(2). https://doi.org/10.3390/pr10020338.

166. Troiano, G., & Nardi, A. (2021). Vaccine hesitancy in the era of COVID-19. *Public Health, 194*. https://doi.org/10.1016/j.puhe.2021.02.025.

167. Vahedifard, F., & Chakravarthy, K. (2021). Nanomedicine for COVID-19: The role of nanotechnology in the treatment and diagnosis of COVID-19. *Emergent Materials, 4*(1). https://doi.org/10.1007/s42247-021-00168-8.

168. Vandervoort, J., & Ludwig, A. (2007). Ocular drug delivery: Nanomedicine applications. *Nanomedicine, 2*(1). https://doi.org/10.2217/17435889.2.1.11.

169. Wan, Y., Deng, W., Su, Y., et al. (2011). Carbon nanotube-based ultrasensitive multiplexing electrochemical immunosensor for cancer biomarkers. *Biosensors and Bioelectronics, 30*(1). https://doi.org/10.1016/j.bios.2011.08.033.

170. Wang, M., Cao, R., Zhang, L., et al. (2020). Remdesivir and chloroquine effectively inhibit the recently emerged novel coronavirus (2019-nCoV) *in vitro*. *Cell Research, 30*(3). https://doi.org/10.1038/s41422-020-0282-0.

171. Wang, X., Zhang, H., & Chen, X. (2019). Drug resistance and combating drug resistance in cancer. *Cancer Drug Resistance, 2*(2). https://doi.org/10.20517/cdr.2019.10.

172. Wang, Z. G., Liu, S. L., & Pang, D. W. (2021). Quantum dots: A promising fluorescent label for probing virus trafficking. *Accounts of Chemical Research, 54*(14). https://doi.org/10.1021/acs.accounts.1c00276.

173. Wen, T., Huang, C., Shi, F. J., et al. (2020). Development of a lateral flow immunoassay strip for rapid detection of IgG antibody against SARS-CoV-2 virus. *Analyst, 145*(15). https://doi.org/10.1039/d0an00629g.

174. Wolfram, J., Zhu, M., Yang, Y., et al. (2015). Safety of nanoparticles in medicine. *Current Drug Targets, 16*(14). https://doi.org/10.2174/1389450115666140804124808.

175. World Health Organization. (2020). *Clinical Management of Severe Acute Respiratory Infection When Novel Coronavirus (nCoV) Infection Is Suspected*. https://iris.who.int/handle/10665/330893.

176. Wouters, O. J., Shadlen, K. C., Salcher-Konrad, M., et al. (2021). Challenges in ensuring global access to COVID-19 vaccines: Production, affordability, allocation, and deployment. *The Lancet, 397*(10278). https://doi.org/10.1016/S0140-6736(21)00306-8.

177. Xu, X., Han, M., Li, T., et al. (2020). Effective treatment of severe COVID-19 patients with tocilizumab. *Proceedings of the National Academy of Sciences of the United States of America, 117*(20). https://doi.org/10.1073/pnas.2005615117.

178. Yao, H. P., Lu, X., Chen, Q., et al. (2020). Patient-derived mutations impact pathogenicity of SARS-CoV-2. *SSRN Electronic Journal*. https://doi.org/10.2139/ssrn.3578153.

179. Yewdell, J. W. (2021). Antigenic drift: Understanding COVID-19. *Immunity, 54*(12). https://doi.org/10.1016/j.immuni.2021.11.016.

180. Yit, J. E., Chew, B. T., & Yau, Y. H. (2020). A review of air filter test standards for particulate matter of general ventilation. *Building Services Engineering Research and Technology, 41*(6). https://doi.org/10.1177/0143624420915626.

181. Younes, N., Al-Sadeq, D. W., AL-Jighefee, H., et al. (2020). Challenges in laboratory diagnosis of the novel coronavirus SARS-CoV-2. *Viruses, 12*(6). https://doi.org/10.3390/v12060582.

182. Zainol Rashid, Z., Othman, S. N., Abdul Samat, M. N., Ali, U. K., & Wong, K. K. (2020). Diagnostic performance of COVID-19 serology assays. *Malaysian Journal of Pathology, 42*(1).

183. Zhai, Z., Li, H., Bahl, R., & Trace, K. (2021). Application of portable air purifiers for mitigating COVID-19 in large public spaces. *Buildings, 11*(8). https://doi.org/10.3390/buildings11080329.

184. Zhang, R. X., Ahmed, T., Li, L. Y., Li, J., Abbasi, A. Z., & Wu, X. Y. (2017). Design of nanocarriers for nanoscale drug delivery to enhance cancer treatment using hybrid polymer and lipid building blocks. *Nanoscale, 9*(4). https://doi.org/10.1039/c6nr08486a.

185. Zhou, Y., Lu, X., Wang, X., Ying, T., & Tan, X. (2023). Potent therapeutic strategies for COVID-19 with single-domain antibody immunoliposomes neutralizing SARS-CoV-2 and Lip/cGAMP enhancing protective immunity. *International Journal of Molecular Sciences, 24*(4). https://doi.org/10.3390/ijms24044068.

186. Zu, Z. Y., Di Jiang, M., Xu, P. P., et al. (2020). Coronavirus disease 2019 (COVID-19): A perspective from China. *Radiology, 296*(2). https://doi.org/10.1148/radiol.2020200490.

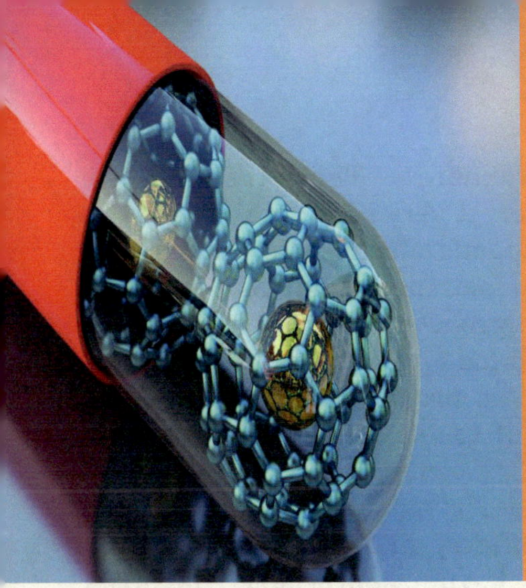

Chapter 9

NANOMEDICINE IN NUTRACEUTICALS

Contents

Manisha Khatri,[1,*] Vanshika Makol,[1] and Harsh Kashyap[2]

[1]*Department of Biomedical Sciences, Shaheed Rajguru College of Applied Sciences for Women, University of Delhi, Vasundhara Enclave, Delhi, India*

[2]*Amity Institute of Biotechnology, Amity University, Noida, Uttar Pradesh, India*

**Corresponding author.*

Abstract

Nanomedicine in nutraceuticals refers to the integration of nanotechnology into the development and delivery of nutritional supplements and functional foods. This innovative approach involves the use of nanoscale techniques and materials to better the bioavailability, stability, and targeted delivery of bioactive compounds present in nutraceutical products. Nanomedicine in nutraceuticals holds promise for improving the absorption of essential nutrients, promoting controlled release, and enhancing the overall effectiveness of these health-promoting compounds.

9.1. Introduction to Nanomedicine

Nanomedicine includes the use of nanotechnology, study and engineering of functional systems at an atomic or molecular scale, in the field of medicine. It mainly focuses on developing new nanostructured materials, of size ranging from 1–100 nm. The biodegradability and biocompatibility of these nanoparticles make them suitable for use in biological systems. Additionally, the increased surface area makes them more durable and conductive.

Nanomedicine has revolutionized therapeutics and diagnosis. Over the recent years, nanotechnology has found its use in an array of medical aspects like drug delivery, biosensors, tissue engineering, imaging, and sensing. The most remarkable is the application of nanomedicine in the field of nutraceuticals. Nutraceutical has recently emerged as an alternative to the conventional medicine, which is associated with many side effects or chronic toxicity. Their palatability and nutrition value makes them suitable as dietary supplements. But a major challenge with nutraceuticals is poor bioavailability. Thus, they require supplementation at very high doses to achieve complete therapeutic effect. Globally, many large FoodTech companies invest millions in research in order to improve the nutrition-profile of their processed food, to increase the shelf-life, prevent microbial proliferation and avoid the accumulation of toxins (Magne, Alencar, and Carneiro, 2023). Nanoparticles offer a great solution to these common problems as they have higher efficacy and lower side effects. They are also having appreciable industrial scalability (Magne, Alencar, and Carneiro, 2023). Hence, nanomaterials (NMs) find a great deal of usage in food and pharmaceutical sector as they offer enhanced bioavailability, with improved pharmacological activity, better solubility, increased encapsulation efficiency, better stability, targeted and sustained drug delivery, protection against microbial degradation and contamination with bio-based packaging (Singh et al., 2022).

9.2. Nanoparticle Formulations

Small size, large surface area and consequently increased surface energy are some of the characteristics of a variety of nanoparticles, which make them be used in the drug packaging or delivery. Furthermore, their electrical, optical, and magnetic properties can be altered by electron confinement. These properties make NMs quite reactive; thus, they tend to absorb biomolecules easily (Soares et al., 2018). While lipid soluble nanoparticles, like liposomes, can easily cross the hydrophobic cell membrane, water-soluble nanoparticles rely on facilitated diffusion assisted by transporter proteins. For charged nanoparticles, only those ranging from 10 to 30 nm can cross-using ion channels (Magne, Alencar, and Carneiro, 2023) (Figure 9.1).

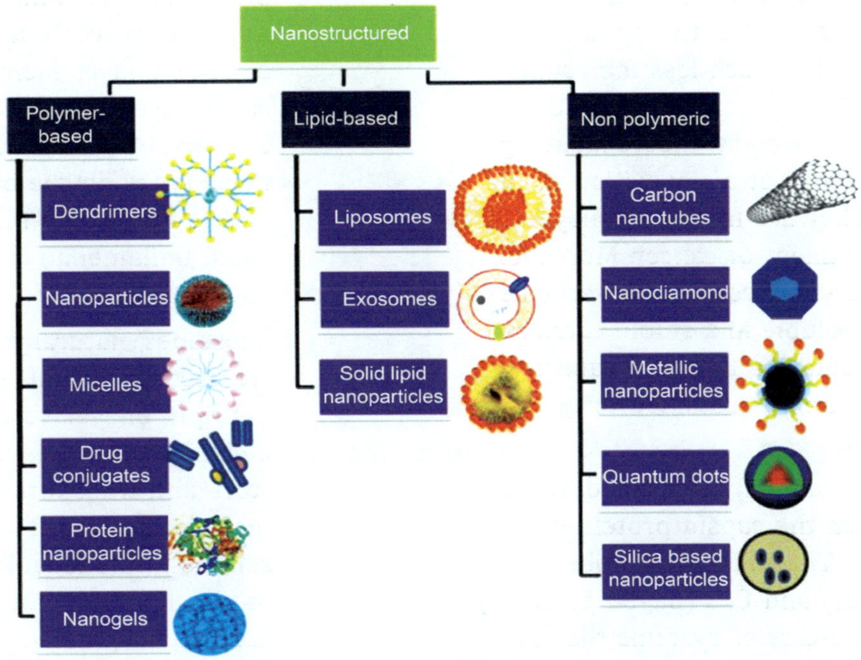

Figure 9.1. Types of nanoparticles (Yetisgin et al., 2020).

Out of all the different types of nanoparticles available to us, a few find their use in medicine owing to the properties described above. The ones mostly used for the therapeutic purpose fall under the category of polymer-based and lipid-based.

9.2.1. Polymer-Based Nanoparticles

- Dendrimers are hyperbranched, compartmentalized structures with high monodispersity. They have a size range of 1–5 nm. As they are fabricated by polymerizing in spherical shape, resulting in cavities, this results in high entrapment efficiency, which makes them very efficient for the delivery of therapeutic agents. Additionally, their target-specific delivery can be improved by conjugating free-end groups to biocompatible compounds. This also results in high bio-permeability and reduced cytotoxicity.
- Nanoparticles can be synthetically made, like polycaprolactone (PCL), polylactic acid (PLA), or can be naturally occurring, like chitosan (CH), gelatin, albumin, and alginate. They are generally non-immunogenic and non-toxic. They are composed of a matrix system and therapeutic agent can either be enclosed in polymer membrane (nanocapsule) or can be directly and uniformly distributed throughout the matrix (nanospheres). This allows high amounts of therapeutic agent to be delivered to the target site. Moreover, specific recognition ligand can be used to improve specificity.
- Micelles are generally present as aggregates in solution. They have a hydrophobic core, which can be covalently linked to water insoluble agents for their delivery. This structural organization offers low rate of dissolution and versatile loading capacity.

- Drug conjugates are used for the delivering the therapeutic agents with much less molecular mass. Conjugation increases the molecular weight, thus enhancing pharmacokinetic disposition in the cells. They are mostly employed in the treatment of cancer. Moreover, polymer-drug conjugates serve as highly soluble and stable carriers, which enhance the drug capacity and results in sustained drug release.
- Protein nanoparticles are designed based on the capsid protein of viruses. The VLPs (Virus-like particles) and CPs (Caged proteins) are nano-carrier systems that can lead to antigen-specific immune responses against certain cell types and are thus used for the development of cancer vaccines. Moreover, protein nanoparticles can also be derived from self-assembling protein polymers like gelatin, collagen, albumin, silk, elastin, and soy isolated from plants or animals.
- Nanogels are composed of chemically or physically cross linked natural or synthetic polymers. They swell up when in contact with water. The most extensively researched applications of nanogels include the delivery of therapeutics like nucleic acids, vaccines, cytokines, and nasal vaccines.

9.2.2. Lipid-Based Nanoparticles

- Liposomes are small artificial vesicles, spherical in shape, mostly composed by hydration of dry phospholipids, like phosphatidylcholine, and cholesterol. As their structure is similar to that of cell's bilayer membrane, they can easily fuse with the cell for drug delivery. They can be classified into three types on the basis of based on the number of bilayers present: small unilamellar, large unilamellar and multilamellar.
- Exosomes, naturally formed and released by various cell types, are lipid bilayer vesicles (like cell membrane), which can be used to store and transport cargo. Since they are derived from patient's own cell, no immunogenicity is observed. Studies on their potential of being used as drug delivery carriers are being conducted.
- Solid lipid nanoparticles (SLNs) are colloidal dispersions in aqueous media, consisting of a lipid matrix that is soluble either at room temperature or body temperature. They are versatile drug delivery vehicles as they can deliver high amounts of both hydrophobic and hydrophilic drugs. They are purposed as effective carriers for oral, cancer, and pulmonary drug delivery.

9.2.3. Methods for Nanoparticle Formulations

- Comminution (top-down approach) includes the breaking down of the bulk/heavy material into small nanosized particles or structures by industrial milling or natural weathering. It is generally inefficient for the production of very small nanoparticles.

- Pyrolysis, forms aggregate and agglomerates instead of singleton primary particles formulation, is the process in which a precursor which is vaporous (liquid or gas) is forced with high pressure through a hole or opening and burned.
- Sol-gel synthesis (bottom-up approach) is a chemical method for the synthesis of metal oxide nanoparticles from metal alkoxide precursor. In this, monomers are typically dissolved in alcohol or water and are converted to a gel by hydrolysis or alcoholysis, involving heating and stirring.

Some of the nanoparticles produced using the above formulation techniques include titania nanoparticles for sunscreens from the minerals anatase and rutile, fullerenes or fumed silica and synthetic silica.

9.3. Bioactive Compounds in Nutraceuticals

Nutraceuticals are dietary supplements used to enhance health by delivering a biologically active component of food in concentrated form. They differ from functional food in the aspect that they provide much higher concentration of usually only one biologically active component along with therapeutic effects like preventing or curing diseases. Nutraceuticals include dietary fiber, green tea, soy, antioxidant vitamins, and so on (Table 9.1).

Table 9.1. Bioactive Compounds Present in Nutraceuticals

Nutraceuticals	Active Compound(s)
Dietary fiber	Cellulose, hemicelluloses, and lignin (Lattimer and Haub, 2010)
Fish oil	Eicosapentaenoic acid (EPA) and docosahexaenoic acid (DHA)
Vitamin E	α-Tocopherol (Michael and Power, n.d.)
Vitamin D	Calcitriol (1,25-dihydroxycholecalciferol)
Vitamin B12	Methylcobalamin and 5-deoxyadenosylcobalamin
Antioxidants	Free oxygen radicals
Green tea	Polyphenol (EGCG) (Kochman et al., 2020)
Soy	Glycinin and β-conglycinin (Shahruzzaman et al., 2022)

Yet, the major challenges faced with nutraceuticals like poor bioavailability and adverse side effects prevent their widespread use. The use of nanoparticles can be quite effective in overcoming these challenges. Most nutraceuticals follow oral route of drug administration as it is patient compliant, but in this route the rate of dissolution and rate of drug permeability through the membrane is quite low due to their larger particle size. Reducing the size of these therapeutic agents to nm could solve this, such that they can be easily dissolved and absorbed simply by the virtue of their small size. This improves bioavailability and reduces the required dose. Furthermore, many surface modifications can be made to the nanoparticles to improve their target specificity. These modifications include attachment of polymers or surfactants, use of PEGylated PLGA-based nanoparticles and many others. Such modifications can alter the hydrophobicity, solubility, and retention of the drug, thus overall impacting the pharmacodynamic and pharmacokinetic properties (Gunasekaran et al., 2014).

9.4. Bioavailability Enhancement

So far, we have seen that the use of nanoparticles improves the absorption and bioavailability of the therapeutic agents. But how do these nanoparticles cross the biological barriers so easily? Due to their variable size, shape, and chemical composition, NMs can easily pass through biological membranes, actively or passively, and interact with the target site. The most common mechanisms of uptake are endocytic and non-endocytic pathway.

Receptor-mediated endocytosis depends on ligand and surface protein interaction for the vesicular uptake of target molecules. The major types of receptor-mediated endocytosis include clathrin-dependent endocytosis, clathrin-independent endocytosis (which is further divided into two types—endophilin mediated/dynamin-dependent, and glycosylphosphatidylinositol-anchored protein-enriched (GEEC)), macropinocytosis, phagocytosis, and caveolin-dependent endocytosis. Out of these, clathrin-dependent endocytosis is primarily utilized for capturing nanoparticles within intracellular vesicles that are approximately of size 100 nm (Niaz et al., 2022). It begins with the attachment of nanoparticle ligands to the receptor (EGFR: epidermal growth factor receptor), followed by clathrin-coated pit formation consisting of receptor bound to the nanoparticle. Then invagination occurs which results in vesicle formation (Figure 9.2).

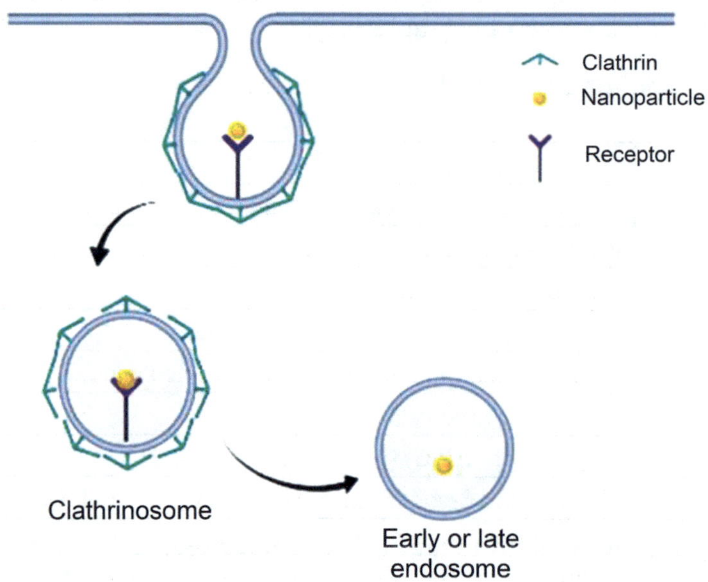

Figure 9.2. Clathrin-dependent endocytic uptake of nanoparticles (Niaz et al., 2022).

Caveolin-dependent endocytosis is another type of receptor-mediated endocytosis in which flask-like membrane invagination (caveolae) occurs. It involves membrane protein caveolin which is essential for forming the flask-like structure in caveolae. Detachment of caveolae from the membrane then results in the formation of caveosome. It is utilized for smaller cargos, with vesicles of approximately 60 nm in size. Nanoparticles with surface ligands such as folic acid, albumin, or cholesterol typically prefer caveolin-dependent endocytosis (Niaz et al., 2022) (Figure 9.3).

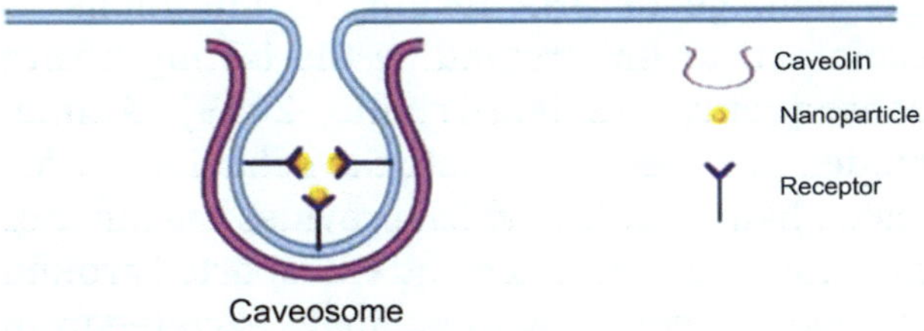

Figure 9.3. Caveolin-dependent endocytic uptake of nanoparticles (Niaz et al., 2022).

In these ways, nanomedicine improves the bioavailability and efficacy of drugs. The most notable usage of nanomedicine is in the treatment of Parkinson's disease (PD). The drugs available for treatment (levodopa) have poor efficacy and delivery because of the presence of blood–brain barrier (BBB). Nanoparticles, including metal nanoparticles, quantum dots (QDs), cerium oxide nanoparticles, organic nanoparticles, liposomes, and so on, are employed for the efficient delivery of drugs. Ropinirole (RP), a dopamine agonist, is loaded onto a solid lipid nanoparticle. It is incorporated into a hydrogel formulation, which results in better oral and topical distribution (Afzal et al., 2022).

9.5. Targeted Delivery

Nanoparticles need to cross many physical and physiological barriers in order to reach the target site while avoiding any non-specific interactions. The specificity can be achieved by surface modification, functionalization, receptor interaction or exploiting the physiological environment of certain cell types, like tumor cells (acidic environment).

Fundamental characteristics a nanoparticle must have for targeted delivery includes:

- Stability in the vascular system (blood);
- Escaping the reticuloendothelial system (RES) clearance;
- Escaping the mononuclear phagocyte system (MPS);
- Penetrating and accumulating in the target site.

Generally, there are two types of targeting mechanisms, active and passive. Passive targeting does not rely on specific receptor-ligand interaction but is based on the size, vascularity or leakiness of the target site. Intracellular pressure and physiochemical nature of the target site are also contributing factors to this type of delivery. Contrary, active targeting depends on specific receptor-ligand interactions. It greatly improves cell penetration and specificity. Receptors that are over-expressed under certain conditions are most commonly targeted for treatment (Figure 9.4).

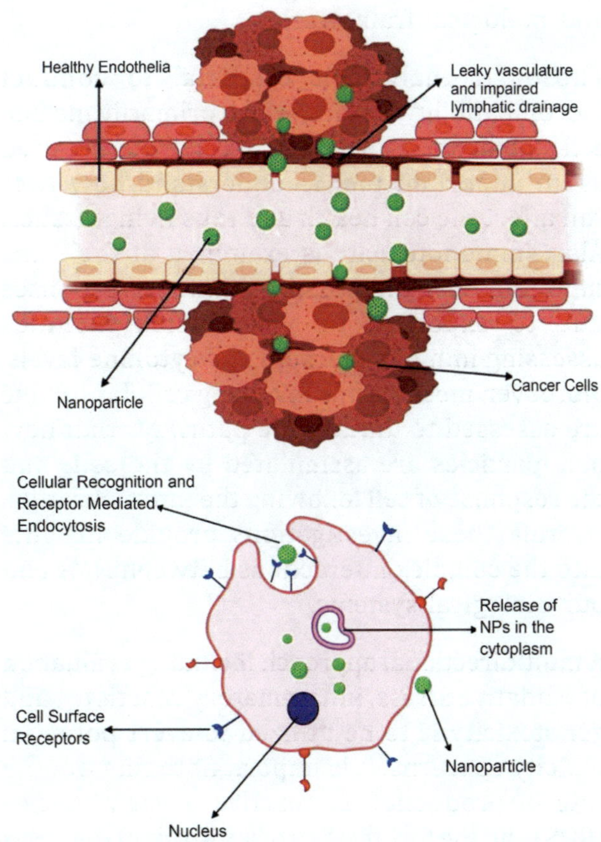

Figure 9.4. Passive versus active targeting (Gavas, Quazi, and Karpiński, 2021).

Thus, nanoparticles can be used to target drugs at specific tissue or cell types only. This targeted delivery minimizes non-specific drug interactions, thereby reducing side effects and the required doses, which ultimately lowers the cost of treatment.

9.6. Safety and Toxicity Considerations

The thorough assessment of NMs in the domain of nutraceuticals is mandatory and requires a thorough assessment protocol to be followed to ascertain safety and efficacy for consumer utilization. This evaluative paradigm follows a multifaceted methodology, to understand the intricate dynamic interaction between the NMs and biological frameworks.

Thorough analysis is essential to conduct biocompatibility studies, which primarily include cell viability tests. A variety of cell types are used as an important tool to understand how NMs can affect the cell health and thus living tissues. Also, immunotoxicity is examined at the same time to assess the possible immune responses due to exposure to NMs, which includes assessing immune markers and cytokine levels. Moreover, mechanisms involving cellular uptake are assessed to unravel the pathways that how nanoparticles are assimilated by the cells and the response of cell following the internalization. Overall, these investigations provide insights into the complex interactions between NMs and our biological systems.

A multidirectional approach including evaluation of oxidative stress, inflammatory reactions, and genotoxicity is to be utilized to avert potential toxicity concerns. It is important to find out the rate of production of reactive oxygen species (ROS) and the fortification of antioxidant defenses to assess the impact of NM on cellular oxidative balance. Additionally, ability of the substance in provoking any inflammatory reaction or any damage to DNA leading to mutations, is examined to understanding the lasting health consequences (Salvia-Trujillo, 2019). Animal models are used to validate the behavior of NMs inside living bodies, which provides the kinetics that how they are taken and transported around the body, broken down, and finally excreted from the system (Ma, 2021). This study is important and crucial to understand the journey of NM inside the biological organism and predict wide range of effect over a long period of time. Although quite challenging but necessary to understand this area for the development and use of nanotechnology in future.

9.6.1. Mitigating Risks and Complying with Regulatory Protocols

A careful consideration, judicious strategy and adherence to regulatory standards are required for incorporating NMs into nutritional supplements to reduce conceivable harms and dangers. Various important pathways are key to this effort, addressing risks and improving the safety of combining the nanoparticles with nutraceuticals.

The very first step involves selecting the NMs and modifications of their characteristics, in order to decrease the natural risks and maximize the essential functionalities that are aimed at specific applications within the supplement formulas. Adjustments/modifications in the surface and encapsulation ways are remarkable strategies in increasing biocompatibility and reducing unfavorable impacts (National Institute for Occupational Safety and Health [NIOSH], 2016).

Customization of NM surfaces includes change in their chemical make up or coatings lead to better interaction of NM with the biological system. Such modifications usually increase the stability, biodegradability, and reduce the potential for toxicity hence enhances safety profiles. Sequestration strategies, such as nanostructuring, or the sequestration within protective systems protect fragile bioactive compounds. Thus, sensitive compounds are with the setting of discharge characteristics and protection against environmental degradation or premature reactions, hence bringing about increased effectiveness within the assurance of safety. It is important to understand safe dose limits and potential combined effects. Accurate dosing schedules help prevent overexposure and reduce the risk of unwanted effects (NIOSH, 2016). Careful studies are required to understand the effect of NMs on biological systems and their long-term effect.

9.7. Regulatory Frameworks and Recent Advancements in Nutraceutical Nanomedicines

9.7.1. Navigating the Regulatory Landscape for Nanotechnology Integration

Organization like Food and Drug Administration (FDA) in USA and Food Safety and Standards Authority of India (FSSAI) in India regulate the use of nanoparticles in health boosting foods and make rules and strict standards to be followed diligently (European Union Observatory for Nanomaterials [EUON], 2023; FSSAI, 2023; United States Environmental Protection Agency [EPA], 2021). This process involves careful safety checks, testing its effects, and clear labeling ensuring a complete safety review. These checks help in building people's trust in using these nutraceuticals modified using nanotechnology.

Recent progress in health food studies sees careful use of nanotechnology. This changes the ways these foods are made for better results and accuracy. Nanocarriers like liposomes, nanoparticles, and nanogels are the most promising methods for enhancing the solubility, bioavailability, stability, and functionality of nutraceuticals (Chaudhary, 2020; Singh, 2019).

9.7.2. Revolutionary Nanocarriers: Bioavailability and Nanoencapsulation

1. **Increasing Bioavailability through Nanocarriers:** Liposomes, nanogels, and nanoparticles designed at the nanoscale are extremely effective in encapsulating and delivering nutraceutical components. This encapsulation improves stability, solubility, and enhances solubility, while ensuring precise and targeted delivery (Singh, 2019).
2. **Evolution in Nanoencapsulation Techniques:** Novel nano-encapsulation methods such as nano-emulsions, SLNs, and polymeric nanoparticles are leading the research (International Standard Organization [ISO], 2021). They preserve delicate bioactive elements, ensuring controlled and sustained release mechanisms for prolonged efficacy (ISO, 2021).

9.7.3. Ongoing Research: Tailoring Nutraceutical Interventions

Ongoing nutraceutical research focuses on using nanotechnology, in designing nanoformulations designed to improve the absorption of vital nutrients. Nanolipid carriers and nanosuspensions are promising solutions, to address the issue of poor solubility and bioavailability (Singh and Sharma, 2017). To overcome the barriers obstructing efficient nutrient absorption, nanolipid carriers and nanosuspensions are designed at the nanoscale. They facilitate the assimilation of essential nutrients, highlighting their potential to improve nutritional efficacy (Singh and Sharma, 2017).

Ongoing studies are exploring how to customize nanoparticles for specific nutraceutical treatments. Modification of their surfaces and conjugation of ligands can precisely target certain cells or tissues, making treatments more effective and reducing side effects (McClements, 2018). How NMs interact with biological systems is a key focus area in nanomedicine. Detailed research examines their compatibility, potential toxicity, and long-term effects to ensure they meet strict safety standards and regulations.

A new development is the combination of artificial intelligence (AI) and nanotechnology, which has the potential to revolutionize personalized nutraceutical formulations (Kumar and Katare, 2018). Customization of nanostructures and effective delivery systems are changing the landscape of preventive healthcare by leading to efficient, tailored, and patient-centric nutraceutical interventions.

9.8. Challenges and Future Directions

The intersection of nanomedicine and nutraceuticals is promising but at the same time challenging too. This will play a key role in shaping the future of health interventions.

9.8.1. Complexity in Formulation and Scale-Up

A major challenge n combining the nanomedicine and nutraceuticals pertains to the complexity in creating the nanostructures. The major struggle is in achieving the consistency and scalability in production methods while keeping the integrity of nanostructures (Sahoo, 2016). Innovative methods are required for standardizing and scaling these formulations to keep the unique properties of NMs, adding on to complexity of the production process. Another challenge is to improving the bioavailability and stability of bioactive compounds in nanocarriers. Effective and meticulous research is required to achieve the best release profiles, ensuring these compounds remain effective after production. Continuous innovation is also warranted in balancing effectiveness, stability, and bioavailability.

Complex regulations possess a significant obstacle too, especially safety concerns related to the use of NMs in nutraceuticals. Balancing these safety requirements with consumer confidence is essential.

9.8.2. Futuristic Trajectories and Exploration Avenues

The future trajectory indicates development in personalized nutraceutical formulations designed using nanomedicine. This paradigm shift has the potential to create personalized formulations to suit individual nutritional needs, leading to a revolution in preventive healthcare.

9.8.3. Precision Targeting and Controlled Release

Future advancements in nanomedicine could lead to highly targeted and controlled release systems for nutraceuticals. These smart nano-delivery systems would respond to specific signals in the body, improving treatment accuracy and reducing side effects. These innovations promise more effective and precise health interventions (Kaul and Beg, 2021).

9.8.4. Sustainable and Scalable Production

For the sustainable development of nanomedicine-based nutraceuticals, it is important to ensure green processes in parallel with improving scalability. Synergy between efficacy and environmental impact is the key to fostering industry growth, leading to a future where sustainable practices merge seamlessly with scalability.

9.9. Regulatory Landscape

The regulations and guidelines for combining nanomedicines and nutraceuticals are complex and constantly changing, with important oversight from various regulatory bodies. This section discusses the key role of these bodies, the need to meet safety standards, and the specific regulations and transparency requirements involved. Regulatory bodies like the FDA, EFSA (European Food Safety Authority), and FSSAI play a crucial role in ensuring the safety and effectiveness of nutraceuticals that include nanomedicines (Akbarzadeh, 2013; EFSA, 2021). Their guidelines involve careful scrutiny, assessment, and approval processes to protect consumers. It is important to follow safety standards for confirming the safety of NMs in nutraceuticals. Manufacturers must conduct thorough safety assessments that meet regulatory standards, involving detailed evaluations to determine safety limits and potential risks of using NMs (Fritz, 2019).

9.9.1. Regulations and Guidelines

1. **Specific Guidelines for Nanomaterials (NMs):** Some regions have pioneered specific guidelines for using NMs into food and supplements. These guidelines include detailed safety evaluations, strict labeling requirements, and rules for reporting NM usage in products (Fritz, 2019). This approach enables consumers to make informed decisions ensuring transparency.
2. **Clear Labeling Practices:** Regulatory bodies promote clear labelling practices, which clearly shows the presence of NMs in nutraceuticals. It is important for building the consumer's trust in these personalized nutraceutical products along with empowering the consumers to make informed decisions (Fritz, 2019).

9.10. Conclusion

The integration of nanomedicine into nutraceuticals is a groundbreaking in the sector of healthcare and nutrition, offering great advancements and better therapeutic outcomes. Combining nanotechnology with medicine has transformed different areas of medicine, ranging from diagnostics to therapeutics. A major step forward in improving human health and well-being is inclusion of NMs in nutraceuticals.

One of the ways of exploiting nanomedicine in nutraceuticals could be through nanostructured materials typically ranging from 1–100 nanometers in size, which offers unparalleled advantages. The very concept of augmented surface area, improved stability, and biocompatibility redefines the common perception of "drug delivery, imaging, tissue engineering, and biosensors" in the context of nutraceuticals. This change addresses the challenges such as poor bioavailability and limited therapeutic efficacy generally encountered in conventional medicine. A variety of nanoparticle formulations, including polymer-based and lipid-based particles, are leading the way in innovative DDS. These nanoparticles are quite intricately designed and tailored in accordance with the efficiency of the therapeutic agents for the delivery at the target sites. These different formulations, from dendrimers and nanogels to liposomes and exosomes, increases bioavailability while ensuring targeted and controlled release, and enhances the precision and effectiveness of nutraceutical therapies.

Furthermore, the easy blend of nanotechnology and nutraceuticals is a sure way to achieve improved health conditions in a cost-effective manner. The poor bioavailability and side effects still limits the use of nutraceuticals for global application, despite having a bright future. In this scenario, nanoparticles offer solutions for most of the drawbacks, by improving absorption, reducing required doses, and improving target specificity through surface modifications. By traversing biological barriers adeptly, nanomedicine paves the way for efficient and targeted drug delivery, thereby minimizing side effects and optimizing therapeutic outcomes. The future looks bright for integrating nanomedicine into nutraceuticals. Customized formulations, precise targeting, and sustainable production methods are expected to advance preventive healthcare and treatments.

In conclusion, combining nanomedicine and nutraceuticals marks a new era in healthcare, bringing unique opportunities for innovation, precision, and better patient outcomes. As research and technology advance, nanotechnology will keep transforming nutraceuticals, shaping the future of modern medicine and ensuring better health and sustainability for future generations.

KEY TERMS FROM THIS CHAPTER

bioavailability
drug delivery
nanocarriers
nanoencapsulation
nanomedicine
nutraceuticals
personalized healthcare
regulatory bodies

References

1. Afzal, O., Altamimi, A. S. A., Nadeem, M. S., Alzarea, S. I., Almalki, W. H., Tariq, A., Mubeen, B., Murtaza, B. N., Iftikhar, S., Riaz, N., & Kazmi, I. (2022). Nanoparticles in drug delivery: From history to therapeutic applications. *Nanomaterials (Basel), 12*(24), 4494. https://doi.org/10.3390/nano12244494.

2. Akbarzadeh, A. (2013). Liposome: Classification, preparation, and applications. *Nanoscale Research Letters, 8*(1), 102. https://doi.org/10.1186/1556-276X-8-102.

3. Chaudhary, A. (2020). Application of nanotechnology in nutraceuticals and functional foods. *Nanobiotechnology, 18*(1), 1–20. https://doi.org/10.1002/nbt.414.

4. European Food Safety Authority (EFSA). (2021). Guidance on the risk assessment of nanomaterials to be applied in the food and feed chain: Human and animal health. *EFSA Journal, 19*(6), e06628. https://doi.org/10.2903/j.efsa.2021.6628.

5. European Union Observatory for Nanomaterials (EUON). (2023). *Regulation and Legislation.* https://euon.echa.europa.eu/regulation.

6. Food Safety and Standards Authority of India (FSSAI). (2023). *Guidelines for the Use of Nanotechnology in Food Products.* https://www.fssai.gov.in/ (accessed on 8 May 2025).

7. Fritz, A. (2019). The coming era of nanomedicine. *The American Journal of Bioethics, 9*(10), 3–11. https://doi.org/10.1080/15265161.2019.1671190.

8. Gavas, S., Quazi, S., & Karpiński, T. M. (2021). Nanoparticles for cancer therapy: Current progress and challenges. *Nanoscale Research Letters, 16*(1), 173. https://doi.org/10.1186/s11671-021-03580-x.

9. Gunasekaran, T., Haile, T., Nigusse, T., & Dhanaraju, M. D. (2014). Nanotechnology: An effective tool for enhancing bioavailability and bioactivity of phytomedicine. *Asian Pacific Journal of Tropical Biomedicine,* S1–S7. https://doi.org/10.1016/S2221-1691(14)60259-3.

10. International Organization for Standardization (ISO). (2021). *ISO/TS 13830:2021 Nanotechnologies–Guidance on Voluntary Labelling for Consumer Products Containing Manufactured Nano-Objects.* https://www.iso.org/standard/72978.html (accessed on 8 May 2025).

11. Kaul, A., & Beg, S. (2021). Nanotechnology-based nutraceuticals: Prospects and perspectives. *Nano Today, 36,* 101021. https://doi.org/10.1016/j.nantod.2020.101021.

12. Kochman, J., Jakubczyk, K., Antoniewicz, J., Mruk, H., & Janda, K. (2020). Health benefits and chemical composition of matcha green tea: A review. *Molecules, 26*(1), 85. https://doi.org/10.3390/molecules26010085.

13. Kumar, P., & Katare, O. P. (2018). Nano nutraceuticals: A review. *International Journal of Pharmaceutics, 539*(1, 2), 1–17. https://doi.org/10.1016/j.ijpharm.2018.01.057.

14. Lattimer, J. M., & Haub, M. D. (2010). Effects of dietary fiber and its components on metabolic health. *Nutrients, 2*(12), 1266–1289. https://doi.org/10.3390/nu2121266.

15. Ma, Q. (2021). Advanced nanoparticulate systems for delivering polyphenols: How far are we? *Journal of Controlled Release, 330,* 1118–1138. https://doi.org/10.1016/j.jconrel.2021.02.019.

16. Magne, T. M., Alencar, L. M. R., & Carneiro, S. V. (2023). Nano-nutraceuticals for health: Principles and applications. *Revita Brasileira de Farmacognosia, 33*, 73–88. https://doi.org/10.1016/j.bjp.2023.01.005.
17. McClements, D. J. (2018). Nanotechnology for increased bioavailability and targeted delivery of nutraceuticals. *Food Engineering Reviews, 10*(2), 133–142. https://doi.org/10.1007/s12393-018-9152-1.
18. Michael, L., & Power, L. K. (n.d.). *Chapter 4–Marmoset Nutrition and Dietary Husbandry.*
19. National Institute for Occupational Safety and Health (NIOSH). (2016). *Approaches to Safe Nanotechnology: Managing the Health and Safety Concerns Associated with Engineered Nanomaterials* (DHHS Publication No. 2016-102). https://www.cdc.gov/niosh/docs/2016-102/ (accessed on 8 May 2025).
20. Niaz, S., Forbes, B., & Raimi-Abraham, B. T. (2022). Exploiting endocytosis for non-spherical nanoparticle cellular uptake. *Nanomanufacturing, 2*(1), 1–16. https://doi.org/10.1007/s42800-022-00102-y.
21. Sahoo, A. K. (2016). Nanotechnology: A boon to nutraceuticals industry. *Heliyon, 2*(12), e00259. https://doi.org/10.1016/j.heliyon.2016.e00259.
22. Salvia-Trujillo, L. (2019). Nano emulsions as delivery systems of hydrophobic nutraceuticals: Strategies for encapsulation and gastrointestinal digestion studies. *Food Research International, 115*, 519–531. https://doi.org/10.1016/j.foodres.2018.10.010.
23. Shahruzzaman, M., Hossain, S., Ahmed, T., Kabir, S. F., Islam, M. M., Rahman, A., Islam, M. S., Sultana, S., & Rahman, M. M. (2022). Chapter 7–Biological macromolecules as antimicrobial agents. *Biological Macromolecules* (pp. 165–202).
24. Singh, A. R., Desu, P. K., Nakkala, R. K., Kondi, V., Devi, S., Alam, M. S., Hamid, H., Athawale, R. B., & Kesharwani, P. (2022). Nanotechnology-based approaches applied to nutraceuticals. *Drug Delivery and Translational Research, 12*(3), 485–499. https://doi.org/10.1007/s13346-022-01045-7.
25. Singh, M. (2019). Nanotechnology in nutraceuticals: A paradigm shift in efficacy standards. *Current Pharmaceutical Design, 25*(18), 2066–2076. https://doi.org/10.2174/1381612825666190521161805.
26. Singh, R. P., & Sharma, G. K. (2017). Nanoencapsulation of bioactive compounds for nutraceutical applications. In *Nanotechnology in Nutraceuticals: Production to Consumption* (pp. 145–168).
27. Soares, S., Sausa, J., Pais, A., & Vitorino, C. (2018). Nanomedicine: Principles, properties, and regulatory issues. *Frontiers in Chemistry, 6*, 360. https://doi.org/10.3389/fchem.2018.00360.
28. United States Environmental Protection Agency (EPA). (2021). *Nanotechnology Regulation Under TSCA.* https://www.epa.gov/reviewing-new-chemicals-under-toxic-substances-control-act-tsca/control-nanoscale-materials-under.
29. Yetisgin, A. A., Cetinel, S., Zuvin, M., Kosar, A., & Kutlu, O. (2020). Therapeutic nanoparticles and their targeted delivery applications. *Molecules, 25*(9), 2193. https://doi.org/10.3390/molecules25092193.

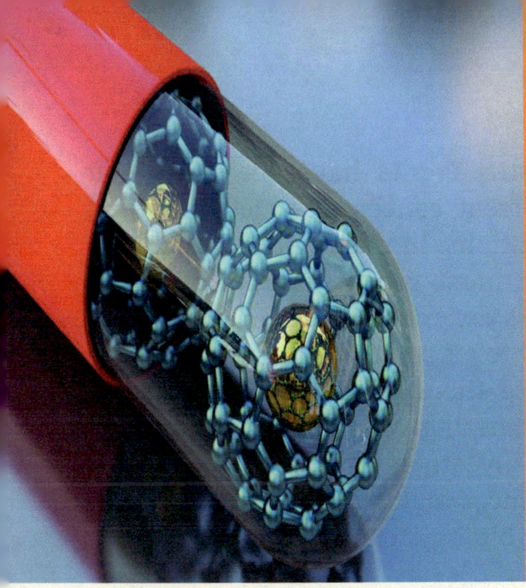

Chapter 10

NANOTOXICITY AND RISK ASSESSMENT OF NANOMEDICINE

Contents

Viswanath Pratap Singh, Puspendra Kumar Rajput, Meenakshi Mishra, Umesh Kumar, and Pankaj Kishor Mishra*

Department of Paramedical Sciences, Subharti Medical College, Swami Vivekanand Subharti University, Meerut, Uttar Pradesh, India

**Corresponding author.*

Abstract

In the 21st century, nanotechnology is rapidly developing. The commercial usage of nanomaterials (NMs) for innovative applications is fast rising. NMs have a large surface area per unit volume and are incredibly tiny. So, nanoparticles have special biological and chemical properties. It is very useful in the fields of industry, agriculture, medicine, text tiles, cosmetics, and food, and is also used in the healthcare sector. NMs are divided into several categories., including silica, metal, metal oxide, and so on. Nanotoxicity is the negative impact of nanoparticles on both human health and the environment. This chapter delves into the composition of NMs and the risks associated with them, as well as the toxicity mechanisms of NM testing. This chapter also focuses on the toxic effects of nanoparticles on systems and the secure use of nanomedicine.

10.1. Nanomaterials (NMs)

10.1.1. Introduction of Nanomaterials (NMs)

The word originates from the Greek word nanos, which means dwarf. It is a prefix that refers to 1 billionth of something, or 0.000000001; the prefix signifies extremely, very small. Nanomaterials (NMs) are frequently employed in medical and pharmaceuticals due to their unique mechanical, optical, and electrical properties. NMs are used in the detection of biological molecules, imaging of sick tissues, and novel therapies. Nano-based particles (1–100 nm) provide miniaturization of biosensors, allowing for smaller samples for biochemical analysis and point-of-care (POC) diagnostics. Nano-pharmaceutics are optimized in medication delivery systems to boost the drug's bioavailability at the target site. Nanoparticle-based diagnostic agents have recently been introduced to treat cancer, allergies, diabetes, and other conditions. In this review chapter, we summarize the most recent breakthroughs in NMs that are less toxic and more efficient, making them suitable for use in diagnosis, imaging systems, disease therapy, drug administration, and tissue engineering. Nanoscience is a branch of science that investigates small objects, and it includes all sciences that deal with the extremely small, such as biology, chemistry, and physics (Bayda et al., 2020).

10.1.2. Types of Nanomaterials (NMs)

Nanomaterials (NMs) are classified depending on their structural configuration or content:

i. Inorganic-based nanomaterials;
ii. Carbon-based nanomaterials;
iii. Organic-based nanomaterials;
iv. Composite-based nanomaterials.

10.1.2.1. Inorganic-Based Nanomaterials (NMs)

Inorganic nanoparticles include a wide variety of compounds such as elemental metals, metal oxides, and metal salts. Silver nanoparticles (AgNPs) are employed as bactericides in various products, whilst gold nanoparticles (AuNPs) are being investigated for a variety of potential applications due to their catalytic activity. Inorganic nanoparticles have outstanding optical characteristics and greatly boost the electric field on their surface. Inorganic nanoparticles are metal oxide or metallic particles that have an inorganic core and an organic outer shell. Some inorganic NMs have been employed for cancer detection, treatment, and immunotherapy. MSNs, AgNPs, CNTs, QDs, and AuNPs are some of the most common inorganic NMs used in biomedicine. Inorganic nanoparticles are typically made up of metal-based or metal oxide-based NMs (Abera, 2023) (Figure 10.1).

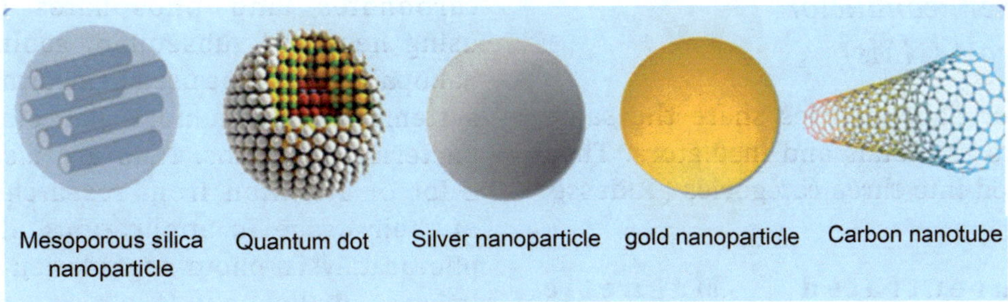

Figure 10.1. Inorganic nanomaterials (NMs).

10.1.2.1.1. Metal-Based Nanoparticles

Metal-based nanoparticles can be created by either destructive or constructive techniques. Metals commonly utilized in nanoparticle synthesis include aluminum (Al), cadmium (Cd), cobalt (Co), copper (Cu), gold (Au), iron (Fe), lead (Pb), silver (Ag), and zinc (Zn). Because of their quantum effects and huge surface-to-volume ratio, metal nanoparticles have excellent ultraviolet-visible sensitivity, as well as electrical, catalytic, thermal, and antibacterial properties. Metal nanoparticles are used in a wide range of scientific domains due to their exceptional optical characteristics (Figure 10.2).

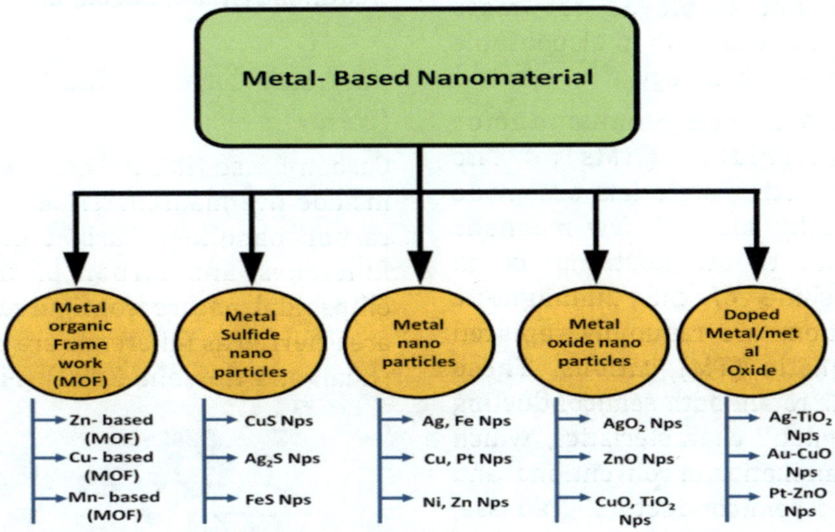

Figure 10.2. Metal-based nanomaterials (NMs).

10.1.2.1.2. Metal Oxide Nanoparticles

Metal oxide nanoparticles, also known as metal oxide NMs, are composed of positive metallic ions and negative oxygen ions. Examples of metal oxide nanoparticles that are frequently synthesized include silicon dioxide (SiO_2), titanium oxide (TiO_2), zinc oxide (ZnO), and aluminum oxide (Al_2O_3). These nanoparticles exhibit remarkable properties compared to their metal analogs (Khan et al., 2022).

10.1.2.1.3. Semiconductor Nanomaterials (NMs)

Semiconductor nanoparticles share the same characteristics as metals and insulators. They are categorized into three categories (Tadesse, 2006):

1. **Concentrated Magnetic Semiconductor Nanomaterials (NMs):** It exhibits spontaneous magnetic order and can be a binary compound such as Europium telluride (EuTe).
2. **Non-Magnetic Semiconductor Nanomaterials (NMs):** Nonmagnetic semiconductors, which lack magnetic ions and are utilized for information processing and communications, have had considerable success due to the charge of electrons in semiconductors, but are not employed for mass storage of information in dispensable information technology.
3. **Diluted Magnetic Semiconductor Nanomaterials (NMs):** The semiconducting materials are made magnetic by adding a few magnetic impurities to the host matrix, in which some of the diamagnetic host cations are randomly replaced by magnetic (TM) cations. These materials retain both semiconducting and magnetic characteristics, which are a combination of conventional and magnetic semiconductors (Tadesse, 2006; Zhang et al., 2016).

10.1.2.1.4. Ceramic Nanomaterials (NMs)

Ceramic NMs are inorganic solids made up of carbides, carbonates, oxides, carbides, Ceramic nanoparticles are inorganic solids composed of carbides, carbonates, oxides, carbides, carbonates, and phosphates synthesized using heat and subsequent cooling. Ceramic nanoparticles can be used in medication delivery systems to target tumors, glaucoma, and some bacterial infections. NMs are also garnering a lot of attention from researchers because of their usage in applications like catalysis, photocatalysis, photo degradation of dyes, and imaging applications (Khan, Saeed, and Khan, 2019).

10.1.2.1.5. Lipid-Based Nanomaterials (NMs)

Lipid-based nanoparticles are typically spherical, with sizes ranging from 10 to 100 nm. It is made up of a lipid-rich solid core and a soluble lipophilic matrix. Lipid-based nanoparticles have medicinal applications, such as medication delivery and RNA release therapy in cancer treatment (Khan, Saeed, and Khan, 2019).

10.1.2.2. Carbon-Based Nanomaterials (NMs)

Carbon-based NMs are composed of carbon and include five main materials, namely, graphene, carbon nanofiber, carbon nanotubes (CNTs), fullerenes, and carbon black. Spherical and ellipsoidal nature configured of carbon NMs are referred as fullerenes are called Bucky balls (Khan and Hossain, 2022) (Figure 10.3).

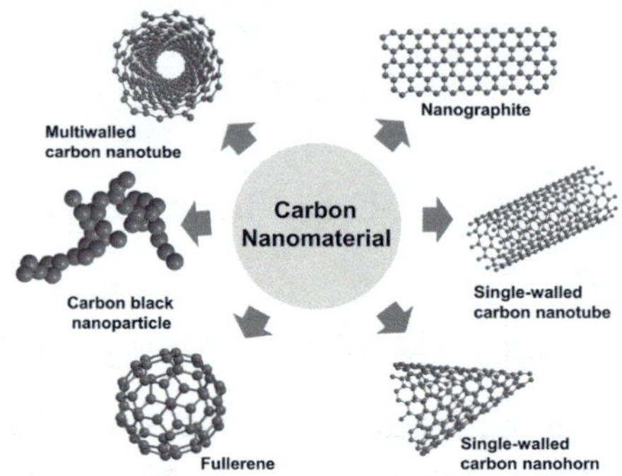

Figure 10.3. Carbon-based nanomaterials (NMs).

10.1.2.3. Organic-Based Nanomaterials (NMs)

On the nanoscale, organic molecules are transformed into organic NMs. Some examples of organic nanoparticles or polymers are liposomes, dendrimers, micelles, and ferritin. Nanocapsule micelles and liposomes are non-toxic biodegradable nanoparticles with hollow interiors that respond to heat, electromagnetic radiation, and light (Figure 10.4).

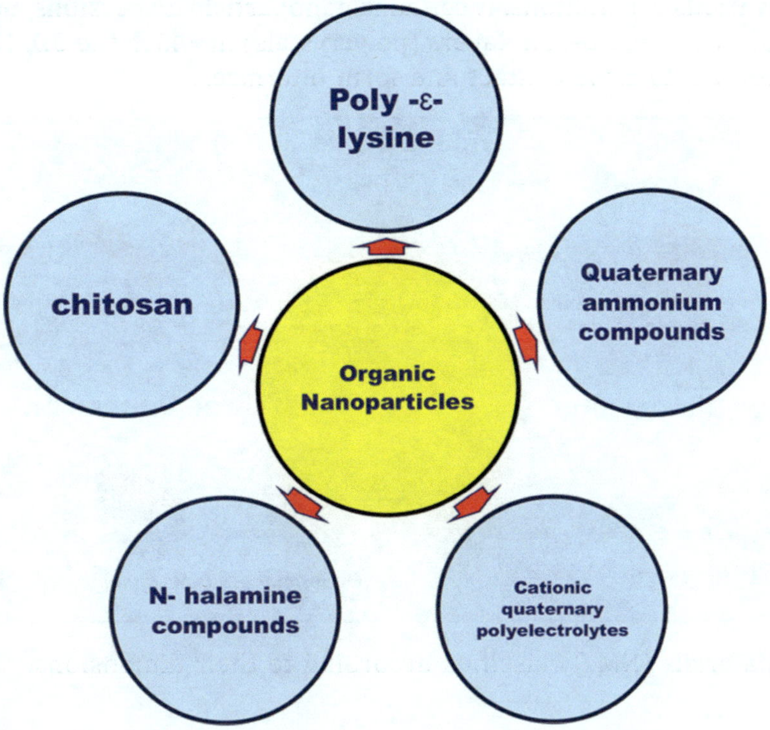

Figure 10.4. Organic nanomaterials (NMs).

10.1.2.4. Composite-Based Nanomaterials (NMs)

Composites NMs are formed by combining nanoparticles with other nanoparticles, nanoparticles with larger-scale materials, and NMs with bulk-type materials. NMs are already being employed to improve mechanical, thermal, and flame-retardant qualities in a wide range of items, including automobile parts and packaging materials.

10.1.2.5. Classification of Nanomaterials (NMs) Based on Dimensions

According to Siegel, nanostructured materials are classified as (Figure 10.5):

1. **Zero-Dimensional Nanomaterials (NMs):** All dimensions (x, y, and z) are at the nanoscale, meaning that no dimension is larger than 100 nm. These include nanospheres and nanoclusters.
2. **One-Dimensional Nanomaterials (NMs):** Two dimensions (x, y) are at the nanoscale, while the other is outside of it. This results in needle-shaped NMs. It comprises nanofibers, nanotubes, nanorods, and nanowires.

3. **Two-Dimensional Nanomaterials (NMs):** One dimension (x) is at the nanoscale, while the other two are larger. These 2D NMs have plate-like shapes and include nanofilms, nanolayers, and nanocoatings with nanometer thickness.
4. **Three-Dimensional Nanomaterials (NMs):** These are nanoparticles that do not belong to the nanoscale in any dimension. These materials have three arbitrary dimensions that exceed 100 nm. The bulk (3D) NMs are made up of several arrangements of nanosized crystals in various orientations. It contains nanoparticle dispersions, bundles of nanowires and nanotubes, and multi-nanolayers (polycrystals) in which the 0D, 1D, and 2D structural elements come into close contact and form interfaces.

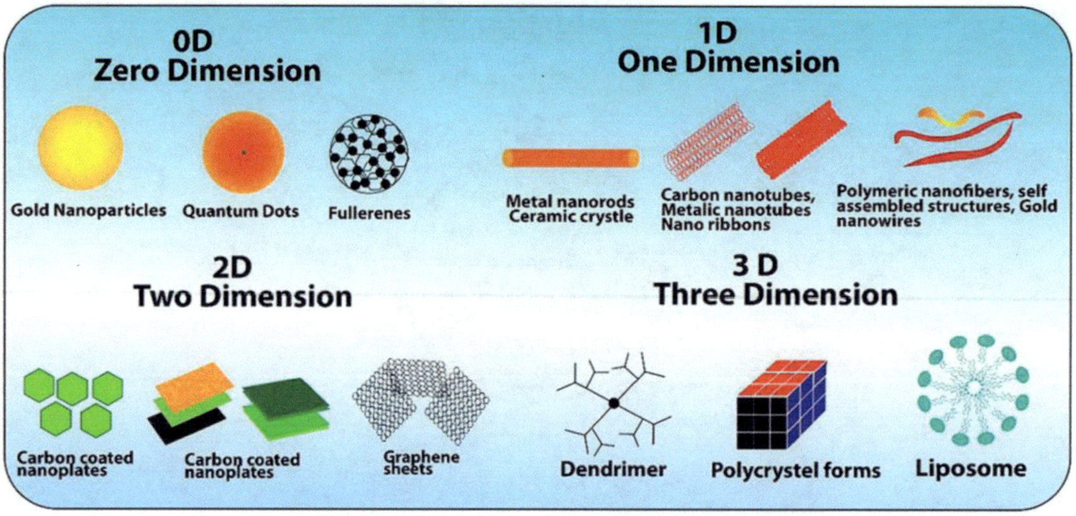

Figure 10.5. Nanomaterials (NMs) classified according to their dimensions.

10.1.2.6. Classification of Nanomaterials (NMs) Based on Their Origin

Nanoparticles are classified into two types based on their origin: natural and artificial:

1. **Natural Nanomaterials (NMs):** These can take many forms, including viruses, protein molecules, minerals like clay, natural colloids like milk and blood (liquid colloids), fog (aerosol type), gelatin (gel type), mineralized natural materials like shells, corals, and bones, insect wings and opals, spider silk, lotus leaves, gecko feet, volcanic ash, and sea spray.
2. **Artificial Nanomaterials (NMs):** CNTs and semiconductor nanoparticles like quantum dots (QDs) are examples of artificial NMs that are made consciously using precise mechanical and manufacturing procedures. NMs are categorized as metal-based materials, dendrimers, or composites depending on their structural makeup.

10.2. Nanotoxicity

Nanotoxicology studies the harmful effects of nanoparticles on human health and the environment. Nanotoxicology seeks to define and identify the risks of manmade NMs, necessitating a multidisciplinary team approach that includes toxicology, biology, chemistry, physics, material science, geology, exposure assessment, pharmacokinetics, and medicine. On the one hand, while it is utilised in biomedicine to diagnose and cure ailments, there is growing concern that it may cause disease. Humans' terrible experiences with carcinogenic items such as tobacco and asbestos, which they once assumed were benign, raised concerns about NPs. Because some NPs have a long, thin, fibrous structure like asbestos, they demonstrate fibrogenic and toxic consequences. "Can nanoparticles be the future asbestos?" prompted the query. Exposure period, dose, aggregation, and concentration, particle size and shape, surface area, and charge are all important considerations in assessing NM toxicity (Klaassen and Watkins, 2015).

10.2.1. Factors

1. **Size:** A nanoparticle's size can influence its toxicity in a number of ways. For example, lowering the size of NMs increases the particle surface area. This permits more molecules to adhere to the surface area, increasing the detrimental effects. Particles of varied sizes may accumulate in different parts of the lungs and escape at different rates (Chithrani, Ghazani, and Chan, 2006).
2. **Particle Surface, Surface Chemistry, and Charge:** The NMs' extended surface area and fine surface structure facilitate biological interaction between the microenvironment and NMs. NMs are coated and can be positively or negatively charged depending on their function. Topographic characterization can be achieved using electron and atomic force microscopes, allowing surface chemistry to be examined. Studies have shown that several parameters can influence nanoparticle toxicity (Ismail et al., 2007).
3. **Dosage:** Inhaling NMs has been linked to dose-dependent harmful consequences, as documented in numerous papers. Recent research suggests that relying just on mass concentration measurements for toxicological dosing yields inaccurate results and fails to fully describe the connection between nanoparticles and exposed tissue (Maynard et al., 2006).

10.3. Entry Route of Nanoparticle in Human Body

The most common way to become exposed to NMs is through inhalation. Additionally, they can enter the body through the skin, ingestion, or injection. Nanoparticles may contribute to the development of some diseases by influencing the lungs and other systems through a variety of mechanisms.

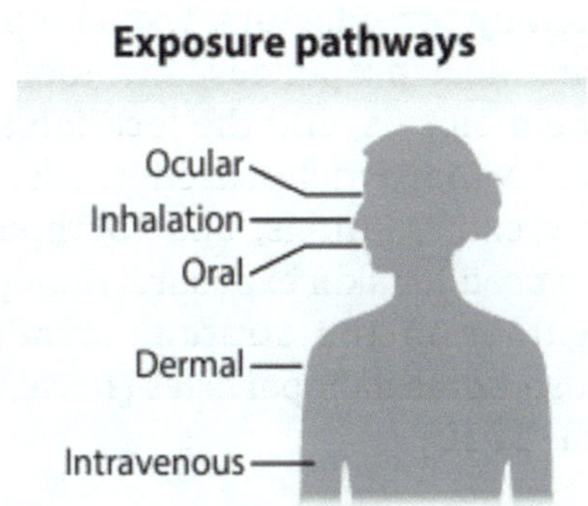

Figure 10.6. Representation of various entry routes.

Respiratory units can carry particles as tiny as 0.1 μm into the distal airways. Inhaled nanoparticles reach the respiratory epithelium and pass through the alveoli-capillary membrane to the interstitium before entering the systemic circulation via blood and lymphatic arteries. Humans, as social organisms, will engage naturally with NMs. Numerous studies have discovered that nanoparticles can affect a variety of body regions. NMs often enter the body via the respiratory tract and make intimate contact with the lungs. NMs frequently enter the body via skin contact or the gastrointestinal tract. Furthermore, implants and injections allow NMs into the body (De Matteis, 2017) (Figure 10.6).

10.3.1. Inhalation Exposure

Nanoparticles settle in the respiratory system according to their size, gravity resistance, and distribution pattern. Nanoparticles enter the body via the respiratory tract and are cleared by mucociliary cells and macrophages. They can also form clusters in the lungs and spread throughout the body via blood circulation. Inhaled nanoparticles can enter a variety of organs, including the brain. A potential link with prostate cancer has been investigated (Sharifi et al., 2012).

10.3.2. Dermal Exposure

Nanoparticle absorption from the skin is determined by three factors: the nanoparticle's physicochemical properties, the tool used to scatter the molecule, and the location and skin conditions. Nanoparticle-based goods, such as cosmetic creams, lotions, and toothpaste, are frequently used for skin exposure. Nanoparticles usually gather in the stratum corneum and dermis. Also, some nanoparticles (Desai, Patlolla, and Singh, 2010).

10.3.3. Ingestion Exposure

Nanoparticles can be absorbed directly from the digestive tract or indirectly via inhaled particles. Nanoparticles such as metal compounds and pesticides provide a significant danger of inadvertent ingestion. This is frequently missed because it is considered to be deliberate or caused by gross negligence. Poor nanoparticle absorption from the intestines, along with liver metabolism, exacerbates the problem (Bouwmeester et al., 2018).

10.4. Use of Nanoparticle in Medicine

Nanomedicine is a growing field in medical sciences, coinciding with advances in nanotechnology. Nanoparticles' flexibility to be changed makes them useful in a variety of applications. Nanoparticles are used and explored in many medical domains, such as illness therapy, surgery, medical implants, smart drug delivery, gene delivery, diagnosis/imaging, tissue engineering, regenerative medicine, and antibiotic resistance.

10.4.1. Cancer Diagnosis and Treatment

Nanoparticles are increasingly being used for cancer detection, imaging, and treatment. QDs are used in magnetic resonance imaging (MRI) to improve the accuracy of cancer detection. Nanoparticle-based test chips, such as lab-on-a-chip (LOC), can detect cancer biomarkers and enable early detection without invasive procedures. CNTs can reveal DNA mutations and detect biomarkers. Dendrimers and nanoparticles can be employed as contrast agents in imaging and for targeted medicine delivery. AuNPs functionalized with lanthanides (Gd^{3+} and Yb^{3+}) were employed *in vivo* for imaging (MRI and CT) and photothermal therapy (PTT). Ion-doped NMs are used in bioimaging and medicinal applications (Zheng et al., 2005).

10.4.2. Gene Therapy

It is a well-studied subject that aims to prevent and treat genetic illnesses by correcting faulty genes. Various ways can be used to deliver or replace the repaired or corrected gene. This strategy provides the potential to treat cancer, infections, cardiovascular diseases, autoimmune disorders, and monogenic diseases like hemophilia.

10.4.3. Treatment Neural Degeneration

Treatment for degenerative diseases and posttraumatic disorders involves regenerating and protecting neural tissue, as well as guiding axon growth, similar to other approaches. Nanomedical applications show promise for treating Parkinson's and Alzheimer's disorders, as well as regenerating axonal damage. Nanoparticles with high affinity for circulating Aβ subtypes may reduce Alzheimer's disease (AD) symptoms (Biju et al., 2011).

10.4.4. Tissue Engineering

This is a widely discussed topic among regenerative medicine, nanomedicine, and biomedical engineers. Biocompatible and biodegradable NM-based bio-scaffolds can be utilized to repair or duplicate damaged tissues while causing minimum harm.

10.4.5. Antimicrobial Activities

Metallic nanoparticles have antibacterial properties and can be used with other drugs to minimize antibiotic resistance. Nanoparticles of ZnO, gold, silver, and other materials are among these agents. Nanoparticles are used to create various surgical or implanted devices for the body (Banoee et al., 2010).

10.4.6. Orthopedic Implants

Orthopedic procedures use a variety of implants, including bone tissue engineering, nanostructured, and surface-modified/coated materials. Polymers, both synthetic and natural, are commonly employed in tissue engineering for bone and cartilage. Examples include collagen, hyaluronic acid (HA), chitosan (CH), titanium alloys, ceramic-coated metal oxides (e.g., alumina, zirconia, titania), hydroxyapatites, and carbon NMs such as graphene and diamond. Carbon nanocomposites with ceramic or polymer matrix are used to enhance the bioactivity, mechanical properties, and osteoconductivity, resulting in faster and more successful healing (Zhou et al., 2015).

10.4.7. Dental Implants

NMs are commonly utilized in dentistry as antibacterial, medicinal, or reinforcing materials. They are also used for polishing the enamel surface, fillings, and dental implants. Composites include CNTs, graphene, hydroxyapatite, iron oxide, zirconia, silica-based NMs, titanium, and AgNPs (Priyadarsini, Mukherjee, and Mishra, 2018).

10.5. Toxic Effects of Nanoparticles on Various Human Systems

The nanoparticles can produce harmful effects in several systems as they enter the body through three primary pathways. This section explores the harmful effects of NMs on systems, primarily through tests on animals.

10.5.1. Circulatory System

Clinical and experimental investigations clearly demonstrate that breathing nano- and micro-particles may have cardiovascular repercussions. Although there appears to be an intuitive link between inhaled nanoparticles and poor respiratory outcomes, the causal relationship between particles in the lung and cardiovascular effects is not entirely understood. It was hypothesized that particle-induced lung inflammation induces systemic cytokine release, culminating in serious cardiovascular repercussions. The cardiovascular effects of injected or inhaled nanoparticles, however, can be directly linked to their presence within the organism, as evidenced by recent studies on humans and animals that show nanoparticles diffuse from the lungs into the systemic circulation before being transported to the organs (Magaye et al., 2014).

10.5.2. Digestive System

In rats, exposure to 100 ppm zirconia oxide nanoparticles causes liver injury. Iron oxide nanoparticles have been shown to cause liver damage in mice (Bellusci et al., 2014).

10.5.3. Endocrine System

Oral iron oxide nanoparticles disrupt thyroid hormones in rats (Babadi et al., 2013).

10.5.4. Immune System

TiO_2 nanoparticles in mice significantly increased the quantity of white blood cells. Iron oxide nanoparticles increase the quantity of white blood cells, mostly affecting the liver and spleen (Xu et al., 2013).

10.5.5. Respiratory System

Nanoparticles are linked to negative outcomes such as decreased macrophage clearance, inflammation, particle buildup, and epithelial cell proliferation, followed by fibrosis, emphysema, and tumor formation (Cai et al., 2017).

10.5.6. Urinary System

Zinc oxide, copper, and iron oxide nanoparticles are harmful to kidney cells in monkeys, pigs, and cows (Saranya et al., 2017).

10.5.7. Reproductive System

Injecting ZnO nanoparticles intraperitoneally in mice resulted in a loss of seminiferous tubule cells (Kong et al., 2014).

10.6. Toxicity Testing

In vitro tests are more common than *in vivo* ones, and dose is crucial in determining toxicity. The toxicity test includes an *in vitro* sedimentation diffusion and dosimeter model. The model distinguishes between exposure (concentration in the cell environment), dose accumulation on the cell surface, and cellular dose (Thomas et al., 2018).

10.6.1. Methods for Evaluating Nanotoxicity and Risk Assessment

Methods for evaluating nanotoxicity and conducting risk assessments in the context of nanomedicine encompass a wide range of experimental, computational, and regulatory approaches. Here are some key methodologies used in this field (Kumar, Dasgupta, and Ranjan, 2018).

10.6.2. In Vitro Models for Nanotoxicity Assessment

The toxicity test utilizes an in vitro sedimentation, diffusion, and dosimetry model, which differentiates among exposure (the concentration in the cellular environment), dose accumulation on the cell surface, and the actual cellular dose. Dose rate can be evaluated as a factor of response by knowing how long it takes to deliver a particular dose. To test toxicity, *in vitro* procedures such as cell viability and proliferation are commonly utilized. Other approaches include gene expression analysis, genotoxicity detection, and *in vitro* hemolysis, Imaging techniques include SEM-EDX, TEM, AFM, VEDIC, and fluorescence spectroscopy.

Combining these assays improves the ability to detect nanotoxicity.

10.6.3. In Vivo Approaches in Assessing Nanotoxicity and Risks

In vivo toxicity tests are typically performed on animal models such as mice and rats. *In vivo* toxicity assessments include bio-distribution, clearance, hematology, serum chemistry, and histopathology. Biodistribution studies look into how nanoparticles go to tissues or organs. Radiolabels detect nanoparticles in both deceased and living animals. The clearance of nanoparticles is accomplished by examining their excretion and metabolism at various time periods following exposure. Another way for assessing *in vivo* toxicity is to examine changes in serum chemistry and cell type following exposure to nanoparticles. To measure the toxicity level caused by a nanoparticle, histopathology is performed on the cell, tissue, or organ following exposure.

10.6.4. Computational Simulations and Predictive Models

Nanotoxicity, the have a look at of the potential detrimental effects of nanoparticles on living organisms, is a vital issue of nanomedicine studies. As nanomedicine maintains to advance, understanding, and assessing the dangers related to nanoparticles turn out to be increasingly vital. Computational simulations and predictive fashions play a substantial role on this system.

1. **Simulation of Nanoparticle Behavior:** Computational simulations can version the conduct of nanoparticles within organic structures, consisting of their interplay with cells, tissues, and organs. These simulations help researchers recognize how nanoparticles circulate, gather, and doubtlessly reason harm in the frame.
2. **Predictive Toxicology Models:** Predictive fashions are advanced based totally on experimental information to forecast the ability toxicity of nanoparticles. These models often contain parameters together with nanoparticle length, form, floor chemistry, and dose to expect their biological effects. Machine getting to know algorithms, such as assist vector machines or neural networks, can be trained on large datasets to enhance the accuracy of predictions.
3. **Quantitative Structure-Activity Relationship (QSAR) Models:** QSAR fashions correlate the physicochemical houses of nanoparticles with their organic activities or toxicities. By analyzing the shape-belongings relationships, QSAR fashions can predict the toxicity of new nanoparticles based totally on their structural characteristics.
4. ***In Silico* ADME (Absorption, Distribution, Metabolism, and Excretion) Modeling:** Understanding the ADME homes of nanoparticles is important for assessing their potential toxicity and therapeutic efficacy. In silico ADME modeling uses computational techniques to simulate the ADME of nanoparticles in organic systems, providing insights into their fate within the frame.
5. **Multi-Scale Modeling:** Nanotoxicity is a complex phenomenon prompted by means of interactions at multiple scales, from molecular interactions to whole organism responses. Multi-scale modeling integrates statistics and computational tactics across one-of-a-kind ranges of organic employer to provide a complete expertise of nanotoxicity mechanisms.

6. **High-Throughput Screening:** Computational fashions can facilitate high-throughput screening of huge numbers of nanoparticles to prioritize people with decrease toxicity for in addition experimental validation. This method quickens the identification of safer nanomedicines even as reducing the need for tremendous animal trying out.
7. **Risk Assessment Frameworks:** Integrating computational simulations and predictive fashions into threat assessment frameworks allows regulators and policymakers to assess the safety of nanomedicines more efficaciously. These frameworks consider elements inclusive of exposure ranges, hazard potential, and dose-reaction relationships to decide desirable degrees of risk.

Overall, computational simulations and predictive models play a critical role in nanotoxicity evaluation and hazard management in nanomedicine, helping in the development of more secure and greater effective nanoparticle-based totally healing procedures (Kumar, Dasgupta, and Ranjan, 2018).

10.7. Conclusion

In conclusion, the burgeoning field of nanomedicine holds immense promise for revolutionizing healthcare through targeted drug delivery, diagnostics, imaging, and therapy. However, alongside these advancements come potential risks associated with the use of nanoparticles in medical applications. Nanotoxicity, the finding of adverse effects induced by nanoparticles, is a critical concern that requires thorough assessment to ensure the safety and efficacy of nanomedicines. The comprehensive evaluation of nanotoxicity and risk assessment of nanomedicine involve interdisciplinary approaches that integrate experimental studies, computational simulations, and predictive models. Through these methodologies, researchers can elucidate the complex interactions between nanoparticles and biological systems, predict potential hazards, and guide the design of safer nanomedicines. Key findings from nanotoxicity studies and risk assessments underscore the importance of considering various factors such as nanoparticle physicochemical properties, dose-response relationships, biodistribution, biocompatibility, and long-term effects. Furthermore, the development and validation of computational models enable researchers to expedite the screening of NMs, prioritize candidates for further evaluation, and optimize their design for improved safety profiles.

KEY TERMS FROM THIS CHAPTER

gene therapy
nanomaterials
pharmacokinetics
semiconductor
graphene
nanotoxicity
risk assessment

References

1. Abera, B. M. B. (2023). Nanomaterials: An overview of synthesis, classification, characterization, and applications. *Nano Select, 4*(1), 486–501.
2. Babadi, V. Y., Najafi, L., Najafi, A., Gholami, H., Zarji, M. E. B., et al. (2013). Evaluation of iron oxide nanoparticles effects on tissue and enzymes of thyroid in rats. *International Research Journal of Biological Sciences, 2*(7), 67–69.
3. Banoee, M., Seif, S., Nazari, Z. E., Jafari-Fesharaki, P., Shahverdi, H. R., et al. (2010). ZnO nanoparticles enhanced antibacterial activity of ciprofloxacin against *Staphylococcus aureus* and *Escherichia coli*. *Journal of Biomedical Materials Research Part B: Applied Biomaterials, 93*(2), 557–561.
4. Bayda, S., Adeel, M., Tuccinardi, T., Cordani, M., & Rizzolio, F. (2020). The history of nanoscience and nanotechnology: From chemical–physical applications to nanomedicine. *Molecules, 25*(1), 112.
5. Bellusci, M., La Barbera, A., Padella, F., Mancuso, M., Pasquo, A., et al. (2014). Biodistribution and acute toxicity of a nanofluid containing manganese iron oxide nanoparticles produced by a mechanochemical process. *International Journal of Nanomedicine, 9*(1), 1919–1929.
6. Biju, D., Lopes-Benjamin, D., Journeay, N., Sadeghi, H., Wu, L. P., et al. (2011). Nanotechnologies for Alzheimer's disease: Diagnosis, therapy and safety issues. *Nanomedicine: Nanotechnology, Biology and Medicine, 7*(5), 521–540.
7. Bouwmeester, H., Van der Zande, M., & Jepson, M. A. (2018). Effects of food-borne nanomaterials on gastrointestinal tissues and microbiota. *Wiley Interdisciplinary Reviews: Nanomedicine and Nanobiotechnology, 10*(1), e1481.
8. Cai, X., Lee, A., Ji, Z., Huang, C., Chang, C. H., et al. (2017). Reduction of pulmonary toxicity of metal oxide nanoparticles by phosphonate-based surface passivation. *Particle and Fiber Toxicology, 14*(1), 1–11.
9. Chithrani, B. D., Ghazani, A. A., & Chan, W. C. (2006). Determining the size and shape dependence of gold nanoparticle uptake into mammalian cells. *Nano Letters, 6*(4), 662–668.
10. De Matteis, V. (2017). Exposure to inorganic nanoparticles: Routes of entry, immune response, biodistribution and *in vitro/in vivo* toxicity evaluation. *Toxics, 5*(4), 29.
11. Desai, P., Patlolla, R. R., & Singh, M. (2010). Interaction of nanoparticles and cell-penetrating peptides with skin for transdermal drug delivery. *Molecular Membrane Biology, 27*(7), 247–259.
12. Ismail, F. S., Rohanizadeh, R., Atwa, S., Mason, R. S., & Ruys, A. J., et al. (2007). The influence of surface chemistry and topography on the contact guidance of MG63 osteoblast cells. *Journal of Materials Science: Materials in Medicine, 18*(5), 705–714.
13. Khan, H. S. Y., Shah, S. Z. A., Khan, M. N., & Shah, A. A. (2022). Classification, synthetic, and characterization approaches to nanoparticles, and their applications in various fields of nanotechnology: A review. *Catalysts, 12*(11), 1386.
14. Khan, I., Saeed, K., & Khan, I. (2019). Nanoparticles: Properties, applications and toxicities. *Arabian Journal of Chemistry, 12*(7), 908–931.
15. Khan, S., & Hossain, M. K. (2022). In *Nanoparticle-Based Polymer Composites*. Woodhead Publishing.

16. Klaassen, C. D., & Watkins, J. B. (2015). *Casarett & Doull's Essentials of Toxicology* (3rd ed.). McGraw Hill Education–Lange.
17. Kong, L., Tang, M., Zhang, T., Wang, D., Hu, K., et al. (2014). Nickel nanoparticles exposure and reproductive toxicity in healthy adult rats. *International Journal of Molecular Sciences, 15*(11), 21253–21269.
18. Kumar, V., Dasgupta, N., & Ranjan, S. (2018). *Nanotoxicology: Toxicity Evaluation, Risk Assessment and Management.* Springer.
19. Magaye, R. R., Yue, X., Zou, B., Shi, H., Yu, H., et al. (2014). Acute toxicity of nickel nanoparticles in rats after intravenous injection. *International Journal of Nanomedicine, 9*(1), 1393–1402.
20. Maynard, A. D., Aitken, R. J., Butz, T., Colvin, V., Donaldson, K., et al. (2006). Safe handling of nanotechnology. *Nature, 444*(7117), 267–269.
21. Priyadarsini, S., Mukherjee, S., & Mishra, M. (2018). Nanoparticles used in dentistry: A review. *Journal of Oral Biology and Craniofacial Research, 8*(1), 58–67.
22. Saranya, S., Vijayaranai, K., Pavithra, S., Raihana, N., & Kumanan, K. (2017). *In vitro* cytotoxicity of zinc oxide, iron oxide and copper nano powders prepared by green synthesis. *Toxicology Reports, 4*, 427–430.
23. Sharifi, S., Behzadi, S., Laurent, S., Forrest, M. L., Stroeve, P., & Mahmoudi, M. (2012). Toxicity of nanomaterials. *Chemical Society Reviews, 41*(6), 2323–2243.
24. Tadesse, G. (2006). *The Study of Antiferromagnetic in Diluted Magnetic Semiconductor "CDMNTE"* (Master's thesis). Addis Ababa University.
25. Thomas, D. G., Smith, J. N., Thrall, B. D., Baer, D. R., Jolley, H., et al. (2018). ISD3: A proterokinetic model for predicting the combined effects of particle sedimentation, diffusion and dissolution on cellular dosimetry for *in vitro* systems. *Particle and Fiber Toxicology, 15*(1), 1–22.
26. Xu, J., Shi, H., Ruth, M., Yu, H., Lazar, L., et al. (2013). Acute toxicity of intravenously administered titanium dioxide nanoparticles in mice. *PLoS ONE, 8*(8), 1–6.
27. Zhang, X. F., Liu, Z. G., Shen, W., & Gurunathan, S. (2016). Silver nanoparticles: Synthesis, characterization, properties, applications, and therapeutic approaches. *International Journal of Molecular Sciences, 17*(9), 1534.
28. Zheng, G., Patolsky, F., Cui, Y., Wang, W. U., & Lieber, C. M. (2005). Multiplexed electrical detection of cancer markers with nanowire sensor arrays. *Nature Biotechnology, 23*(10), 1294–1301.
29. Zhou, C., Deng, C., Chen, X., Zhao, X., Chen, Y., et al. (2015). Mechanical and biological properties of the micro-/nano-grain functionally graded hydroxyapatite bio ceramics for bone tissue engineering. *Journal of the Mechanical Behavior of Biomedical Materials, 48*, 1–11.

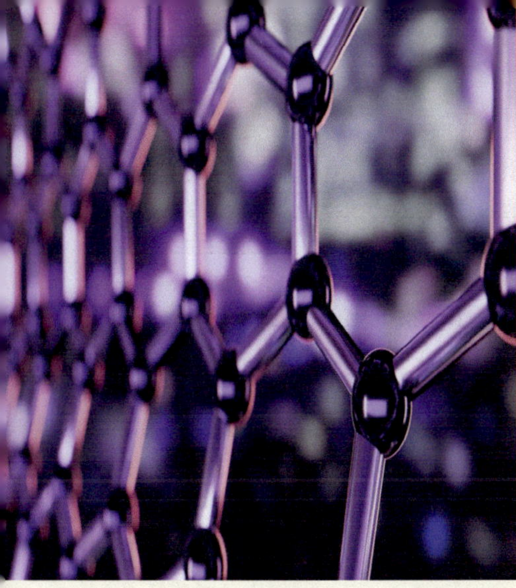

Chapter 11

IMPACT OF NANOMATERIAL ON ENVIRONMENT: FATE OF NANOMATERIAL

Contents

Swati, Sakshi, and Archana Gupta*

Department of Biotechnology and Microbiology, Faculty of Science and Humanities, SRM University Delhi-NCR, Sonepat, Haryana, India

**Corresponding author.*

Abstract

Nanotechnology has sparked widespread attention due to the requirements and applications of nanoparticles in human endeavors, including industry, agriculture, business, medicine, public health and a wide variety of sectors having the human reach. A number of research evaluating the potential ecotoxicity of nanomaterials (NMs) has increased over the previous decade which raises the question of providing complete acceptance to the nanoparticles. This chapter provides a glance at the matter to evaluate whether despite their benefits, nanoparticles should be considered as potential improvers or danger to health. Overview of the environmental destiny of commonly utilized nanoparticles (NPs) such as Ag-NPs, ZnO-NPs, and TiO_2-NPs, based on current findings.

11.1. Nanomaterials (NMs)

11.1.1. Introduction to Nanomaterials (NMs)

Nanomaterials (NMs) contain at least one structural dimension at the nanoscale (one nanometer is a billionth of a meter or 10^{-9} of a meter) and have attracted intense research interest due to their application potential in various fields of science and technology (Kabir et al., 2018). NMs are utilized to detect biological molecules, image diseased tissues, and develop innovative therapeutics. Nano-based particles (1–100 nm) can miniaturized biosensors, enabling smaller samples for biochemical analysis and point-of-care (POC) diagnosis (Bayda et al., 2020). Today's scientists are able to create a wide range of materials at the nanoscale, including graphene, carbon nanotubes (CNTs), nanofibers, and nanoclays, all of which have greater chemical reactivity and are lighter, stronger, and have more control over the light spectrum. Nanoparticles can be engineered from a variety of materials, including metals, metal oxides, polymers, and carbon-based materials. Despite these technological advancements in NMs, there is still a lack of knowledge on the potential impacts of NMs on human health. Understanding the behavior and interactions of nanoparticles is essential for calculating their potential benefits while ensuring their safe and responsible use in different applications. One exciting area of research in NMs involves the development of smart or responsive NMs that can exhibit dynamic responses to external stimuli such as light, temperature, pH, or mechanical forces. These responsive NMs could be used in sensors that detect environmental pollutants and trigger a signal in the presence of specific contaminants. But as a two-faced sword, a detailed impact study needs to be done in order to provide them with assent. If a remediation strategy is not established, NMs can cause a variety of difficulties applied on environment too as they may not be identifiable after being released into the environment (Khan, Abdalla, and Qurashi, 2017). In this chapter we summarize the impact of NM on aqueous ecosystem, effect on soil and agriculture, and wildlife and biodiversity.

11.1.2. Methods of Synthesis

The two basic methodologies commonly used for NP synthesis are top-down and bottom-up approaches (Figure 11.1(a)).

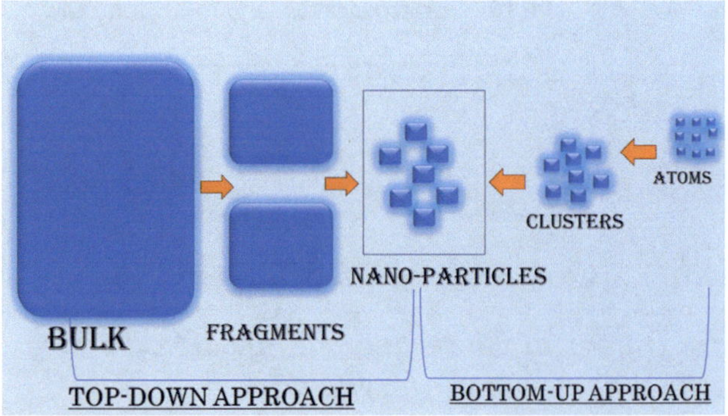

Figure 11.1(a). Methods of synthesis of nanomaterials (NMs).

These two approaches combine three different synthetic methods: chemical, physical, and biological. The physical method uses a top-down approach, while the other two methods are based on a bottom-up approach (Arole and Munde, 2014). It is a top-down approach that uses the entire analog as a starting point and gradually removes them one by one to produce a good NP. Photolithography, milling procedures, electron beam lithography, and ion plasma etching are some of the top-down techniques frequently used for large-scale production of NPs (Fu et al., 2018). It is a bottom-up approach where atoms and molecules combine to create a series of NPs. Sol-gel processing, laser pyrolysis (Abid et al., 2021), plasma or flame sputter synthesis, chemical vapor deposition, self-assembly of monomer molecules, electrochemical or chemical nanostructure deposition and bio-assisted synthesis are examples of bottom-up methods (Parashar, Shukla, and Singh, 2020) (Figure 11.1(b)).

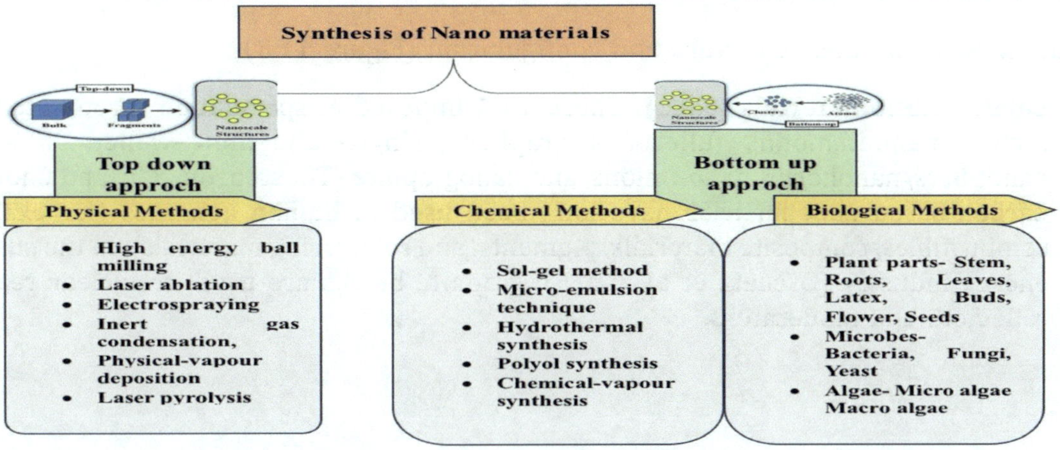

Figure 11.1(b). Methods of synthesis of nanomaterials (NMs).

11.1.3. Types of Nanomaterials (NMs)

Since NMs come from a wide variety of sources, it is necessary to classify and categorize them in order to comprehend them better. The classification of NMs can be done according to their dimensionality, origin, composition, porosity, phases, and dispersion.

Classification based on their dimensionality (Figure 11.2):

1. **Zero-Dimensional (0D) Nanomaterials (NMs):** NMs that are zero-dimensional (0D) possess all three dimensions at the nanoscale (less than 100 nm). Graphene quantum dots (GQDs), carbon quantum dots (CQDs), and fullerenes are a few examples (Wang et al., 2020).
2. **One-Dimensional (1D) Nanomaterials (NMs):** Materials classified as one-dimensional (1D) NMs have just one dimension larger than 100 nm. Electrons can be emitted in a low electric field from metal, metal oxides, and carbon-based 1D NMs with a high aspect ratio, such as nanotubes, nanowires, and nanofibers (Barhoum et al., 2021).
3. **Two-Dimensional (2D) Nanomaterials (NMs):** Two dimensions more than 100 nm characterize two-dimensional (2D) NMs. Their geometries resemble plates, and their thin layers are at least one atomic layer thick. Silicate clays, graphene, graphene oxide, and reduced graphene oxide are some examples of 2D NMs.

4. **Three-Dimensional (3D) Nanomaterials (NMs):** These substances have three dimensions greater than 100 nm. This class includes, but is not limited to, bundles of nanowires, nanotubes, and box-shaped graphene nanostructures (Zhao and Lei, 2020).

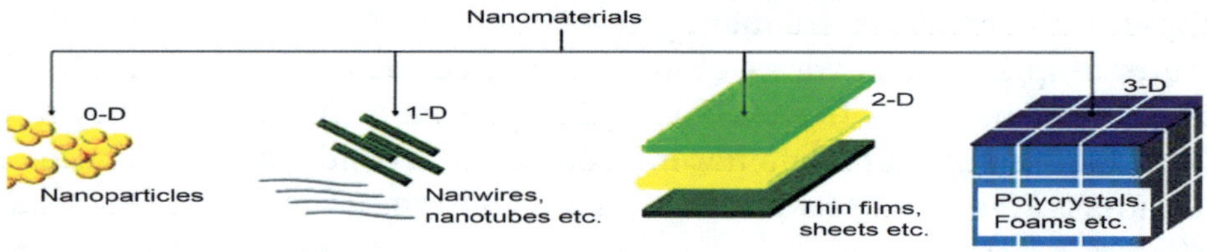

Figure 11.2. Nanomaterials (NMs) categorized based on their dimensionality.

Classification based on their structure and configuration (Figure 11.3):

1. **Carbon Nanomaterials (NMs):** These are composed of sp^2-bonded carbon atoms. They include nanodiamonds, fullerenes, graphene, single- and multi-walled CNTs, carbon nanofibers, nanohorns, nano-onions, and nanographite (Thostenson, Ren, and Chou, 2001). Carbon-based nanoparticles have long been used in human activities (for example, as combustibles, composite materials, pigments, and reinforcing materials). In the sustainable energy industry (Oschatz et al., 2016), graphite blocks are used in nuclear reactors as reflectors and moderators.

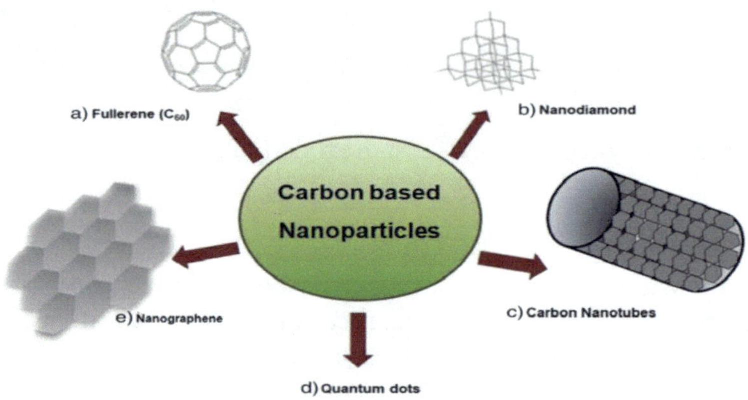

Figure 11.3. Carbon-based nanomaterials (NMs).

2. **Organic Nanomaterials (NMs):** These have functional qualities as a result of the chemical interaction of its main constituent (carbon) with other elements, which bestow unique functions and reactivity to the nanostructured architecture. This category contains lipid and polymer nanoparticles. Typically, both nanoparticle kinds are nanospheres or have a nano-encapsulated shape spanning from 10 to 1000 nm (Ramsden, 2011).
3. **Inorganic Nanomaterials (NMs):** These are formed by non-carbon components such as metals, metal oxides, and metal salts. They take on various shapes (spheres, cylinders, oblates, ellipsoids, cubes, and stars) depending on the atom packing, but preserve the crystallinity of metal-based compounds. However, there are amorphous inorganic nanoparticles. MSNs, AgNPs, CNTs, QDs, and AuNPs are some of the most widely utilized inorganic NMs in biomedicine (Figure 11.4).

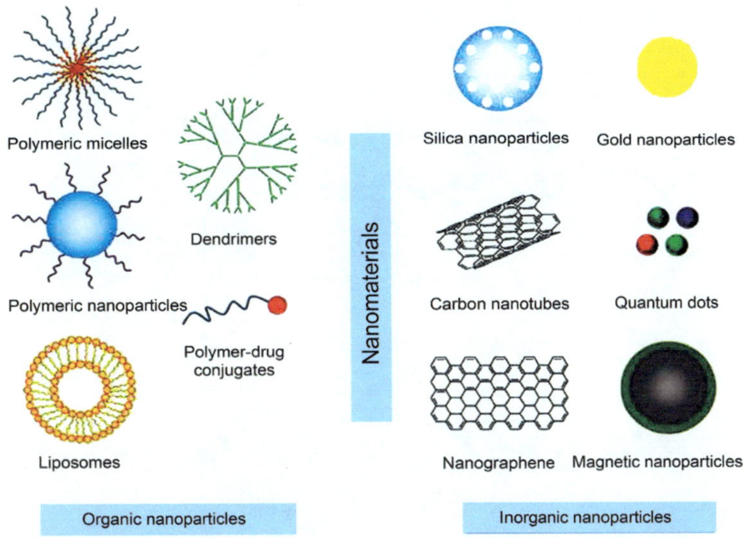

Figure 11.4. Organic and inorganic nanomaterials (NMs).

4. **Hybrid Nanomaterials (NMs):** These are multiphase materials that contain at least one nanosized component (1–100 nm) or have nanometric phase separation (Zhang, 2014). Hybrid nanocomposites are matrix-based, which can be polymer, ceramic, hydrogel, or metal.

Classification based on their porosity (Figure 11.5):

1. **Mesoporous Materials (Super-Nanoporous):** Nanoporous materials containing pores with diameters between 2 and 50 nm.
2. **Microporous Material:** Nanoporous materials with pores smaller than 2 nm in diameter include examples such as zeolites and metal–organic frameworks.
3. **Macroporous Material:** Nanoporous materials with pores larger than 50 nm in diameter.

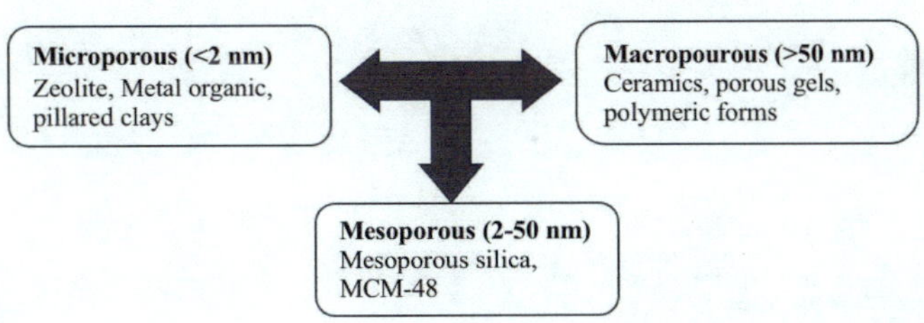

Figure 11.5. Classification of nanomaterials (NMs) based on porosity.

11.2. Applications of Nanomaterials (NMs)

Nanomaterials (NMs) have diverse applications across medical, environmental, and industrial fields, as illustrated in Figure 11.6. These include uses in drug delivery, biosensors, cosmetics, pollution control, and more.

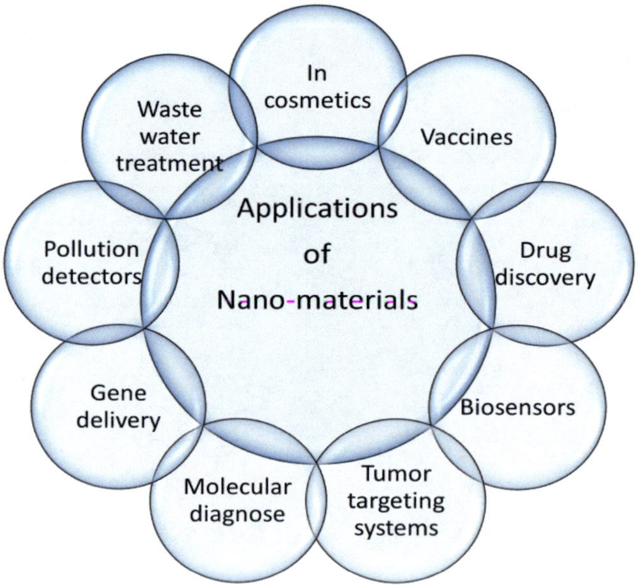

Figure 11.6. Applications of nanomaterials (NMs).

11.3. Fate and Behavior of Nanomaterials (NMs) in the Environment

The growing rates of NM synthesis, the potential for their release into the environment, and the resultant effects on ecosystem health is also increasing. The fate of NMs in the environment is determined by their physicochemical properties and interactions with other contaminants. NMs discovered in the environment can be the result of natural processes or intentional/unintentional human activities (Smita et al., 2012) (Figure 11.7).

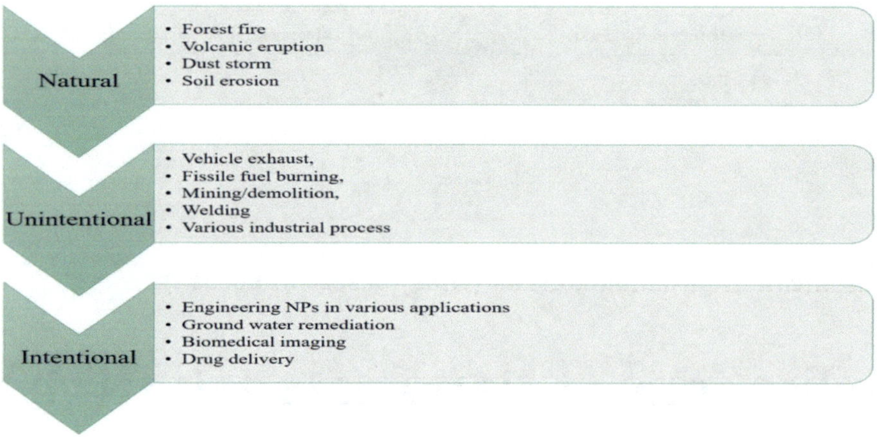

Figure 11.7. Common sources of nanomaterials (NMs) in the environment.

Nanoparticles can either stay intact or go through one or more of the following changes after entering the environment: Agglomeration/deagglomeration settling, full mineralization (to carbon dioxide and water), biological or chemical change to other chemicals, and/or dissolution speciation (i.e., interaction with other ionic or molecular dissolved chemical compounds). After being discharged into the environment, NMs accumulate in several environmental matrices such as air, water, soil, and sediments (Figure 11.8).

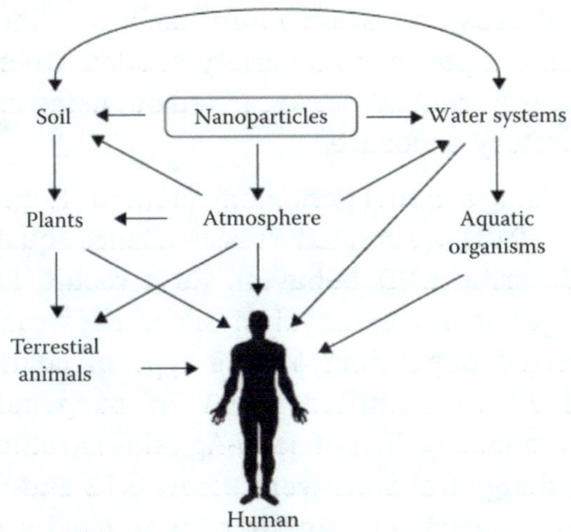

Figure 11.8. Possible pathways of nanomaterials (NMs) in the environment.

11.3.1. Soil

Soil is a multilayered and complicated interface of various substances (e.g., gases, solids, water, organic/inorganic components) and organisms. Engineered NMs can enter soils from a variety of sources and pathways, including fertilizers and plant protection products, biosolids, sewage water, and floodplains (Batley, Kirby, and McLaughlin, 2013). NMs have the potential to impact soil quality and ecosystem health through various mechanisms, depending on their properties, interactions, and concentrations in the environment. NMs penetrate through soil pores and bind to soil particles because of their large surface area. Sedimentation, filtration, or straining in finer pores can also immobilize large NM aggregates (Mukhopadhyay, 2014). Certain NMs may exhibit toxic effects on soil organisms such as earthworms, bacteria, fungi, and plants. Nanoparticles can penetrate cell membranes and disrupt cellular functions. The mobility of NMs in soils is determined by a variety of factors, like nanoparticle physical-chemical properties, soil and environmental features, and interactions with natural colloidal material. It was previously shown that silver NMs can act as a soil-based sink for Ag ions and that silver NM concentrations have a significant influence on their aggregation. Nanoparticles may adsorb onto soil particles, affecting nutrient uptake by plants. Previous research has also shown that plants may take up and translocate NMs from the soil, which may influence germination and growth and discover the harmful impacts of TiO_2 and ZnO NMs on the biodiversity of soil microbial populations.

11.3.2. Water

Nanoparticles can quickly reach aquatic environments by surface runoff from soils, industrial releases, and the disposal of wastewater treatment effluents. Thus, a variety of activities, such as accumulation, disaggregation, diffusion, interaction with other elements and aquatic animals, biological degradation (aerobic and anaerobic), and abiotic degradation (including photolysis and hydrolysis), influence the fate of NMs in the aquatic system (Vale et al., 2015). Nanoparticles can have both positive and negative impacts on water quality and aquatic ecosystems, depending on their properties, concentrations, and interactions with the environment. The combined impacts of particle size and coating material type were found to be critical in determining the fate of citrate and polyvinylpyrrolidone-coated silver nanoparticles (AgNPs) in water in a prior study (Rocha et al., 2015).

On a positive note, nanoparticles can be proven as much awaited boon by giving solutions to some common problems including:

1. **Water Treatment:** Nanoparticles such as silver, titanium dioxide, and iron oxide have been used in water treatment technologies for disinfection, pollutant removal, and catalytic reactions. These nanoparticles can help remove contaminants, pathogens, and organic pollutants from water, improving water quality and safety.
2. **Nanoremediation:** Nanoparticles can be used in various technologies to clean up contaminated water bodies by degrading or immobilizing pollutants. Nanoparticles like zero-valent iron (ZVI) can help remediate groundwater contaminated with heavy metals and chlorinated solvents.
3. **Sensor Technology:** Nanoparticles are used in sensor technologies for detecting pollutants and pathogens in water. Nanoparticle-based sensors offer high sensitivity, selectivity, and real-time monitoring capabilities for early detection of water quality issues.

But, just like coin has two sides there is and will always be chances of threat to the environment by the use of nanoparticles as:

1. **Ecotoxicity:** Some nanoparticles may show toxic effects on aquatic organisms such as fish, algae, zooplankton, and bacteria. They can disrupt cellular functions, induce oxidative stress, or interfere with metabolic processes in aquatic biota, leading to adverse effects on their growth, reproduction, and even on survival.
2. **Environmental Persistence:** Some nanoparticles can persist in water environments for extended periods due to their stability and low degradation rate and later may accumulate in sediments or water columns, impacting ecosystem dynamics.
3. **Bioaccumulation:** Nanoparticles can build up in aquatic organisms through food chains, creating risks of biomagnification and long-term exposure to higher trophic levels.

The negative consequences of NMs exposure on aquatic organisms, such as DNA damage, death, oxidative stress, and growth loss, have been documented in a few studies (Baker, Tyler, and Galloway, 2014). However, organisms in actual ecosystems are more likely to undergo chronic exposure to a variety of NMs, whereas these experiments were carried out using acute laboratory exposure.

Using a model parsimony method (Hendren et al., 2013), we created a mass-balance equation to describe END behavior. As a result, large changes in the removal of silver NMs can be expected depending on the type of coatings utilized to stabilize them in suspension. Approximately 95% of nano-Ag values in effluent and sludge fractions were below 0.12 and 0.35 μg L^{1}, respectively. Another study used a life-cycle approach to forecast ambient quantities of ENM-containing products in the US, Europe, and Switzerland. Surface water concentrations of fullerenes and nano-TiO_2 were 0.003 and 21 ng L^{1}, respectively, while sewage treatment effluents had values of 4 ng L^{1} and 4 μg L^{1}. According to O'Brien and Cummins (2010), Irish WWTPs have an average NM removal efficiency ranging from 59.8% to 70.2%, while water treatment plants have efficiencies ranging from 0% to 96.95%. The proposed model aims to predict the behavior of NMs such as TiO_2, Ag (metal and ionic forms), and CeO_2 in surface water and human exposure.

11.3.3. Air

There are still significant knowledge gaps about NMs' environmental destiny, particularly after emission into the atmosphere. Each stage of an engineered NMs life cycle, from generation to end-of-life, can result in discharge into the environment. Atmospheric NMs are created by automobile traffic exhaust, combustion, explosion, and oxidation of atmospheric gases (John et al., 2017). Engineered NMs released into the atmosphere are exposed to sunlight and UV wavelengths at substantially higher levels than those released into other compartments. Nanoparticles in the atmosphere can contribute to visibility reduction by scattering and absorbing light, leading to haze, smog, and decreased visual clarity. Ultrafine particles with sizes in the nanoscale range can penetrate into lungs and enter the bloodstream, leading to respiratory problems, cardiovascular conditions. There is a good chance that this exposure will also increase the potential for photochemical alterations to NMs. In the atmosphere, NMs can undergo a variety of changes, including the condensation of low volatility chemicals and the dissipation of adsorbed water or other volatiles, which results in a decrease in size. Therefore, deviations in particle size distributions are possible without affecting total numerical concentrations. Moreover, gravitational settling velocities—which correlate to molecule size are necessary for the deposition of NMs from air. The composition of trash incineration plants has a significant impact on the emissions of ENMs. Organic and carbonaceous ENMs often burn entirely, but nanoclays seem to linger in combustion leftovers. In many applications including cleaning, packing, sonication, mixing, and spraying, NMs are frequently released in huge aggregates rather than at the nanoscale. Moreover, significant amounts and concentrations of NMs could be discharged into air by explosion, fire, and carrier leakage (Hartmann et al., 2014).

11.3.4. Impact on Humans and Other Mammals

The toxicity and exposure of NMs, which can penetrate and absorb into mammalian cell membranes, are becoming increasingly concerning. Inhalation of airborne nanoparticles can lead to respiratory inflammation, oxidative stress, impaired lung function. Oral, cutaneous, inhalation, and/or gastrointestinal tract exposure are among the many ways that NMs might come into contact with goods including sunscreen, skin care products, paints and coatings, food and health supplements, food additives, and food colorings (Binderup et al., 2013). Furthermore, ENMs are occasionally purposefully injected into the human body for therapeutic purposes. Negative health consequences are caused by NMs through oxidative damage and the production of reactive oxygen species (ROS). NMs can interact with immune cells and modulate immune responses, leading to inflammation, allergic reactions and autoimmune responses. Researchers have discovered links between exposure to NMs in the neonatal period (the first month following birth) and increased aggravation of asthma, reduced lung function, and coughing and wheezing without illness (Meldrum et al., 2017). Moreover, long-term exposure to NMs may lower forced vital capacity (FVC) and forced expiratory volume (FEVI). According to Becker, CNTs and nanoscale TiO_2 particles have the potential to cause malignancies in animal models (Becker et al., 2011).

11.4. What Makes Nanomaterials (NMs) Active After Release?

Animal respiratory or digestive systems or plant roots are the most likely pathways for biota uptake. Additionally, uptake via epithelial surfaces is conceivable. The cell walls of plants and fungi serve as a first line of defense against the entry of NMs. Certain NMs may bind to natural organic matter (NOM) preferentially in terrestrial (and aquatic) environments, decreasing its bioavailability. These nanoparticles might be able to be absorbed by sediment feeders. In fact, if they are linked to NOM, they might preferentially consume them and strip or de-associate them in the gastrointestinal system. There have been prior reports of decreased antibacterial activity due to decreased bioavailability resulting from increased sorption of C_{60} to soil organic matter. According to Kennedy the stabilization of aquatic systems by NOM may keep NMs in the water column, increasing their bioavailability to aquatic species. However, this relationship to NOM may also lessen or even completely eradicate antibacterial activity (Bhatnagar and Sillanpää, 2017).

11.5. Environmental Effects

Because of their unique qualities (e.g., extremely small size and high surface-volume ratio), the effects and toxicity of NMs on the environment in terms of their interaction with biological substances remain little understood. Increasing the use of NMs in commercial and consumer items raises the risk of direct and indirect human exposure (Pattan and Kaul, 2014). Concerns have also been raised about whether the production of NMs may result in new dangers. The subsections address both the good and negative consequences of nanotechnology on the environment in light of their significance.

11.5.1. Positive Effects

There are substantial financial, social, and environmental benefits that nanotechnology offers. Eventually, nanotechnology might be used to create breakthroughs that are more energy-efficient and reduce the impact of humans on the environment. Energy-saving and energy-efficient devices have been developed through the application of nanotechnology in a variety of applications. Researchers have worked extremely hard to create "scrubbers" made of CNTs that can separate carbon dioxide from emissions from power plants. Using adsorption, filtration, and oxidation methods, NMs have been effectively used to purify air and water more effectively than with traditional methods. NMs have a unique ability to respond to pollutants and convert them into harmless particles. Nano-material coatings can withstand contaminants and have self-cleaning properties. NMs are also employed in sensing technology to detect low-level pollution. Nanotechnology can improve the efficiency and sustainability of batteries. Furthermore, by converting oil into biodegradable molecules, NMs can effectively clean up oil spills (Patel and Mahajan, 2017).

11.5.2. Negative Effects

It is very difficult to draw any conclusions about the ecological effects and environmental stability of NMs because the environmental impacts of NMs cannot be accurately diagnosed and there are too many variables to take into account (e.g., NMs identification, low detection limits, and unknown environmental concentrations). A small alteration to NMs' chemical structure could have a significant impact on their characteristics and transform them into hazardous substances. It was discovered that, if nanosilver was present in the soil, plants (such as monocotyledonous wheat and dicotyledonous cucumber) may absorb it. Plant growth was reduced as a result of the activation of genes linked to the ethylene signaling pathways caused by the uptake of nanoparticles. Additionally, NMs promoted the defense system's upregulation in plants, which likewise decreased plant growth. Nanoparticles like TiO_2 can have a genotoxic effect on plants like Allium cepa and Nicotiana tabacum causing

DNA damage at low doses of 0.25 mM found that nano-Zn and nano-ZnO had a negative impact on seed germination and growth in ryegrass/corn (Ghosh, Bandyopadhyay, and Mukherjee, 2010). Multi-walled CNTs, aluminum, and alumina had minimal effect on seed germination and plant growth. According to toxicological studies, NMs may damage unicellular aquatic organisms and creatures (such as fish and Daphnia). The effect of nano-Cd on Daphnia magna was studied to determine its toxicity.

11.6. Method of Assessment In Vitro

Assessment techniques *in vitro* have been modelled after studies in the field of mammalian toxicity. For instance, oxidative assessment has been studied using a variety of methodologies, while work in the fields of proteomics and genomes is progressing more slowly. Other techniques, taken from research on mammals, may be applied as well.

For example, the effects of NMs on fish hepatocyte function could be assessed using the enzyme lactate dehydrogenase (LDH) as a marker for cell toxicity, or the stability of the lysosome in mollusk hemocyte cells could be assessed. In order to better understand how some hazardous effects may arise and to assess possible long-term repercussions, it is crucial to link effects at various organizational levels (González, Barrera, and Martinez, n.d.). A thorough method for evaluating impacts is provided by *in vivo* exposures, which are followed by evaluation of particular endpoints at the organ and organelle levels as well as biochemical endpoints. Studies like the ones mentioned above that are conducted *in vitro* provide a targeted evaluation of the mechanistic impacts at a particular organizational level.

11.7. Method of Assessment In Vivo

There is still substantial dispute in the literature about what may be regarded as optimal approaches to exposures. A variety of methodologies have been used to assess the risk of nanoparticles to environmental organisms. The methodologies were chosen based on the species being examined. Laboratory studies have examined the impact of various NMs on reference species used in ecotoxicology. Endpoints including mortality, growth, eating, and reproduction are frequently used in ecotoxicology studies (Parashar et al., 2022). Furthermore, specific biomarkers, such as methods of assessing oxidative stress (in a specific organ or throughout the body, e.g., lipid peroxidation), genetic damage, CYP450 levels, gene expression, and damage to specific cell organelles (e.g., mitochondria or nucleus), are all widely used in the assessment of NMs. Cytological responses, including cellular apoptosis and necrosis, have also been employed.

11.8. Risk Assessment

The way that nanoparticles are employed in the workplace, how they are divided into various media (such as air and water), how mobile they are in each of these media, and how stable they are all affect how they interact with the environment. To evaluate the risks associated with nanoparticles, some basic information about their behavior and toxicity is needed. However, this information alone cannot be used to make a realistic assessment; rather, some data on the expected concentration of nanoparticles in environmental systems would be required, and there is currently no accurate information regarding such concentrations. The resources, environmental pathways, and applications of nanoparticles, together with the plants and animals that are sensitive to them, must be determined as a foundation for the environmental risk assessment of nanoparticles (Reijnders, 2006).

11.9. Regulations

New technology or products must undergo extensive testing for negative environmental and health effects before being used described the precautionary principles of environmental decision-making as follows:

- Taking preventive measures in the face of uncertainty.
- Shifting the burden of proof to the proponents of the action.
- Exploring potentially harmful alternatives and measures.
- Increasing public participation in decision-making has become more common, but before the introduction of NM, such principles were not followed, leaving uncertainty about the risks and benefits of NM (Kriebel et al., 2001).

However, some organizations have proposed preliminary occupational limits (OEL) for NMs. For example, the US National Institute for Occupational Safety and Health (NIOSH) proposed a recommended exposure limit (REL) for CNTs of 1 $\mu g/m^3$ for an 8-hour time-weighted average (TWA). NIOSH also proposed ultrafine (nanoscale) and pigment (> 100 nm) titanium dioxide RELs of 0.3 and 2.4 mg/m^3 for a 10-hour TWA per day. In addition, manufacturers must submit detailed information (e.g., specific chemical identification data, production methods, processing, production volume, exposure and release data, use area, and available health and safety data) about NM to the US Environmental Protection Agency check that the products do not pose a danger to people and/or the environment. The British Standards Institution (BSI) proposed NM reference levels for insoluble, highly soluble, and hazardous substances as 0.066, 0.5, and 0.1×OEL for micro-sized material, respectively (NIOSH, 2013; OECD Environment Directorate, 2014). In addition, the BSI reference level for fibrous NM is 0.01 fibers/mL. According to the German Institute for Occupational Safety and Health (IFA), the reference level for metals, metal oxides, and bio-persistent granular NM (density > 6000 kg/m^3) is 20,000 particles/cm^3, and for bio-persistent granular NM (density < 6000 kg/m^3), it is 40,000 particles/cm^3. However, such NM-OEL values are not necessarily sufficient to protect against health risks. Therefore, it is better to keep exposure limits as low as possible by implementing appropriate control measures such as safety data sheets, labels, and tags. However, such NM-OEL values are not necessarily sufficient to protect against health risks.

Therefore, it is recommended to keep the exposure limit as low as possible by applying appropriate control measures such as safety data sheets, labels, and tags. According to the European Union (EU) Regulation 1272/2008, NMs considered hazardous must be classified and labelled accordingly.

Through the Cefic-LRI project, mapped the nanotechnology governance environment considering existing regulatory frameworks, reporting systems, standardization, and best practice guidelines. In addition, voluntary NM reporting systems in European countries help to collect information on toxicity levels and to understand production and market distribution (Hermann et al., 2014).

11.10. Conclusion

NPs emissions into the environment can occur at any point during their life cycle, but the impact is more difficult to assess when the goods are used by consumers. Transformations influence the physicochemical properties of NPs, resulting in an environmental impact that differs from that of the original NPs. As a result, they should carefully analyze the toxicity research. Although toxicity mechanisms vary depending on the type of the NPs, the majority of them are based on oxidative stress processes, which cause ROS production and damage to cell structures. There are several *in vivo* and *in vitro* studies that back up the evidence of NPs' potential toxicity in a wide range of living creatures, changing cell structure in various ways. The effects of NP toxicity vary depending not just on the NM's properties, but also on the target organism. It is challenging to generalize about the environmental impact of NPs emissions due to the way that species experience this impact and the response that is triggered, which mostly relies on how they are exposed to the harmful agents. Thus, studies have demonstrated that the best method for assessing this impact is to analyze each pollution instance with a specific focus. However, depending on how they are used, some NPs have qualities that have a positive effect on the environment, reducing pollution, energy waste, and the greenhouse effect. Lastly, it is critical to emphasize that the laws pertaining to these contaminants are out of date. A balance between scientific advancement and sustainable growth must be maintained, even while the creation of new, exact legislation that carefully restricts NPs emissions is vital.

KEY TERMS FROM THIS CHAPTER

- carbon nanotubes
- environmental impacts
- nanomaterials
- recommended exposure limit
- decision-making
- environmental risk management
- nanoscale
- risk assessment

References

1. Abid, N., et al. (2021). Synthesis of nanomaterials using various top-down and bottom-up approaches, influencing factors, advantages, and disadvantages: A review. *Advances in Colloid and Interface Science, 300,* 102597.
2. Arole, V. M., & Munde, S. V. (2014). Fabrication of nanomaterials by top-down and bottom-up approaches—An overview. *Journal of Materials Science, 1,* 89–93.
3. Baker, T. J., Tyler, C. R., & Galloway, T. S. (2014). Impacts of metal and metal oxide nanoparticles on marine organisms. *Environmental Pollution, 186,* 257–271.
4. Barhoum, A., Favre, T., Sayegh, S., Tanos, F., Coy, E., Iatsunskyi, I., Razzouk, A., Cretin, M., & Bechelany, M. (2021). 3D self-supported nitrogen-doped carbon nanofiber electrodes incorporated Co/CoOx nanoparticles: Application to dyes degradation by electro-Fenton-based process. *Nanomaterials, 11,* 2686.
5. Batley, G. E., Kirby, J. K., & McLaughlin, M. J. (2013). Fate and risks of nanomaterials in aquatic and terrestrial environments. *Accounts of Chemical Research, 46*(3), 854–862.
6. Bayda, S., Adeel, M., Tuccinardi, T., Cordani, M., & Rizzolio, F. (2020). The history of nanoscience and nanotechnology: From chemical–physical applications to nanomedicine. *Molecules, 25,* 112.
7. Becker, H., Herzberg, F., Schulte, A., & Kolossa-Gehring, M. (2011). The carcinogenic potential of nanomaterials, their release from products and options for regulating them. *International Journal of Hygiene and Environmental Health, 214,* 231–238.
8. Bhatnagar, A., & Sillanpää, M. (2017). Removal of natural organic matter (NOM) and its constituents from water by adsorption: A review. *Chemosphere, 166,* 497–510.
9. Binderup, M. L., Bredsdorff, L., Beltoft, V. M., Mortensen, A., Loeschner, K., Larsen, E. H., & Eriksen, F. D. (2013). Systemic absorption of nanomaterials by oral exposure. *Environmental Project No. 1505.* Danish Environmental Protection Agency.
10. Fu, X., Cai, J., Zhang, X., Li, W. D., Ge, H., & Hu, Y. (2018). Top-down fabrication of shape-controlled, monodisperse nanoparticles for biomedical applications. *Advanced Drug Delivery Reviews, 132,* 169–187.
11. Ghosh, M., Bandyopadhyay, M., & Mukherjee, A. (2010). Genotoxicity of titanium dioxide (TiO_2) nanoparticles at two trophic levels: Plant and human lymphocytes. *Chemosphere, 81,* 1253–1262.
12. González Castro, F., Barrera, M., & Martinez, C. R. (n.d.). A dynamic tension has developed in prevention science regarding two imperatives.
13. Hartmann, N. I. B., Skjolding, L. M., Hansen, S. F., Baun, A., Kjølholt, J., & Gottschalk, F. (2014). Environmental fate and behavior of nanomaterials: New knowledge on important transformation processes. *Environmental Project No. 1594.* Danish Environmental Protection Agency.
14. Hendren, C. O., Badireddy, A. R., Casman, E., & Wiesner, M. R. (2013). Modelling nanomaterial fate in wastewater treatment: Monte Carlo simulation of silver nanoparticles (nano-Ag). *Science of the Total Environment, 449,* 418–425.
15. Hermann, A., Diesner, M. O., Abel, J., Hawthorne, C., & Greßmann, A. (2014). Assessment of impacts of a European register of products containing nanomaterials. *Umweltbundesamt, Text 23/2014.* Germany.

16. John, A. C., Küpper, M., Manders-Groot, A. M. M., Debray, B., Lacome, J. M., & Kuhlbusch, T. A. J. (2017). Emissions and possible environmental implication of engineered nanomaterials (ENMs) in the atmosphere. *Atmosphere, 8*(5), 84.

17. Kabir, E., Kumar, V., Kim, K. H., Yip, A. C. K., & Sohn, J. R. (2018). Environmental impacts of nanomaterials. *Journal of Environmental Management.*

18. Khan, A., Abdalla, A., & Qurashi, A. (2017). Synthesis of hierarchical WO_3 and Bi_2O_3/WO_3 nanocomposite for solar-driven water splitting applications. *International Journal of Hydrogen Energy, 42*, 3431–3439.

19. Kriebel, D., Tickner, J., Epstein, P., Lemons, J., Levins, R., & Loechler, E. L. (2001). The precautionary principle in environmental science. *Environmental Health Perspectives, 109*, 871–876.

20. Meldrum, K., Guo, C., Marczylo, E. L., Gant, T. W., Smith, R., & Leonard, M. O. (2017). Mechanistic insight into the impact of nanomaterials on asthma and allergic airway disease. *Particle and Fiber Toxicology, 14*, 45–53.

21. Mukhopadhyay, S. S. (2014). Nanotechnology in agriculture: Prospects and constraints. *Nanotechnology, Science and Applications, 7*, 63–71.

22. NIOSH. (2013). Occupational exposure to carbon nanotubes and nanofibers. *National Institute for Occupational Safety and Health.*

23. OECD Environment Directorate. (2014). Ecotoxicology and environmental fate of manufactured nanomaterials: Test guidelines. *Expert Meeting Report, Series on the Safety of Manufactured Nanomaterials.*

24. Oschatz, M., Borchardt, L., Hippauf, F., Nickel, W., Kaskel, S., & Brunner, E. (2016). Interactions between electrolytes and carbon-based materials—NMR studies on electrical double-layer capacitors, lithium-ion batteries, and fuel cells. In *Annual Reports on NMR Spectroscopy* (Vol. 87, pp. 237–318). Elsevier.

25. Parashar, M., Shukla, V. K., & Singh, R. (2020). Metal oxides nanoparticles via sol–gel method: A review on synthesis, characterization and applications. *Journal of Materials Science: Materials in Electronics, 31*(5), 3729–3749.

26. Parashar, P., Singh, N., Alka, Maurya, P., & Saraf, S. A. (2022). An assessment of *in-vitro* and *in-vivo* evaluation methods for theragnostic nanomaterials. *Current Pharmaceutical Design, 28*(2), 78–90.

27. Patel, V., & Mahajan, Y. R. (2017). *Techno-Commercial Opportunities of Nanotechnology in Wind Energy*. Wiley-VCH Verlag GmbH & Co. KGaA.

28. Pattan, G., & Kaul, P. (2014). Health hazards associated with nanomaterials. *Toxicology and Industrial Health, 30*, 499–519.

29. Ramsden, J. J. (2011). The impacts of nanotechnology. *Nanotechnology Perceptions, 7*, 28–66.

30. Reijnders, L. (2006). Cleaner nanotechnology and hazard reduction of manufactured nanoparticles. *Journal of Cleaner Production, 14*, 124–133.

31. Rocha, T. L., Gomes, T., Sousa, V. S., Mestre, N. C., & Bebianno, M. J. (2015). Ecotoxicological impact of engineered nanomaterials in bivalve mollusks: An overview. *Marine Environmental Research, 111*, 74–88.

32. Smita, S., Gupta, S. K., Bartonova, A., Dusinska, M., Gutleb, A. C., & Rahman, Q. (2012). Nanoparticles in the environment: Assessment using the causal diagram approach. *Environmental Health, 11*, 1–13.

33. Thostenson, E. T., Ren, Z., & Chou, T. W. (2001). Advances in the science and technology of carbon nanotubes and their composites: A review. *Composites Science and Technology, 61*, 1899–1912.

34. Vale, G., Mehennaoui, K., Cambier, S., Libralato, G., Jomini, S., & Domingos, R. F. (2015). Manufactured nanoparticles in the aquatic environment—Biochemical responses on freshwater organisms: A critical overview. *Aquatic Toxicology, 170*, 162–174.

35. Wang, Z., Hu, T., Liang, R., & Wei, M. (2020). Application of zero-dimensional nanomaterials in biosensing. *Frontiers in Chemistry, 8*, 320.

36. Zhang, C. (2014). Understanding the wear and tribological properties of ceramic matrix composites. In *Advances in Ceramic Matrix Composites* (pp. 312–339). Elsevier.

37. Zhao, H., & Lei, Y. (2020). 3D nanostructures for the next generation of high-performance nanodevices for electrochemical energy conversion and storage. *Advanced Energy Materials, 10*, 2001460.

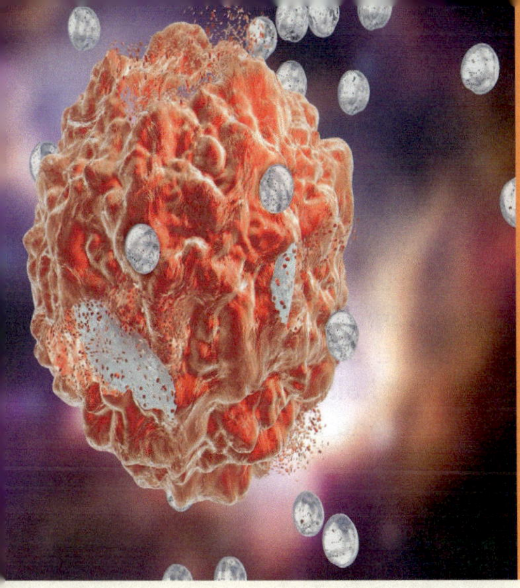

Chapter 12

NANOMEDICINE: CHALLENGES AND FUTURE PERSPECTIVES

Contents

Priyanka Yadav,[1] Khushboo Bhutani,[1] Amisha Singh,[2] Rashmi Tyagi,[3] Vandana Dahiya,[4] and Manoj Kumar Yadav[5,*]

[1]*Department of Biotechnology, SRM University Delhi-NCR, Sonepat, Haryana, India*

[2]*Department of Biotechnology, JAIN University, Bangalore, Karnataka, India*

[3]*Department of Pharmacy, GNIT College of Pharmacy, Greater Noida, Uttar Pradesh, India*

[4]*Department of Biomedical Engineering, ASET, Amity University, Haryana, India*

[5]*Department of Biomedical Engineering, SRM University Delhi-NCR, Sonepat, Haryana, India*

**Corresponding author*

Abstract

The chapter "Nanomedicine: Challenges and Future Perspectives" delves into the multifaceted landscape of nanotechnology in healthcare, exploring the challenges it faces and the promising avenues for future development. Nanomedicine, leveraging the unique properties of nanoparticles, offers transformative potential in diagnostics, therapeutics, and personalized medicine. This chapter provides a comprehensive overview of the hurdles faced by this evolving field and prospects for its advancement.

The introductory segment lays the groundwork by elucidating the pivotal role of nanotechnology in healthcare and emphasizes the imperative of addressing challenges while exploring future avenues. The fundamentals of nanomedicine, spanning nanoparticle-based drug delivery, targeted therapy, and diagnostic applications, form the core discussion, providing insights into its versatile applications.

Challenges in nanomedicine, including concerns about nanoparticle toxicity, barriers in drug delivery, and the complex regulatory landscape, are meticulously explored. The chapter delves into disease-specific applications, emphasizing the use of nanotechnology in cancer therapy, infectious disease management, and interventions in neurodegenerative diseases.

Moreover, the narrative progresses to envision the future of nanomedicine by discussing innovations in nanoparticle design, personalized medicine approaches, and emerging applications that aim to revolutionize healthcare. Ethical and societal considerations, including ethical implications and societal acceptance, are examined within the context of nanomedicine's rapid advancements.

Additionally, the chapter addresses commercialization challenges, scaling up production, and discusses international collaborations and research initiatives that aim to propel nanomedicine into a global and accessible healthcare solution. In conclusion, this chapter provides a comprehensive assessment of the challenges, current achievements, and future prospects of nanomedicine. By navigating through the hurdles and opportunities in this field, the chapter offers a holistic understanding of the exciting potential and considerations for the future of nanomedicine in revolutionizing healthcare.

12.1. Introduction

12.1.1. Overview of Nanomedicine

Since ancient times, natural plant-based products have been widely used to effectively treat a wide range of illnesses. It is a fact that the majority of modern medications are derived from plants, owing to their proven efficacy and safety (Swamy and Sinniah, 2016). Nearly, 25% of the main pharmaceutical chemicals and their derivatives currently available on the market are sourced from natural resources. The statistics mentioned above represents the power of natural remedies that they continue to play a significant role in modern medicine (Mohanty et al., 2017). Despite the numerous benefits of investments in natural products-based medicines, pharmaceutical companies have shown reluctance in investing more in medication delivery and discovery processes that are based on natural products. One of the main challenges associated with employing natural chemicals as medication are concerned with issues related to their toxicity and biocompatibility (Bonifácio et al., 2014).

There are several challenges when it comes to large-sized material distribution and drug delivery, but there are also promising solutions on the horizon. By exploring novel drug delivery techniques, such as nanotechnology, researchers and companies may be able to overcome some of the limitations that have traditionally made medication delivery more difficult

(Jahangirian et al., 2017). Nanotechnology has emerged as a promising avenue for the production of nanomedicines, leveraging therapeutic substances at the nanoscale level. Nanoparticles have played a pivotal role in advancing biomedicine, facilitating medication delivery, tissue engineering, nanobiotechnology, and biosensors (Omietimi et al., 2023). It is worth noting that nanoparticles typically consist of small nanospheres composed of materials produced at the atomic or molecular level. This unique feature confers greater mobility within the human body compared with bulkier materials, making them an attractive option for biomedical applications. Through the use of nanoparticles' special qualities, nanomedicine provides revolutionary possibilities for customized, therapeutic, and diagnostic medical care (Rudramurthy et al., 2016). One of the best therapeutic options associated with nanoparticles are nanomedicines.

Nanomedicine is a rapidly developing field that applies information and methods from nanoscience to medical biology with the aim of preventing and treating diseases. This interdisciplinary field involves the use of materials of nanoscale dimensions, such as actuating materials in living cells, as well as nanosensors and robots for sensing, delivery, and diagnosis. The potential of these materials is being actively explored in order to create new and innovative solutions to the challenges of modern medicine (Patra et al., 2018).

12.1.2. Importance of Nanotechnology in Healthcare

Nanomedicine has depicted various promising applications in various areas of medicine, including drug delivery, therapeutics, regenerative medicine, gene therapy, oncology, dentistry, and diagnostics. Researchers are exploring ways to leverage nanotechnology for illness prevention, diagnosis, and treatment, as well as designing medical instruments and procedures for the next generation of medical scientists. This chapter compiles the various facets of nanomedicine and includes the most recent information about the use of nanotechnology in medicine and treatments from reputable scientific sources (Malik et al., 2023).

12.1.2.1. Nanotechnology in Diagnostics

In current era, nanodevices currently revolutionizes the diagnostic sciences by enabling the early and precise identification of several diseases. By utilizing nanotechnology to study diseases at the molecular and cellular level, researchers can gain valuable insights into potential treatment methods. The technology has the potential to completely transform the diagnostics industry by enhancing the precision, sensitivity, and speed of medical examinations. It is clear that nanotechnology is set to become the cornerstone of modern medicine, and its impact cannot be overstated (Malik et al., 2023).

Nanomedicine is enabling more accurate disease prediction in *in vitro* diagnostic sciences. Using nanodevices that operate at the subcellular level, samples from human tissue and bodily fluids can be analyzed with unprecedented precision. This technology has the potential to revolutionize diagnostics by enhancing the speed and accuracy of medical examinations (Dang and Guan, 2020).

12.1.2.2. Nanotechnology in Pharmacy

Nanoscience has transformed the pharmaceutical industry by improving the efficacy and reducing the toxicity of therapeutic medications. Nanoparticles enhance medication properties by increasing solubility, stability, and bioavailability. This has greatly benefited patients. Nanoscience has transformed the pharmaceutical industry by improving medication properties and reducing toxicity. However, the dosage of nanoparticles depends on various factors, such as size, form, surface characteristics, and mode of administration. Careful dosing regimen planning is necessary to maximize therapeutic benefits while minimizing side effects (Mazayen et al., 2022) (Figure 12.1).

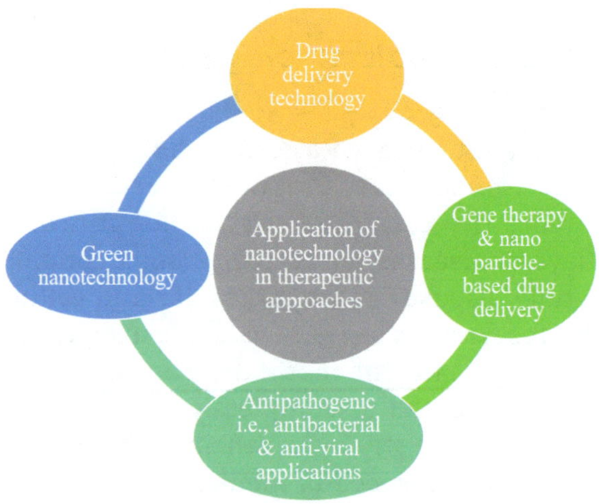

Figure 12.1. Various applications of nanotechnology in the healthcare sector.

12.1.2.3. Nanotechnology and Regenerative Medicines

Nano-assemblies potent tissue regeneration capabilities have significantly improved tissue repair. These technologies are targeted towards mechanical aspects that induce tissue regeneration, migration, adhesion of cells, and differentiation. Research is now being conducted in the area of nanomedicine to create materials at the nanoscale, including gold and silver nanoparticles (AgNPs), dendrimers, nanorods, carbon buckyballs, nanoshells, nanocubes, and numerous other types of nanoparticles. Each has unique attributes that are connected and can be applied directly to the tissues and organs that are their intended use. Research on the antiviral, antifungal, therapeutic, diagnostic, and, most critically, anticancer effects of these nano-agents are being conducted by numerous groups across the globe (Tang et al., 2019).

12.1.2.4. Nanotechnology-Based Surgical Applications

Medicine could undergo a transformation with the potential to enhance patient outcomes through both surgical nanorobotics as well as nanobioelectric medicine. To fully realize these technologies, promise and guarantee their efficacy and safety, however, a great deal of study is still required. A surgical nanorobot that operates via the vascular system is being developed via interdisciplinary collaborations in the domains of biology, engineering, and programming. The multifunctional objective of these small-scale gadgets is to search for lesions and pathogens and provide treatments against them (Wang et al., 2022) (Figure 12.2).

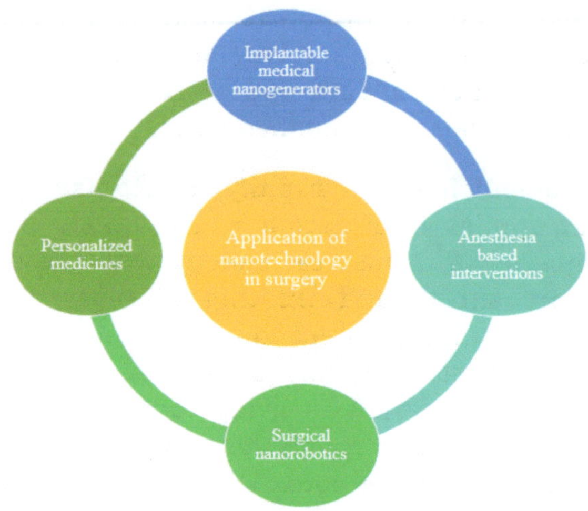

Figure 12.2. Different sectors of applications based on surgical interventions.

Nanobioelectric medicine and surgical nanorobotics both hold the potential to transform medicine and enhance patient outcomes. There is also a new wave of bioelectric medicine on the market that sticks to biological components for better therapeutic and diagnostic outcomes. This nanobioelectronic is being used to treat cardiovascular conditions, cancer, and other human body abnormalities (Zhang et al., 2022). As the name suggests, nanogenerators are an implantable kind of medical nanosensors that are self-powered. They operate on the tenet that mechanical energy from motion of the body can be transformed into an electric spark.

In dental surgeries and other delicate medical procedures, such brain surgery, induction of anesthesia is an essential phase. Researchers are developing nanorobotic suspension combinations that produce a colloidal suspension containing millions of nanoscale active analgesic nanoparticles for use in such anesthesia induction treatments (Zhang et al., 2022).

A crucial first step in delicate medical procedures including brain surgery and dental surgeries is inducing anesthesia. Researchers are developing nanorobotic suspension mixtures that combine millions of nanoscale active analgesic nanoparticles to create a colloidal fluid for use in such anesthesia induction treatments. These nanoparticles penetrate deeply, achieving the level of loose tissue, and are applied to patients' gingival and other sensitive areas. The method by which these nanomaterials (NMs) transit is by the combination of positional navigation, chemical and temperature gradients, and on-site nanocomputer monitoring and control (Zhang et al., 2023).

12.1.3. Significance of Addressing Challenges and Exploring Future Directions

Nanomedicine can combat incurable diseases and achieve treatment goals with nano-pharmaceuticals and nanotherapeutics. It requires a global effort to translate laboratory innovations into clinical applications. Nanomedicines can minimize side effects, improve diagnosis and therapies, and enhance quality of life while maximizing healthcare cost-effectiveness (Mandal et al., 2021).

Nanomedicine is still in its infancy, despite its potential benefits to bypass biological barriers, administer hydrophobic active substances efficiently, and selectively target infection areas. A comparatively small number of nanoparticle-based medications have been approved for clinical usage due to various obstacles and impediments at various stages of development, and the majority of nanomedicine research and inventions are currently restricted to the laboratory stage (Mandal et al., 2021).

12.2. Fundamentals of Nanomedicine

12.2.1. Nanoparticles in Drug Delivery

Nanotechnology uses nanoparticles, which are small-sized nanospheres made up of materials designed at the atomic or molecular level, to develop curative agents at the nanoscale. This has greatly impacted the field of biomedicine, including areas such as nanobiotechnology, drug delivery, biosensors, and tissue engineering. Nanospheres provide a reliable drug delivery mechanism due to their small size, enabling accurate encapsulation and controlled release of medication (Mirza and Siddiqui, 2014).

In medication delivery systems, a variety of biopolymeric polymers are employed. For instance, one of the essential nanoparticles, chitosan's (CH) muco-adhesive qualities make it ideal for tight epithelial junctions. CH-based nanoparticles provide sustained drug delivery for pulmonary, nasal, intestinal, and buccal regions. Recent research shows the nanoparticles' interaction with mucin results in decreased viscosity, yet their mucoadhesion promotes extended antibiotic release. These nanoparticles could prolong drug half-life in the eyes, making them a good option for sustained ocular drug delivery (Silva et al., 2017).

Nanospheres are a reliable drug delivery mechanism due to their small size, enabling accurate encapsulation and controlled release of medication. Bio-nanomaterials, particularly functionalized nanoparticles are the foundation for many drug delivery system (DDS) designs. The potential for using NM-based drug delivery to target specific sites and eliminate tumors without harming surrounding tissues is generating a lot of interest in the field. Nanospheres provide a reliable drug delivery mechanism due to their small size, enabling accurate encapsulation and controlled release of medication (Wang et al., 2008). Nanospheres were originally developed as vaccination and anticancer drug carriers. However, by altering the biodistribution and toxicodynamic of pharmaceuticals, the nanoscale size ranges may greatly improve drug delivery. This can make the comparatively simple task of delivering many types of medications that present significant delivery challenges *in vivo* (Vauthier et al., 2007).

To reduce the toxicity concerns, nanoparticles have primarily been employed in conjunction with natural ingredients. Because it reduces the amount of potentially dangerous ingredients in the biosynthetic process, the green chemistry approach to developing drug-loaded nanoparticles is strongly supported. However, the negative effects of the drugs can be reduced by utilizing green nanoparticles for drug delivery. Furthermore, these NMs' bioactivity can be further increased by modifying their surface modifications, hydrophobicity, size, and shape (Lam et al., 2017).

Nano-sized colloidal particles as drug carriers are a breakthrough in pharmacotherapy. They transport hormone, anti-cancer, and anti-hypertensive drugs and expand the application of pharmacokinetics. For instance, trans-retinoic acid nanoparticle coated with $CaCO_3$ can re-disperse in water and increase insulin secretion from islets. Nanoparticles offer a new hope for patients, delivering medication to previously inaccessible areas of the body (Yamaguchi and Igarashi, 2006).

12.2.2. Targeted Therapy and Precision Medicine

With enormous promise for improving healthcare, the use of nanotechnology in medicine is opening up new avenues and offering substantial chances for creative, efficient treatments for a wide range of illnesses. The physical characteristics of nanocarriers such as their dimension, form, surface charge, and intrinsic chemical properties as well as the addition of active ligands for the recognition of biological receptors, all have an impact on biological transport processes, which span from external barriers (skin and mucosa) to places of interest at the cellular and subcellular levels (Lammers et al., 2012).

One of the diseases associated with targeted therapy in nanotechnology is cancer. Over the years, a wide range of methods and approaches have been assessed for medication targeting to tumors. Systems that are frequently used include liposomes, polymers, micelles, nanoparticles, and antibodies (Malik et al., 2023). Strategies that are commonly employed include triggered drug delivery, passive drug targeting, active drug targeting to cancer cells, and active drug targeting to endothelial cells. Preclinical and clinical research in this field has advanced significantly, and some nanomedicine formulations (mostly passively targeting tumors) have been licensed for use in humans. The understanding of the (patho-) physiological principles of therapeutic targeting to cancers has also advanced significantly (Lammers et al., 2012).

A new paradigm in therapeutics may be introduced with the ability to insert medications or genes into detectable site-targeted nanosystems, which could lead to the development of image-based drug delivery and dosage. It is possible add complex therapeutic agent payloads to the carriers themselves, such as genes or radionuclides. Substances can be deposited in subterranean oil layers, bound to or dissolved in carrier lipid coatings, or retained inside the carriers themselves (Song et al., 2002).

Numerous drugs have been reported to be transported by nontargeted nanocarriers, such as polymer nanosystems, albumin, and solid lipid particles. But the application of targeted agents ought to concentrate even higher drug concentrations inside particular tissues through particular absorption pathways, suggesting that serum drug levels could be more successfully reduced to lessen detrimental side effects (Wickline and Lanza, 2003).

12.2.2.1. Precision Medicine

Acknowledging individual heterogeneity in genes, environment, and lifestyle, precision medicine promises better health outcomes. The next 10 years will see more transformations in healthcare due to the growth of precision medicine in several domains, including large cohorts, AI, routine clinical genomics, phenomics, and environment, and providing value across a range of people. It is necessary to develop highly modular and adjustable methods of delivering medicines in order to account for the huge variability of biological barriers and disease states within and across patient groups. Precision medicine describes how different NP design choices (architecture, material qualities, targeting, and responsiveness) can overcome obstacles unique to individual patients and diseases. It also highlights the consequences of these NP properties on delivery (Mitchell et al., 2021).

12.2.3. Diagnostic Nanomedicine: Imaging and Sensing

Mostly, target-specific medication delivery using nanocarriers as systems or vehicles has been investigated. These vehicles have mostly been used to deliver anticancer medicines. Iron oxide, liposomes, nanomicelles, nanoparticles, gold, and carbon-based materials are a few examples of nanocarriers. For regulated drug release, such delivery systems can be created (Cholkar et al., 2017).

For pharmacologists and drug delivery scientists, disease diagnostics and molecular imaging present difficult topics. Our understanding of disease prognosis and the development of effective treatments have improved with the advent of nanotechnology and imaging tools. Scientific advancements in anti-aging techniques have been noteworthy. Imaging's sensitivity, specificity, and accuracy were enhanced by the integration of nanotechnology and imaging (Crous and Abrahamse, 2021).

Imaging methods have a significant impact on science research, drug development, and clinical diagnostics. With fluorescence and nanotechnology, accurate localization through contrast viewing is possible. These methods are relevant in research, diagnosis, and illness prognosis. Interest in photoacoustics and ultrasound imaging is increasing. This chapter highlights imaging techniques in molecular biology and clinical settings, nanocarriers with imaging techniques for diagnosis and prognosis, and the latest advancements in fluorescence techniques. Imaging methods are crucial and have the potential to revolutionize medicine (Crous and Abrahamse, 2021).

12.3. Challenges in Nanomedicine

12.3.1. Nanoparticle Toxicity and Safety Concerns

As nanoparticles have prooxidant functional groups on their surface, reactive oxygen species (ROS) are stimulated by them (Khanna et al., 2015; Manke et al., 2013). A lot of ROS production induces oxidative stress which can activate pro-inflammatory response like less mitochondrial membrane potential and antioxidant enzyme activity which results in DNA damage and apoptosis. More nanoparticles toxicity is induced by smaller sized practical as they can penetrate easily through cell membrane (Fu et al., 2014). Besides, nanoparticles induce oxidative stress in cells because of depletion in number of antioxidants which can compensate the oxidative stress of a cell. All these factors lead to mitochondrial membrane damage and apoptosis (Manke et al., 2013). Nanoparticles have been found to involve in providing toxicity in various organ systems (Khanna et al., 2015). A nanoparticle ZNO induce inflammation by endosome formation in macrophages (Roy et al., 2014). It can be inferred that ROS and cell apoptosis from oxidative stress shows various effects like: DNA damage, Lipid peroxidation, Mitochondrial dysfunction, phagocytic oxidative outbreak, cancer, fibrosis, and inflammation. Nanoparticles like PEG coated, and citrate capped Ag induces complement system which in turn stimulate inflammatory response which become uncontrolled in some cases and cause a serious problem. Sometimes complement system activation by nanoparticles may result in allergic reactions (Moghimi, 2014). Poly(2-methyl-2-oxazoline) (PMOXA)-coated Au nanoparticles activated the complement system via the classical pathway. Nanoparticle induced complement system activation shows the effects such as: opsonization, adaptive defense, inflammation, chemotaxis (Tavano et al., 2018). A major impact of nanoparticles toxicity is seen on gastrointestinal pathways which is directly linked to their size and composition (Gago et al., 2023; Ibrahim et al., 2018). Small sized nanoparticles effects liver including steatosis, cytoplasmic degeneration, inflammatory cells infiltration, Kupffer cell activation and hemorrhage while large sized NPs have the potential to damage spleen (Ibrahim et al., 2018). Au nanoparticles and copper oxide show similar effects on liver overall toxicity while kidneys are less effected except a low effect is exhibited by small sized NPs (below 30 nm) on kidney's proximal tubule epithelial cells (Astashkina et al., 2014). Besides it, polystyrene nanoparticles induce intestinal inflammation. Several studies have been carried out about the impact of nanoparticle toxicity on the neurons using blood–brain barrier (BBB) (Kim et al., 2009).

Some *in vivo* studies were made to analyze the changes in biomarker by NP toxicity such as the quantity of an enzyme glutathione peroxidase an antioxidant was decreased in the cell (Siddiqi et al., 2012). It has been found by *in vitro* studies that NP toxicity cause cell death, change in morphology, genotoxicity, oxidative stress and proinflammatory responses (Manke et al., 2013). Nanoparticles enter the circulatory system to reach at the Sertoli cells barriers and induce the toxicity in reproductive cells such as ZnO can bind with estrogen receptor which is responsible for the damage of endocrine balance (Chen and Gao, 2017).

12.3.2. Drug Delivery Barriers

There are various barriers for nanomedicines delivery which effects the efficiency of these drugs. The barriers stability depends on the route of drug administration and disease progression (Kou et al., 2018). For the proper distribution of drug nanoparticle-based drugs should cross all barriers on the way they may be physiological barriers and biological barriers (Cheng et al., 2020). These barriers become more prominent in diseased condition at various levels such as microenvironmental level, cellular level, and patient to patient basis (Nag and Delehanty, 2019). One of the most important barriers to nanomedicine distribution and delivery is blood flow, excretion, coronas, and phagocytic cells. All these factors are affected by circulation time and structural stability of the drug so formulation of NP drugs is manipulated in such a way so that desirable outcomes can be achieved such as nanoparticles with size less than 200 nm were found to be excreted properly through kidneys while NP> 200 nm activates the complement system and cause the inflammation (Hoshyar et al., 2016; Mitchell et al., 2021). There are several physical barriers which prevent the Np delivery to targeted cell. These are tight junctions of the endothelial cell and junction between endothelial cells and epithelial cells of gastrointestinal tract, microglial cells and pericytes of the BBB which come across oral and intravenous administration of the drug while entering the central nervous system (CNS). Drug must cross the BBB endothelial cell using receptor mediated endocytosis and exocytosis system. Around 5% of the NP medicine can reach the CNS and less than 5% reaches the targeted cell (Saraiva et al., 2016). Rapidly growing microbes inside the targeted tissue or body poses a prominent barrier to the NP drug distribution (Guo et al., 2021; Oliva et al., 2015). Biofilms and mucus layer are also the most prominent barriers for respiratory system (Cone, 2009; Ensign et al., 2012). Another very important barrier to NP delivery is the intracellular barrier which come across when drug reaches the targeted cell such as hydrophobicity and charge which affect cellular absorption in macrophage and cancer cell.

12.3.3. Regulatory Hurdles and Approval Processes

Despite highly effective drug delivery and distribution of nanoparticles they impose a various challenge for reaching into clinic which include nanomedicine do not have any unified definition or classification, so they do not have agreed regulations (Allan et al., 2021; Foulkes et al., 2020; Sarwal et al., 2018). There are different analytical methods for each nanoparticle (Leong et al., 2019; Sainz et al., 2015; Soares et al., 2018). Their pharmacokinetic profile is different from standard material (Agrahari and Hiremath, 2017; Limaye et al., 2014) and they show a greater issue for the stability after manufacturing (Mühlebach, 2018; Sainz et al., 2015; Soares et al., 2018). Besides, *in vitro*, and pre-clinical studies for the toxicology of nanoparticles are not able to be validated by *in vivo* complexity (Chen et al., 2021; Edmondson et al., 2014; Flühmann et al., 2019; Paradise, 2019), their Systemic biodistribution with fate is also a challenge (Flühmann et al., 2019). The environmental impact makes nanoparticles drug delivery less efficient (Allan et al., 2021; Foulkes et al., 2020; Gaur et al., 2020) The definition and classification of NM is the main problem in front of regulatory team and the same product show the lack of consensus classification around the globe so regulatory process is hindered (Kelly, 2010).

A recommendation for first suitable definition of "nanomaterial" within the EU (European Union and United Kingdom) for legislative and policy is d used, although this recommendation is not legally imposed yet in European Medicines Union (EMU), EU regulatory bodies has declared that there should be some specific preliminary guidelines to standardize nanomedicine preparation standards but there are no firm official guidelines in published form (Çetintaş et al., 2021; Halamoda-Kenzaoui et al., 2019).

Similarly, the USA (United States of America) do not have specific nanomedicine guidelines, several regulatory frameworks for nanomedicines have been published by Food and Drug Administration (FDA) such as foodstuffs (FDA, 2014), cosmetics (Food and Administration), and animal feed (Committee et al., 2018). Canada also does not have any proper guidelines for nanomedicines they just follow the existing rules of Organization for Economic Co-operation and Development (OECD) Council (Carroll and Kellow, 2021; Woodward, 2009). Some countries like India, Japan, China, and Thailand are now working on creating regulatory guidelines related to nanomedicines (Allan et al., 2021; Dinda, 2019).

12.4. Nanomedicine and Disease Treatment

12.4.1. Cancer Therapy and Nanoparticle-Based Treatments

Nanotechnology is widely being used for the treatment of cancer now a days. Nanomedicines potency depends upon their size shape and composition (Bahrami et al., 2017). For cancer treatment nanoparticles-based medicine must have the size in the range of 10 to 100 nm diameter as they are suitable for delivery and show enhanced permeability and retention (EPR) effect. Another feature a nanomedicine must have for cancer is their hydrophilicity, so that they can remain in the blood circulation for a longer time with the enhanced penetration and accumulation of drug in tumors (Perrault et al., 2009; Wong et al., 2011; Yang et al., 2014). Liposome which is considered as the first nanoparticle is suitable for cancer cure. Liposome is very efficient for the delivery of some cancer drugs such as doxorubicin and paclitaxel (Wang et al., 2017). Liposome based drugs are very common for breast and prostate cancer as well (Tang et al., 2020).

Gold nanoparticles (AuNPs) have the ability to increase drug accumulation in tumors as well as to overcome drug resistance (Cheng et al., 2013), including applications in gene therapy, photothermal therapy (PTT), and immunotherapy (Riley and Day, 2017). Carbon nanotubes (CNTs), a type of tubular material, also have strong potential in drug delivery as they exhibit significant biological, physical, and chemical properties. Important drugs such as doxorubicin, paclitaxel, and methotrexate have been delivered using CNTs. Another potential nanoparticle is a type of mesoporous silica carrier for drug delivery (Gao et al., 2019). They a large pore space to accommodate the more volume of anticancer drugs. They have a very efficient pharmacokinetics and treatment effect, with high stability (Xu et al., 2019). Another category of cancer nanomedicine used to treat prostate and breast cancer is the liposome-silica hybrid (LSH) nanoparticle which is made up of a core particle of silica surrounding by lipid bilayer (Colapicchioni et al., 2015). Magnetic nanoparticles are used as carrier for drug for better stability and biocompatibility they are usually covered by organic materials, such as polymers and fatty acids. For gene therapy for cancer treatment magnetic nanoparticles have proven to be highly efficient (Colapicchioni et al., 2015).

12.4.2. Infectious Disease Management

Infectious diseases like tuberculosis and HIV are being cured using nanomedicines because of their significant potency in delivering the antibiotics in the target cell. Almost all pathogens invade macrophages to destroy immune system, so nanoparticles loaded antibiotics are proved to reach the macrophages more efficiently as compared to bare drug. In a study, it was found that administration of the antiretroviral drug azidothymidine carried by the nanoparticle poly(hexacyanoacrylate) resulted in improved accumulation in organs such as the liver, lungs, and spleen. By *in vivo* study on rats 60% of the nanocarrier drug was recovered from the tissues of the organs like liver, lungs, and spleen while only 12% drug was found to be present after the treatment of soluble drug alone. At the infection site blood vessels become very leaky thereby nanocarriers penetration to the site is enhanced in the organs other than liver spleen and lungs also (Laverman et al., 1999; Löbenberg et al., 1998). In a study of unilateral bacterial infection in the calf muscle of rats, they were provided with radiolabeled liposomes intravenously which resulted into accumulation of high (40 times) liposome concentration inside the abscess. Hence permeability of the nanomedicine into the target tissue is high with longer circulation times which results in to improved targeting efficiency (Siegel et al., 2016). A drug Ciprofloxacin loaded with the nanocarrier, liposomes with functionalized mannose were applied to rats as a pulmonary spray and its outcomes on the alveolar macrophages were analyzed with the findings that it was found to be present 1.5 times in alveolar macrophages than liposome without mannose (Chono et al., 2008). Likewise, when normal drug and nanocarrier based drug (liposome loaded drug) delivery were compared it was exhibited that liposome-based drug showed 23 times more bioavailability in the alveolar macrophages than normal drug. Besides, nanomedicines are proved to be showing better delivery of drug to the site of infection by targeting epitopes of the pathogens. A drug, pentamidine, carried by the nanoparticle PLGA, was used for the treatment of *Trypanosoma brucei*, which causes African sleeping sickness. Another drug, streptavidin coated with magnetic nanoparticles, when administered to cultures of *S. aureus*, resulted in a 2.5-fold increase in binding compared to IgG-coated nanoparticles (Kim et al., 2013).

12.4.3. Neurodegenerative Disease Interventions

The most common neurodegenerative diseases are, Alzheimer's disease (AD), Parkinson's disease (PD), Huntington's disease (HD), and amyotrophic lateral sclerosis (ALS). Nanomedicines have been proved to be efficient delivery system of various type of medicines with phytoconstituents, and biomolecules to the specific targeted tissues of the body including the complex organ like brain (Nguyen et al., 2021; Raja et al., 2023). Using nanoparticles as a drug carrier has improved the efficiency of treatment for neurodegenerative diseases (Mukherjee et al., 2020). Lipid nanoparticles are being widely used for the targeted delivery of drugs to the brain. These systems are proven to be potent technology because of their safety, biocompatibility, and biodegradability. Lipid nanoparticles are working efficiently for delivering the drug to the brain disease because of their similar composition with BBB (both have lipid molecules) so they can penetrate easily into the brain. These LNPs are being researched at high level because they are efficiently used for the management of neurodegenerative diseases (Maqsood et al., 2022; Sohail et al., 2023). The biodegradable PLGA based nanomedicine are used to treat Alzheimer as they can cross BBB and show neuroprotective potential (Aalinkeel et al., 2018).

12.5. Future Directions and Innovations

12.5.1. Advances in Nanoparticle Design and Engineering

Recent advances in nanoparticle design and engineering have led to revolutionary changes across various fields, offering precise control over nanoscale properties and functionalities. These innovations have enabled the development of tailored nanoparticles with specific physicochemical characteristics, enhancing performance in applications like drug delivery, imaging, energy storage, and catalysis. Breakthroughs include multifunctional nanoparticles capable of simultaneous drug delivery and imaging, as well as stimuli-responsive variants releasing payloads triggered by pH, temperature, or light. Novel synthesis methods such as bottom-up assembly and molecular self-assembly have facilitated the creation of complex nanoparticle structures with meticulous control over size, shape, and surface chemistry (Wang et al., 2018). These advancements hold great promise in addressing challenges in nanomedicine, environmental remediation, and renewable energy, paving the way for next-generation technologies with improved efficiency, selectivity, and sustainability. Meanwhile, the interdisciplinary nature of nanoparticle research, spanning chemistry, engineering, physical sciences, molecular engineering, biology, and biotechnology, drives the development of more efficient and targeted DDS (Betz et al., 2023). These systems aim to deliver drugs directly to specific cells or tissues, minimizing side effects and optimizing therapeutic outcomes. Crucially, the unique properties of nanoparticles, such as increased binding affinity, improved bioavailability and compatibility, and controlled drug release profiles, underscore their pivotal role in shaping the future of nanomedicine, ensuring precise and effective treatment strategies tailored to individual patients (Pandey et al., 2024).

12.5.2. Personalized Nanomedicine and Patient-Centric Approaches

Personalized nanomedicine and patient-centric approaches are integral to modern healthcare, enabling tailored treatments for individual patients based on their unique needs and characteristics. The development of nanomedicines, utilizing nanotechnology in medical applications, is a significant aspect of personalized medicine, offering targeted therapies with minimized side effects. Three-dimensional (3D) printing, an emerging technology, has the potential to revolutionize nanomedicine by facilitating the creation of patient-specific structures, leading to improved treatment outcomes and enhanced patient satisfaction (Alzoubi et al., 2023). In cancer therapy, a patient-centric approach is crucial, where nanotheranostics can be tailored to individual patients' needs, enhancing drug response while minimizing side effects (De Maria Marchiano et al., 2021). Similarly, in type 2 diabetes mellitus (T2DM), nanotechnology offers transformative possibilities by improving drug delivery and enabling personalized treatment to better control blood sugar levels (Kyrochristos et al., 2018). Overall, personalized nanomedicine holds promise for revolutionizing healthcare by delivering precise, effective, and patient-centered therapies, although challenges such as regulatory hurdles and interdisciplinary collaboration remain. Nonetheless, ongoing research and innovation offer hope for improved outcomes and quality of life for patients worldwide (Germain et al., 2020).

12.5.3. Emerging Applications and Multidisciplinary Collaborations

Emerging applications and multidisciplinary collaborations are pivotal in driving research and innovation across various fields. These collaborations allow experts from diverse disciplines to pool their knowledge and skills, tackle complex challenges, and forge innovative solutions (Lyall et al., 2011). By integrating insights and methodologies from different domains, researchers can redefine problems and generate novel outcomes that transcend disciplinary boundaries. In higher education, multidisciplinary collaborations are vital for fostering interdisciplinary research, nurturing diversity, and preparing students for global citizenship. Through partnerships across academic disciplines, institutions can foster breakthrough discoveries, create inclusive learning environments, and cultivate a culture where diverse perspectives are valued. Additionally, in areas like neurotechnology, multidisciplinary collaborations have propelled research forward, fostering cross-disciplinary approaches to fields such as neurobiology and pain research. These collaborations have led to the development of new curricula, interdisciplinary projects, and research initiatives spanning faculties such as engineering, medicine, economics, and music, thus significantly contributing to advancements in neurotechnology from diverse perspectives. In summary, emerging applications and multidisciplinary collaborations are driving forces in research and innovation, enabling the exploration of complex challenges and the development of transformative solutions across various domains (Sciences et al., 2018).

12.6. Ethical and Societal Considerations

12.6.1. Ethical Implications in Nanomedicine

The ethical implications of nanomedicine are multifaceted and complex, touching on various key issues. Risk assessment stands out as a critical concern due to the incomplete understanding of potential risks associated with NMs and nanotechnology, compounded by the lack of standardized protocols for assessment and uncertainties surrounding human exposure during clinical trials. Informed consent emerges as another pivotal ethical consideration, demanding full transparency about the risks and benefits of nanomedicine interventions to uphold patients' autonomy in decision-making (Das et al., 2021). Moreover, ethical debates surrounding the enhancement of human capabilities raise questions about the ethical limits of such enhancements and their broader societal implications. Ethical concerns also extend to research involving human embryonic stem cells, prompting reflections on the ethical status of human embryos and implications for human reproduction and identity (Aach et al., 2017). Additionally, the toxicity, self-assembly, and uncontrolled function of nanoparticles and nanosystems pose ethical challenges, demanding a balance between potential benefits and risks. Addressing these ethical complexities requires robust regulatory frameworks, equitable distribution strategies, interdisciplinary dialogue, and public awareness initiatives to ensure responsible innovation and decision-making in the dynamic landscape of nanomedicine (Fisher et al., 2012).

12.6.2. Societal Acceptance and Regulation

Societal acceptance and regulation play pivotal roles in the advancement and oversight of nanomedicine. While nanomedicine products currently fall under conventional regulatory frameworks for medicinal and medical devices, there is a pressing need for enhanced governance, transparency, and effective control due to the technology's rapid development (Bowman and Gatof, 2015). Public perception of nanotechnology, particularly in health and environmental contexts, tends to be favorable, yet concerns persist regarding uncertainty and trust in governmental and industrial entities. Ethical regulation of nanomedicine faces hurdles stemming from uncertainties about potential risks to human health and the environment, industry-sponsored research integrity, and varying levels of societal acceptance (Moos, 2014). As nanomedicine evolves, interdisciplinary research across fields like engineering, medicine, and public health will be pivotal, driving its transformative potential in 21st-century healthcare. The societal response to nanotechnology hinges on perceptions of usefulness, necessity, tangibility, and proximity to end-users, shaping its acceptance across diverse application domains. Achieving a harmonious balance between societal acceptance and regulation requires continual dialogue and adaptation to meet the evolving needs and values of communities (Brown et al., 2015).

12.6.3. Balancing Innovation with Responsibility

Balancing innovation with responsibility in the field of nanomedicine involves several critical considerations. These include ensuring ethical and egalitarian use of new technology, addressing safety and ethical issues, and promoting informed consent, privacy, accountability, bias, safety, regulation, transparency, and ethical decision-making. Legal and ethical issues, including privacy and data protection, compliance with existing standards and regulatory pathways, continuous monitoring and reporting requirements, professional standards for healthcare providers, and intellectual property regulations, are vital for AI-enabled nanomedicine (Ebbesen and Jensen, 2006). Public engagement and consultation requirements are also crucial to ensure diverse perspectives are considered in ethical decision-making processes. This involves developing guidelines for obtaining regulatory approvals and ensuring ongoing compliance, continuous education and training of healthcare professionals on ethical considerations, and robust monitoring mechanisms. Informed consent and autonomy involve establishing clear protocols for obtaining consent from patients and respecting their autonomy. Transparency and accountability involve developing regulations requiring transparency in AI algorithms and accountability for system failures. Bias and fairness involve addressing algorithmic bias and proactively identifying and mitigating biases to ensure fair treatment for diverse patient populations (Ramezani and Faris, 2024). Intellectual property regulations for AI-enabled nanomedicine should balance innovation with accessibility, affordability, and fairness. Public engagement and consultation requirements ensure diverse perspectives are considered in ethical decision-making processes. Education and training on interoperability are essential for healthcare professionals to understand the ethical implications of interoperability in AI-enabled nanomedicine. By addressing these ethical considerations, stakeholders can promote interoperability that respects patient autonomy, enhances collaboration, and prioritizes equitable healthcare outcomes. In summary, balancing innovation with responsibility in nanomedicine involves addressing ethical and safety considerations, promoting informed consent, privacy, accountability, bias, safety, regulation, transparency, and ethical decision-making, and ensuring diverse perspectives are considered in ethical decision-making processes. Intellectual property regulations, public engagement and consultation requirements, education, and training on interoperability, and robust monitoring mechanisms are also crucial to promoting interoperability that respects patient autonomy, enhances collaboration, and prioritizes equitable healthcare outcomes (Mette and Thomas, 2006).

12.7. Challenges in Commercialization and Scaling Up

12.7.1. Economic and Market Challenges

The current age is a "no or low controversy era," in which aversion to or worry about new technology is at an all-time low. As a result, the general attitude is positive toward new technologies such as nanotechnology (Satterfield et al., 2009). However, obtaining technical know-how or a newer technology product does not guarantee successful sales. The technology must be well received by the industry, that is, the industry must believe in its performance before it can harness all of its energies and attempts to gain public support.

Commercialization is the process of transforming novel innovations into successful commercial endeavors, which may involve a diverse group of individuals with scientific, business, and economic backgrounds (Reamer et al., 2003). The process consists of a series of steps that begin with the conception of an idea, technology development, and commercialization; fostering those ideas to technology development; creating a prototype to establish the validity of the idea; developing a new process or optimizing existing processes; and finally supplying proposed deliverables to the market, promoting them, and creating new infrastructures for facilitated supply and purchase.

Because of widespread worry and rejection, nanotech-based pharmaceutical businesses have few financing choices, whereas co-founders of start-ups invest their own money and knowledge. The current status of the global economy is not "nanofriendly," and startups are having problems raising early funds. Given the risk of funding companies prematurely, investors are hesitant to pour large amounts of capital into these companies until they have dependable technologies, ready to commercialize products, defendable patents, growing target markets in sight, the possibility of high profitability, and strong management teams.

Because of the lengthy development time necessary for nanotech-based goods, most patents are likely to expire soon after commercial introduction. As a result, the number of years available for recovering developmental expenditures and earning a reasonable return to promote further research in this specific sector is just insufficient. Companies have refrained from investing in nanotech-based products due to the depressing situation of extremely low expected returns, as well as the uncertainty and risk connected with these initiatives. According to data from the US Patent and Trademark Office (PTO), as of December 2012, over 8000 US nanopatents had been issued by several PTO technological centers (Paradise, 2011).

Inadequate knowledge and communication lead to uncertainty, distrust, and even dread. This may result in not just the cancellation of a specific nanomedical project but also jeopardize the future of nanotechnology as a whole. Several nanomedicine products have been licensed by the US Food and Drug Administration (FDA) and the European Medicines Agency (EMA) for a variety of therapeutic purposes (Anselmo and Mitragotri, 2016; Ragelle et al., 2017; Sainz et al., 2015). High therapeutic efficacy and safety are the two most important requirements for a product to become commercially successful. However, most nanomedicine products fail to meet these conditions, preventing their successful commercialization (Thapa and Kim, 2023).

12.7.2. Scaling Up Nanomedicine Production

Nanomedicines present numerous hurdles for researchers seeking to maximize patient advantages during diagnosis and therapy (Muthu and Wilson, 2010). Various developmental stages precede the market introduction of new nanomedicine products. Industrial scale-up (large-scale industrial manufacturing) is a major upcoming difficulty in the nanomedicine development stages. It is generally known that nanomedicine preparations on the laboratory scale are feasible and thoroughly reported by numerous studies (Kulkarni and Feng, 2011; Muthu et al., 2012). At the same time, industrial factorial design (scale-up) of nanomedicines has received less attention during development. Limited trials and insufficient information on nanomedicine scale-up technologies may impede its market introduction (Saraf, 2009).

During the developmental stage of investigational new drug (IND), a small number of nanodrugs are synthesized with definite achievable reproducibility, accurate and optimized characteristics. But when manufactured at large scale, there are potential issues which affect the quality of nanodrugs which includes (i) lack of developmental guidelines; (ii) inconsistent batch to batch reproducibility; (iii) inadequate developmental pathways for *in vitro* synthesis of drugs; (iv) inefficient infrastructure and in-house expertise of sterilization techniques; and (v) environmental exposure during manufacture of nanomedicines (Kad et al., 2022).

The consequences of scale-up and the process limits of preparative processes are regarded as important obstacles in large-scale production. First, scale-up has been shown to primarily affect nanoparticle properties such as particle size, drug encapsulation, process residual materials, colloidal stability, and surface shape. Colombo et al. found that scaling up the emulsion-based approach from the laboratory scale of 60 mL to the industrial scale of 2 L (almost 33-fold) did not affect encapsulation efficiency (Colombo et al., 2001). However, increasing impeller speed and agitation time resulted in smaller particle sizes. As the polymer content decreased, so did the size of the nanoparticles. Another study by Galindo-Rodriguez et al. revealed that during scale-up from a laboratory batch volume of 60 mL to 1.5 L, increasing the stirring rate decreased particle size in the emulsion-based approach (Galindo-Rodríguez et al., 2005). Furthermore, they discovered that the scale-up approach lowered the drug loading in nanoparticles.

A short consumption duration is always preferred for a single pilot batch. Galindo-Rodriguez et al. examined the process time necessary to produce a pilot batch (Galindo-Rodríguez et al., 2005), and it was revealed that the nanoprecipitation approach took less time (120 min) than the emulsion-based method (350 min) (Charcosset and Fessi, 2005; El-Harati et al., 2006).

Continuously expanding the manufacturing of NPs requires market and economic efficiency. Commercially, the nanomedicine sector is estimated to be worth USD 350.8 billion in 2025. Despite these potentials, the fundamental issues for PNPs in nanomedicine research have shown to be a significant hurdle to pushing PNPs to clinical stages (Albalawi et al., 2021). One issue is to scale up and continuously manufacture NPs on a big scale (Colby et al., 2021; Mughal et al., 2021). There are several interesting alternatives for large-scale NP production: membrane extrusion, supercritical fluid technology, industrial microreactors, and nanobiotechnology. The FDA has asked pharmaceutical firms to convert from batch to continuous processing by 2026. As a result, chemical fluxes are gradually becoming the norm in pharmaceutical production. This will become the new norm for large-scale NP production (Herdiana et al., 2022; Wojnicki et al., 2018).

The success of any product, including nanomedicines, is dependent on large-scale industrial production and commercialization. As a result of their successful laboratory scale development, the scientific community should devote more attention to large-scale industrial manufacturing. Practical experimental designs could give effective solutions to the issues posed by nanomedicine scale-up. Once scale-up is completed, nanomedicines will become more widely available in the market for the treatment of a variety of conditions.

12.7.3. Commercial Success Stories and Case Studies

Nanomedicine is the application of nanotechnology in medicine. Nanomedicine has several commercial successes and case studies demonstrating its potential to revolutionize healthcare. Here are some notable examples:

1. **Abraxane (Albumin-Bound Paclitaxel):** Abraxane, developed by Abraxis BioScience (acquired by Celgene in 2010), is a nanoparticle albumin-bound formulation of paclitaxel approved for the treatment of various cancers, including breast, lung, and pancreatic cancer. Its unique delivery system encapsulates paclitaxel within albumin nanoparticles, enhancing solubility, tumor targeting, and efficacy. Clinical trials have shown superior outcomes these cancers compared to traditional paclitaxel formulations, with reduced toxicity. Regulatory approvals and commercial success have cemented Abraxane's status as a cornerstone in oncology, inspiring further research in nanoparticle-based drug delivery for cancer therapy (Afzal et al., 2022).
2. **Doxil (Liposomal Doxorubicin):** Doxil, developed by Johnson & Johnson, is a liposomal formulation of doxorubicin used in the treatment of ovarian cancer, AIDS-related Kaposi's

sarcoma, and multiple myeloma. Its liposome encapsulation reduces cardiotoxicity while enhancing drug delivery to tumors. Approved for these diseases, Doxil exemplifies the success of nanomedicine in improving therapeutic efficacy and patient outcomes (Gabizon et al., 2003).

3. **NanoKnife (Irreversible Electroporation):** NanoKnife, developed by AngioDynamics, utilizes irreversible electroporation technology to deliver short electrical pulses to target and destroy tumor cells while preserving surrounding tissues. It is used for the treatment of solid tumors. This selective treatment spares critical structures like blood vessels and nerves, making it suitable for tumors in challenging locations. NanoKnife shows promise for treating pancreatic, liver, prostate, and other solid tumors (Martin et al., 2012).
4. **MagForce AG (NanoTherm Therapy):** MagForce AG developed NanoTherm therapy, which utilizes magnetic nanoparticles injected into tumors and activated by an alternating magnetic field to generate heat, leading to localized tumor destruction. It is used for the treatment of brain tumors (Maier-Hauff et al., 2011).
5. **BIND-014 (Docetaxel Nanoparticles):** BIND-014, developed by BIND Therapeutics, is a targeted nanoparticle-drug conjugate containing docetaxel, designed to selectively accumulate in tumor tissue and release the drug, minimizing systemic toxicity. It is being investigated for the treatment of various solid tumors (Davis et al., 2008).
6. **Vaccine:** Lipid nanoparticles have been utilized as delivery systems for mRNA vaccines, such as those developed by Pfizer-BioNTech and Moderna for COVID-19. It serves as carriers for mRNA vaccines, shielding the fragile mRNA molecules and facilitating cellular uptake. LNPs encapsulate the mRNA, protect it from degradation, and help it enter host cells. This innovative delivery system enables efficient translation of the mRNA into viral proteins, eliciting robust immune responses against COVID-19 (Pardi et al., 2018; Sahin et al., 2020).
7. **Gene Therapy:** Nanoparticles are used as carriers for gene editing tools such as CRISPR-Cas9, enabling targeted gene modification for therapeutic purposes. Functionalized nanoparticles protect the CRISPR components from degradation, facilitate cellular uptake, and precisely target desired genomic loci. This approach holds promise for treating genetic disorders, cancer, and other diseases through precise gene modification (Wang et al., 2016; Yin et al., 2014).
8. **Diagnostic Imaging:** Nanoparticles are used as contrast agents in various imaging techniques such as MRI, CT scans, and PET scans to improve sensitivity and specificity. As contrast agents, they enhance imaging modalities by improving signal intensity and targeting specificity. Surface modifications tailor nanoparticles for specific imaging applications, such as tumor detection or vascular imaging. Their small size enables deep tissue penetration and prolonged circulation, offering valuable insights into disease pathology and treatment response in clinical settings (Gao et al., 2009; Jokerst and Gambhir, 2011).

12.8. International Collaboration and Research Initiatives

12.8.1. Global Efforts in Advancing Nanomedicine

Nanomedicine, a burgeoning field at the intersection of nanotechnology and medicine, has garnered significant attention and investment worldwide due to its immense potential in revolutionizing healthcare. Global efforts in advancing nanomedicine have been driven by the quest for more precise diagnostics, targeted drug delivery, and innovative therapeutic strategies, all aimed at enhancing patient outcomes while minimizing side effects (Salamanca-Buentello and Daar, 2021). Across continents, researchers, policymakers, and industry leaders are collaborating to harness the unique properties of nanoparticles and NMs for a wide range of medical applications.

In the United States, the National Institutes of Health (NIH) has been a key proponent of nanomedicine research, funding numerous initiatives through programs like the National Cancer Institute's (NCI) Alliance for Nanotechnology in Cancer and the National Institute of Biomedical Imaging and Bioengineering (https://nano.cancer.gov/). These efforts have led to groundbreaking discoveries in cancer therapeutics, such as the development of nanoparticle-based DDS capable of selectively targeting tumor cells while sparing healthy tissue.

Meanwhile, in Europe, the European Commission has allocated substantial resources to support nanomedicine research and innovation through initiatives like the European Technology Platform on Nanomedicine (ETPN) and the European Nanomedicine Characterization Laboratory (EU-NCL). These collaborative platforms facilitate interdisciplinary collaborations and provide infrastructure for the characterization and standardization of nanomedicine products, essential for their translation into clinical practice (https://etp-nanomedicine.eu/).

In Asia, countries like Japan and China have also made significant strides in nanomedicine research. Japanese institutions such as the National Institute for Materials Science (NIMS) and the University of Tokyo have been at the forefront of developing novel NMs for biomedical applications, including drug delivery, imaging, and regenerative medicine (https://www.nims.go.jp/eng/). In China, the government's strategic investments in nanotechnology have fueled rapid advancements in nanomedicine, with research institutions and industry partners collaborating to address pressing healthcare challenges, such as infectious diseases and chronic conditions (http://www.nanoctr.cn/).

Furthermore, international collaborations and consortia play a crucial role in advancing nanomedicine on a global scale. Initiatives like the International Alliance for Nanotechnology in Cancer (IANC), a collaborative network involving researchers from the United States, Europe, and Asia, facilitate knowledge exchange and resource sharing to accelerate the development of nanomedicine-based cancer therapies (https://ncl.cancer.gov/). Similarly, consortia like the global enterprise for micronutrient and medicine delivery (GEMMeD) bring together stakeholders from academia, industry, and government to tackle global health issues through innovative nanomedicine solutions, particularly in resource-limited settings (https://gemmedproject.org/).

India is also contributing significantly to this field, synergizing academia, research institutions, and industry. Government organizations like the Defense Research and Development Organization (DRDO), the Department of Biotechnology (DBT), as well our country's premier research Institution Indian Council of Medical Research (ICMR) have taken lead in fostering research along and innovation in nanomedicine with active support and involvement of the best of scientific minds at private universities and corporations (Mago et al., 2022).

These global efforts in advancing nanomedicine are underpinned by rapid technological advancements in NM synthesis, characterization, and manufacturing, as well as growing understanding of biological processes at the nanoscale. However, challenges remain, including regulatory hurdles, safety concerns, and ethical considerations surrounding the use of nanotechnology in healthcare. Addressing these challenges will require continued collaboration among stakeholders, as well as robust regulatory frameworks to ensure the safe and responsible development of nanomedicine products.

12.8.2. Collaborative Research and Knowledge Sharing

Collaborative research and knowledge sharing are fundamental to the advancement of nanomedicine, fostering innovation, and accelerating the translation of scientific discoveries into clinical applications. Academic institutions, research organizations, and industry partners worldwide collaborate on interdisciplinary projects to address complex challenges in nanomedicine. International consortia and networks play a pivotal role in promoting collaboration and knowledge sharing in nanomedicine research. The International Consortium for Nanotechnology (http://www.icon-europe.org/), for instance, facilitates collaborative research projects among researchers from different countries, enabling the exchange of expertise, resources, and data. These collaborations leverage diverse perspectives and expertise to overcome barriers and accelerate scientific progress in nanomedicine.

Furthermore, scientific conferences, workshops, and symposiums serve as platforms for researchers to share their findings, discuss emerging trends, and forge collaborations. In addition to in-person gatherings, online platforms and open-access journals contribute to knowledge sharing in nanomedicine. Platforms like NanoHUB (https://nanohub.org/) facilitate virtual collaboration and access to computational tools and resources for nanomedicine research.

12.8.3. International Initiatives for Addressing Global Health Challenges

International initiatives are pivotal in leveraging nanomedicine to tackle global health challenges. The Global Health Innovative Technology (GHIT) Fund exemplifies this collaborative approach, uniting Japan, the United States, the Bill and Melinda Gates Foundation, and pharmaceutical companies to expedite the discovery and development of novel drugs, vaccines, and diagnostics for infectious diseases prevalent in low- and middle-income countries (Slingsby and Kurokawa, 2013). By pooling resources and expertise, the GHIT Fund aims to bridge the gap between scientific innovation and healthcare delivery in resource-limited settings (Hinoshita, 2016). Similarly, the World Health Organization (WHO) plays a vital role in coordinating global efforts to address health disparities through initiatives like the Global Observatory on Health Research and Development. This platform monitors research activities worldwide, including in nanomedicine, to identify emerging trends and prioritize areas for intervention, thereby promoting equitable access to healthcare technologies (WHO, 2019). Moreover, the IANC, spearheaded by the NCI in the United States, fosters collaboration among researchers and institutions worldwide to advance nanotechnology-based solutions for cancer detection, treatment, and prevention (Hartshorn et al., 2019). Through these international partnerships and initiatives, nanomedicine emerges as a promising tool for addressing pressing health challenges on a global scale, emphasizing the importance of collaborative research and innovation in improving healthcare outcomes worldwide.

12.9. Conclusion

Nanomedicine offers numerous applications in diagnosis, therapeutic, and personalized medicine, including drug delivery, therapeutics, regenerative medicine, gene therapy, oncology, dentistry, and diagnostics. The sensing, delivery, and diagnosis involve using nanosensors, nanorobots, and actuating materials in living cells. The use of nanodevices, nanoparticles, and nano-assemblies for diagnosis applications enables early and precise detection of diseases. It improves overall precision by improving solubility, stability, bioavailability, sensitivity, and speed of medical examinations. The unique properties of nanoparticles make them popular in targeted therapy and precision medicine and have the potential to target specific sites and eliminate tumors without harming surrounding tissues. The integration of nanotechnology with other advanced technologies such as imaging tools has enhanced overall accuracy, and sensitivity for disease diagnosis and molecular imaging. However, nanoparticle toxicity and biocompatibility are still major concerns, as they can induce oxidative stress and inflammatory responses inside the living cells. Numerous scientific reports have been studied, that show the toxic effect of nanoparticles on gastrointestinal pathways, liver, kidneys, and reproductive cells. Ethical and social concerns in nanomedicine include risk assessment, informed consent, societal acceptance and regulation. Comprehensive regulatory framework, equitable distribution strategies, multidisciplinary dialogue and public awareness campaigns are crucial for responsible innovation and decision-making in the evolving field of nanomedicine.

In summary, in the process of innovation in nanomedicine, addressing ethical and safety concerns, promoting informed consent, privacy, accountability, bias, safety, regulation, transparency, and ethical decision-making are the necessary steps taken into account. The key to the advancement of this field is a profound understanding of existing barriers, manageable hurdles, and future requirements. For safe and effective nanomedicine solutions it is important to address the issues related to biocompatibility, toxicity, and regulatory obstacles that require collaboration among academics, industry stakeholders, regulatory bodies, and the public to create effective and safe nanomedicine solutions. The ongoing advancement in nanomedicine, with developments in regulatory and ethical frameworks, will facilitate the emergence of a new era in medical care, therefore improving patient outcomes and boosting quality of life.

KEY TERMS FROM THIS CHAPTER

- biocompatibility
- diagnosticsnanomedicine
- nanoparticles
- novel drugs
- open-access journals
- regenerative medicine
- regulation
- toxicity

References

1. Aach, J., Lunshof, J., Iyer, E., & Church, G. M. (2017). Addressing the ethical issues raised by synthetic human entities with embryo-like features. *eLife, 6*, e20674.
2. Aalinkeel, R., Kutscher, H. L., Singh, A., Cwiklinski, K., Khechen, N., Schwartz, S. A., Prasad, P. N., & Mahajan, S. D. (2018). Neuroprotective effects of a biodegradable poly (lactic-co-glycolic acid)-ginsenoside Rg3 nano formulation: A potential nano therapy for Alzheimer's disease? *Journal of Drug Targeting, 26*(2), 182–193.
3. Afzal, O., Altamimi, A. S. A., Nadeem, M. S., Alzarea, S. I., Almalki, W. H., Tariq, A., Mubeen, B., Murtaza, B. N., Iftikhar, S., Riaz, N., & Kazmi, I. (2022). Nanoparticles in drug delivery: From history to therapeutic applications. *Nanomaterials, 12*(24).
4. Agrahari, V., & Hiremath, P. (2017). Challenges associated and approaches for successful translation of nanomedicines into commercial products. *Nanomedicine, 12*(8), 819–823.
5. Albalawi, F., Hussein, M. Z., Fakurazi, S., & Masarudin, M. J. (2021). Engineered nanomaterials: The challenges and opportunities for nanomedicines. *International Journal of Nanomedicine, 16*, 161–184.
6. Allan, J., Belz, S., Hoeveler, A., Hugas, M., Okuda, H., Patri, A., Rauscher, H., Silva, P., Slikker, W., & Sokull-Kluettgen, B. (2021). Regulatory landscape of nanotechnology and nano plastics from a global perspective. *Regulatory Toxicology and Pharmacology, 122*, 104885.
7. Alzoubi, L., Aljabali, A. A., & Tambuwala, M. M. (2023). Empowering precision medicine: The impact of 3D printing on personalized therapeutic. *AAPS Pharm SciTech, 24*(8), 228.
8. Anselmo, A. C., & Mitragotri, S. (2016). Nanoparticles in the clinic. *Bioengineering & Translational Medicine, 1*(1), 10–29.
9. Astashkina, A. I., Jones, C. F., Thiagarajan, G., Kurtzeborn, K., Ghandehari, H., Brooks, B. D., & Grainger, D. W. (2014). Nanoparticle toxicity assessment using an *in vitro* 3-D kidney organoid culture model. *Biomaterials, 35*(24), 6323–6331.
10. Bahrami, B., Hojjat-Farsangi, M., Mohammadi, H., Anvari, E., Ghalamfarsa, G., Yousefi, M., & Jadidi-Niaragh, F. (2017). Nanoparticles and targeted drug delivery in cancer therapy. *Immunology Letters, 190*, 64–83.
11. Betz, U. A., Arora, L., Assal, R. A., Azevedo, H., Baldwin, J., Becker, M. S., Bostock, S., Cheng, V., Egle, T., & Ferrari, N. (2023). Game changers in science and technology—Now and beyond. *Technological Forecasting and Social Change, 193*, 122588.
12. Bonifácio, B. V., Silva, P. B., Ramos, M. A., Negri, K. M., Bauab, T. M., & Chorilli, M. (2014). Nanotechnology-based drug delivery systems and herbal medicines: A review. *International Journal of Nanomedicine, 9*, 1–15.
13. Bowman, D. M., & Gatof, J. (2015). Reviewing the regulatory barriers for nanomedicine: Global questions and challenges. *Nanomedicine, 10*(21), 3275–3286.
14. Brown, J., Fatehi, L., & Kuzma, J. (2015). Altruism and skepticism in public attitudes toward food nanotechnologies. *Journal of Nanoparticle Research, 17*, 1–31.
15. Carroll, P., & Kellow, A. (2021). *The OECD: A Decade of Transformation: 2011–2021*. Walter de Gruyter GmbH & Co KG.

16. Çetintaş, H. C., Tonbul, H., Şahin, A., & Çapan, Y. (2021). Regulatory guidelines of the US Food and Drug Administration and the European Medicines Agency for actively targeted nanomedicines. In *Drug Delivery with Targeted Nanoparticles* (pp. 725–741). Springer.
17. Charcosset, C., & Fessi, H. (2005). A new process for drug loaded nano capsules preparation using a membrane contactor. *Drug Development and Industrial Pharmacy, 31*(10), 987–992.
18. Chen, X., & Gao, C. (2017). Influences of size and surface coating of gold nanoparticles on inflammatory activation of macrophages. *Colloids and Surfaces B: Bio Interfaces, 160*, 372–380.
19. Chen, X., Zhang, Y. S., Zhang, X., & Liu, C. (2021). Organ-on-a-chip platforms for accelerating the evaluation of nanomedicine. *Bioactive Materials, 6*(4), 1012–1027.
20. Cheng, J., Gu, Y. J., Cheng, S. H., & Wong, W. T. (2013). Surface functionalized gold nanoparticles for drug delivery. *Journal of Biomedical Nanotechnology, 9*(8), 1362–1369.
21. Cheng, Y. H., He, C., Riviere, J. E., Monteiro-Riviere, N. A., & Lin, Z. (2020). Meta-analysis of nanoparticle delivery to tumors using a physiologically based pharmacokinetic modeling and simulation approach. *ACS Nano, 14*(3), 3075–3095.
22. Cholkar, K., Hirani, N. D., & Natarajan, C. (2017). Nanotechnology-based medical and biomedical imaging for diagnostics. In A. K. Mitra, K. Cholkar, & A. Mandal (Eds.), *Emerging Nanotechnologies for Diagnostics, Drug Delivery and Medical Devices* (pp. 355–374). Elsevier.
23. Chono, S., Tanino, T., Seki, T., & Morimoto, K. (2008). Efficient drug targeting to rat alveolar macrophages by pulmonary administration of ciprofloxacin incorporated into mannosylated liposomes for treatment of respiratory intracellular parasitic infections. *Journal of Controlled Release, 127*(1), 50–58.
24. Colapicchioni, V., Palchetti, S., Pozzi, D., Marini, E. S., Riccioli, A., Ziparo, E., Papi, M., Amenitsch, H., & Caracciolo, G. (2015). Killing cancer cells using nanotechnology: Novel poly(I:C) loaded liposome–silica hybrid nanoparticles. *Journal of Materials Chemistry B, 3*(37), 7408–7416.
25. Colby, A. H., Liu, R., Doyle, R. P., Merting, A., Zhang, H., Savage, N., Chu, N. Q., Hollister, B. A., McCulloch, W., Burdette, J. E., Pearce, C. J., Liu, K., Oberlies, N. H., Colson, Y. L., & Grinstaff, M. W. (2021). Pilot-scale production of expansile nanoparticles: Practical methods for clinical scale-up. *Journal of Controlled Release, 337*, 144–154.
26. Colombo, A. P., Briançon, S., Lieto, J., & Fessi, H. (2001). Project, design, and use of a pilot plant for nano capsule production. *Drug Development and Industrial Pharmacy, 27*(10), 1063–1072.
27. Committee, E. S., Hardy, A., Benford, D., Halldorsson, T., Jeger, M. J., Knutsen, H. K., More, S., Naegeli, H., Noteborn, H., & Ockleford, C. (2018). Guidance on risk assessment of the application of nanoscience and nanotechnologies in the food and feed chain: Part 1, human and animal health. *EFSA Journal, 16*(7), e05327.
28. Cone, R. A. (2009). Barrier properties of mucus. *Advanced Drug Delivery Reviews, 61*(2), 75–85.
29. Crous, A., & Abrahamse, H. (2021). Innovations in nanotechnology for biomedical sensing, imaging, drug delivery, and therapy. In *Innovations in Nanotechnology for Biomedical Sensing, Imaging, Drug Delivery, and Therapy* (pp. 21–42).
30. Dang, Y., & Guan, J. (2020). Nanoparticle-based drug delivery systems for cancer therapy. *Smart Materials in Medicine, 1*, 10–19.
31. Das, A., Deka, D., Abrar, S. S., Pathak, S., & Banerjee, A. (2021). Ethics in nanomedicine. In *Nanomedicine for Cancer Diagnosis and Therapy* (pp. 203–219). Springer.

32. Davis, M. E., Chen, Z. G., & Shin, D. M. (2008). Nanoparticle therapeutics: An emerging treatment modality for cancer. *Nature Reviews Drug Discovery, 7*(9), 771–782.

33. De Maria Marchiano, R., Di Sante, G., Piro, G., Carbone, C., Tortora, G., Boldrini, L., Pietragalla, A., Daniele, G., Tredicine, M., & Cesario, A. (2021). Translational research in the era of precision medicine: Where we are and where we will go. *Journal of Personalized Medicine, 11*(3), 216.

34. Dinda, A. (2019). Challenges in the development of an Indian guideline for nano pharmaceuticals. *Private communication at Global Summit on Regulatory Science.*

35. Ebbesen, M., & Jensen, T. G. (2006). Nanomedicine: Techniques, potentials, and ethical implications. *BioMed Research International, 2006.*

36. Edmondson, R., Broglie, J. J., Adcock, A. F., & Yang, L. (2014). Three-dimensional cell culture systems and their applications in drug discovery and cell-based biosensors. *Assay and Drug Development Technologies, 12*(4), 207–218.

37. El-Harati, A. A., Charcosset, C., & Fessi, H. (2006). Influence of the formulation for solid lipid nanoparticles prepared with a membrane contactor. *Pharmaceutical Development and Technology, 11*(2), 153–157.

38. Ensign, L. M., Cone, R., & Hanes, J. (2012). Oral drug delivery with polymeric nanoparticles: The gastrointestinal mucus barriers. *Advanced Drug Delivery Reviews, 64*(6), 557–570.

39. Fisher, E., Boenink, M., Van Der Burg, S., & Woodbury, N. (2012). Responsible healthcare innovation: Anticipatory governance of nano diagnostics for theragnostic medicine. *Expert Review of Molecular Diagnostics, 12*(8), 857–870.

40. Flühmann, B., Ntai, I., Borchard, G., Simoens, S., & Mühlebach, S. (2019). Nanomedicines: The magic bullets reaching their target? *European Journal of Pharmaceutical Sciences, 128*, 73–80.

41. Food and Drug Administration. (2014). *Guidance for Industry: Assessing the Effects of Significant Manufacturing Process Changes, Including Emerging Technologies, on the Safety and Regulatory Status of Food Ingredients and Food Contact Substances, Including Food Ingredients that are Color Additives.*

42. Food and Drug Administration. (2014). *Guidance For Industry: Safety Of Nanomaterials in Cosmetic Products.*

43. Foulkes, R., Man, E., Thind, J., Yeung, S., Joy, A., & Hoskins, C. (2020). The regulation of nanomaterials and nanomedicines for clinical application: Current and future perspectives. *Biomaterials Science, 8*(17), 4653–4664.

44. Fu, P. P., Xia, Q., Hwang, H. M., Ray, P. C., & Yu, H. (2014). Mechanisms of nanotoxicity: Generation of reactive oxygen species. *Journal of Food and Drug Analysis, 22*(1), 64–75.

45. Gabizon, A., Shmeeda, H., & Barenholz, Y. (2003). Pharmacokinetics of pegylated liposomal doxorubicin: Review of animal and human studies. *Clinical Pharmacokinetics, 42*(5), 419–436.

46. Gago, L., Quiñonero, F., Perazzoli, G., Melguizo, C., Prados, J., Ortiz, R., & Cabeza, L. (2023). Nanomedicine and hyperthermia for the treatment of gastrointestinal cancer: A systematic review. *Pharmaceutics, 15*(7), 1958.

47. Galindo-Rodríguez, S. A., Puel, F., Briançon, S., Allémann, E., Doelker, E., & Fessi, H. (2005). Comparative scale-up of three methods for producing ibuprofen-loaded nanoparticles. *European Journal of Pharmaceutical Sciences, 25*(4, 5), 357–367.

48. Gao, F., Wu, J., Niu, S., Sun, T., Li, F., Bai, Y., Jin, L., Lin, L., Shi, Q., & Zhu, L. M. (2019). Biodegradable, pH-sensitive hollow mesoporous organosilicon nanoparticle (HMON) with controlled release of pirfenidone and ultrasound-target-microbubble-destruction (UTMD) for pancreatic cancer treatment. *Theragnostic, 9*(20), 6002–6018.

49. Gao, J., Gu, H., & Xu, B. (2009). Multifunctional magnetic nanoparticles: Design, synthesis, and biomedical applications. *Accounts of Chemical Research, 42*(8), 1097–1107.

50. Gaur, N., Sharma, N., Dahiya, A., Yadav, P., Ojha, H., Goyal, R. K., & Sharma, R. K. (2020). Toxicity and regulatory concerns for nano formulations in medicine. In *The ELSI Handbook of Nanotechnology: Risk, Safety, ELSI and Commercialization* (pp. 333–357).

51. Germain, M., Caputo, F., Metcalfe, S., Tosi, G., Spring, K., Åslund, A. K., Pottier, A., Schiffelers, R., Ceccaldi, A., & Schmid, R. (2020). Delivering the power of nanomedicine to patients today. *Journal of Controlled Release, 326*, 164–171.

52. Guo, S., Liang, Y., Liu, L., Yin, M., Wang, A., Sun, K., Li, Y., & Shi, Y. (2021). Research on the fate of polymeric nanoparticles in the process of the intestinal absorption based on model nanoparticles with various characteristics: Size, surface charge and pro-hydrophobics. *Journal of Nanobiotechnology, 19*, 1–21.

53. Halamoda-Kenzaoui, B., Holzwarth, U., Roebben, G., Bogni, A., & Bremer-Hoffmann, S. (2019). Mapping of the available standards against the regulatory needs for nanomedicines. *Wiley Interdisciplinary Reviews: Nanomedicine and Nanobiotechnology, 11*(1), e1531.

54. Hartshorn, C. M., Russell, L. M., & Grodzinski, P. (2019). NCI Alliance for Nanotechnology in Cancer–Catalysing research and translation towards novel cancer diagnostics and therapeutics. *Wiley Interdisciplinary Reviews: Nanomedicine and Nanobiotechnology, 11*(6), e1570.

55. Herdiana, Y., Wathoni, N., Shamsuddin, S., & Muchtaridi, M. (2022). Scale-up polymeric-based nanoparticles drug delivery systems: Development and challenges. *Open Nano, 7*, 100048.

56. Hinoshita, E. (2016). Industry, academia and government partnership through the Global Health Innovative Technology Fund (GHIT). *Yakugaku Zasshi, 136*(2), 237–242.

57. Hoshyar, N., Gray, S., Han, H., & Bao, G. (2016). The effect of nanoparticle size on *in vivo* pharmacokinetics and cellular interaction. *Nanomedicine, 11*(6), 673–692.

58. Ibrahim, K. E., Al-Mutary, M. G., Bakhiet, A. O., & Khan, H. A. (2018). Histopathology of the liver, kidney, and spleen of mice exposed to gold nanoparticles. *Molecules, 23*(8), 1848.

59. Jahangirian, H., Lemraski, E. G., Webster, T. J., Rafiee-Moghaddam, R., & Abdollahi, Y. (2017). A review of drug delivery systems based on nanotechnology and green chemistry: Green nanomedicine. *International Journal of Nanomedicine, 12*, 2957–2978.

60. Jokerst, J. V., & Gambhir, S. S. (2011). Molecular imaging with theragnostic nanoparticles. *Accounts of Chemical Research, 44*(10), 1050–1060.

61. Kad, A., Pundir, A., Arya, S. K., Bhardwaj, N., & Khatri, M. (2022). An elucidative review to analytically sieve the viability of nanomedicine market. *Journal of Pharmaceutical Innovation, 17*(1), 249–265.

62. Kelly, B. (2010). Nanomedicines: Regulatory challenges and risks ahead. *Regulatory Affairs Pharma, 10*, 14–17.

63. Khanna, P., Ong, C., Bay, B. H., & Baeg, G. H. (2015). Nanotoxicity: An interplay of oxidative stress, inflammation and cell death. *Nanomaterials, 5*(3), 1163–1180.

64. Kim, J. H., Kim, J. H., Kim, K. W., Kim, M. H., & Yu, Y. S. (2009). Intravenously administered gold nanoparticles pass through the blood–retinal barrier depending on the particle size, and induce no retinal toxicity. *Nanotechnology, 20*(50), 505101.

65. Kim, M. H., Yamayoshi, I., Mathew, S., Lin, H., Nayfach, J., & Simon, S. I. (2013). Magnetic nanoparticle targeted hyperthermia of cutaneous *Staphylococcus aureus* infection. *Annals of Biomedical Engineering, 41*, 598–609.

66. Kou, L., Bhutia, Y. D., Yao, Q., He, Z., Sun, J., & Ganapathy, V. (2018). Transporter-guided delivery of nanoparticles to improve drug permeation across cellular barriers and drug exposure to selective cell types. *Frontiers in Pharmacology, 9*, 337630.

67. Kulkarni, S. A., & Feng, S. S. (2011). Effects of surface modification on delivery efficiency of biodegradable nanoparticles across the blood-brain barrier. *Nanomedicine (London), 6*(2), 377–394.

68. Kyrochristos, I. D., Ziogas, D. E., & Roukos, D. H. (2018). Precision in personalized prediction-based medicine. *Personalized Medicine, 15*(6), 467–470.

69. Lam, P. L., Wong, W. Y., Bian, Z., Chui, C. H., & Gambari, R. (2017). Recent advances in green nanoparticulate systems for drug delivery: Efficient delivery and safety concern. *Nanomedicine, 12*(4), 357–385.

70. Lammers, T., Kiessling, F., Hennink, W. E., & Storm, G. (2012). Drug targeting to tumors: Principles, pitfalls and (pre-) clinical progress. *Journal of Controlled Release, 161*(2), 175–187.

71. Laverman, P., Boerman, O. C., Oyen, W. J., Dams, E. T. M., Storm, G., & Corstens, F. H. (1999). Liposomes for scintigraphy detection of infection and inflammation. *Advanced Drug Delivery Reviews, 37*(1–3), 225–235.

72. Leong, H. S., Butler, K. S., Brinker, C. J., Azzawi, M., Conlan, S., Dufès, C., Owen, A., Rannard, S., Scott, C., & Chen, C. (2019). On the issue of transparency and reproducibility in nanomedicine. *Nature Nanotechnology, 14*(7), 629–635.

73. Limaye, V., Fortwengel, G., & Limaye, D. (2014). Regulatory roadmap for nanotechnology-based medicines. *International Journal of Drug Regulatory Affairs, 2*(4), 33–41.

74. Löbenberg, R., Araujo, L., von Briesen, H., Rodgers, E., & Kreuter, J. (1998). Body distribution of azidothymidine bound to hexyl-cyanoacrylate nanoparticles after IV injection to rats. *Journal of Controlled Release, 50*(1–3), 21–30.

75. Lyall, C., Bruce, A., Tait, J., & Meagher, L. (2011). *Interdisciplinary Research Journeys: Practical Strategies for Capturing Creativity*. Bloomsbury Academic.

76. Mago, A., Junaid Tahir, M., Arslan Khan, M., Abbasher Hussien Mohamed Ahmed, K., & Usman Munir, M. (2022). Nanomedicine: Advancement in healthcare. *Annals of Medicine and Surgery (London), 79*, 104078.

77. Maier-Hauff, K., Ulrich, F., Nestler, D., Niehoff, H., Wust, P., Thiesen, B., Orawa, H., Budach, V., & Jordan, A. (2011). Efficacy and safety of intertumoral thermotherapy using magnetic iron-oxide nanoparticles combined with external beam radiotherapy on patients with recurrent glioblastoma multiforme. *Journal of Neuro-Oncology, 103*(2), 317–324.

78. Malik, S., Muhammad, K., & Waheed, Y. (2023). Emerging applications of nanotechnology in healthcare and medicine. *Molecules, 28*(18).

79. Mandal, S. D., Mandal, S., Pathak, Y. V., & Patel, J. K. (2021). Current challenges and future directions in nanomedicine. In J. K. Patel & Y. V. Pathak (Eds.), *Emerging Technologies for Nanoparticle Manufacturing* (pp. 575–583). Springer International Publishing.

80. Manke, A., Wang, L., & Rojanasakul, Y. (2013). Mechanisms of nanoparticle-induced oxidative stress and toxicity. *BioMed Research International, 2013.*

81. Maqsood, S., Din, F. U., Khan, S. U., Elahi, E., Ali, Z., Jamshaid, H., Zeb, A., Nadeem, T., Ahmed, W., & Khan, S. (2022). Levosulpiride-loaded nanostructured lipid carriers for brain delivery with antipsychotic and antidepressant effects. *Life Sciences, 311*, 121198.

82. Martin, R. C., McFarland, K., Ellis, S., & Velanovich, V. (2012). Irreversible electroporation therapy in the management of locally advanced pancreatic adenocarcinoma. *Journal of the American College of Surgeons, 215*(3), 361–369.

83. Mazayen, Z. M., Ghoneim, A. M., Elbatanony, R. S., Basalious, E. B., & Bendas, E. R. (2022). Pharmaceutical nanotechnology: From the bench to the market. *Future Journal of Pharmaceutical Sciences, 8*(1), 12.

84. Mirza, A. Z., & Siddiqui, F. A. (2014). Nanomedicine and drug delivery: A mini review. *International Nano Letters, 4*(1), 94.

85. Mitchell, M. J., Billingsley, M. M., Haley, R. M., Wechsler, M. E., Peppas, N. A., & Langer, R. (2021). Engineering precision nanoparticles for drug delivery. *Nature Reviews Drug Discovery, 20*(2), 101–124.

86. Moghimi, S. M. (2014). Cancer nanomedicine and the complement system activation paradigm: Anaphylaxis and tumor growth. *Journal of Controlled Release, 190*, 556–562.

87. Mohanty, S. K., Swamy, M. K., Sinniah, U. R., & Anuradha, M. (2017). *Leptadenia reticulata* (Retz.) Wight & Arn. (Jivanti): Botanical, agronomical, phytochemical, pharmacological, and biotechnological aspects. *Molecules, 22*(6), 1019.

88. Moos, P. (2014). *An Uncertain Business: Industry Responses to The Regulation of Nanotechnologies.* European University Institute.

89. Mughal, B., Zaidi, S. Z. J., Zhang, X., & Hassan, S. U. (2021). Biogenic nanoparticles: Synthesis, characterisation and applications. *Applied Sciences, 11*(6), 2598.

90. Mühlebach, S. (2018). Regulatory challenges of nanomedicines and their follow-on versions: A generic or similar approach? *Advanced Drug Delivery Reviews, 131*, 122–131.

91. Mukherjee, S., Madamsetty, V. S., Bhattacharya, D., Roy Chowdhury, S., Paul, M. K., & Mukherjee, A. (2020). Recent advancements of nanomedicine in neurodegenerative disorders theragnostic. *Advanced Functional Materials, 30*(35), 2003054.

92. Muthu, M. S., & Wilson, B. (2010). Multifunctional radio nanomedicine: A novel nanoplatform for cancer imaging and therapy. *Nanomedicine (London), 5*(2), 169–171.

93. Muthu, M. S., Kulkarni, S. A., Raju, A., & Feng, S. S. (2012). Theranostic liposomes of TPGS coating for targeted co-delivery of docetaxel and quantum dots. *Biomaterials, 33*(12), 3494–3501.

94. Nag, O. K., & Delehanty, J. B. (2019). Active cellular and subcellular targeting of nanoparticles for drug delivery. *Pharmaceutics, 11*(10), 543.

95. National Academy of Sciences, Division of Behavioral and Social Sciences, Board on Science Education, Division of Engineering and Applied Sciences, Board on Mathematical Sciences,

Committee on Science and Technology, & Board on Health Sciences Policy. (2018). *Envisioning the Data Science Discipline: The Undergraduate Perspective: Interim Report.* National Academies Press.

96. Nguyen, T. T., Nguyen, T. T. D., Vo, T. K., Nguyen, M. K., Van Vo, T., & Van Vo, G. (2021). Nanotechnology-based drug delivery for central nervous system disorders. *Biomedicine & Pharmacotherapy, 143*, 112117.

97. Oliva, N., Carcole, M., Beckerman, M., Seliktar, S., Hayward, A., Stanley, J., Parry, N. M. A., Edelman, E. R., & Artzi, N. (2015). Regulation of dendrimer/dextran material performance by altered tissue microenvironment in inflammation and neoplasia. *Science Translational Medicine, 7*(272), 272ra211.

98. Omietimi, H. B., Afolalu, S. A., Kayode, J. F., Monye, S. I., Lawal, S. L., & Emetere, M. E. (2023). An overview of nanotechnology and its application. *E3S Web of Conferences, 391*, 01079.

99. Pandey, A., Singh, B. K., Gayathiri, E., Balasubramani, S., Duraisamy, S. M., Kothari, A., & Patel, D. K. (2024). Nanoparticles in biomedical and clinical research: A current perspective and future implications. In *Nanomaterials for Biomedical and Bioengineering Applications* (pp. 415–457). Springer.

100. Paradise, J. (2011). Claiming nanotechnology: Improving USPTO efforts at classification of emerging nano-enabled pharmaceutical technologies. *Northwestern Journal of Technology and Intellectual Property, 10*, 169.

101. Paradise, J. (2019). Regulating nanomedicine at the Food and Drug Administration. *AMA Journal of Ethics, 21*(4), 347–355.

102. Pardi, N., Hogan, M. J., Porter, F. W., & Weissman, D. (2018). mRNA vaccines–A new era in vaccinology. *Nature Reviews Drug Discovery, 17*(4), 261–279.

103. Patra, J. K., Das, G., Fraceto, L. F., Campos, E. V. R., Rodriguez-Torres, M. P., Acosta-Torres, L. S., Diaz-Torres, L. A., Grillo, R., Swamy, M. K., Sharma, S., Habtemariam, S., & Shin, H. S. (2018). Nano-based drug delivery systems: Recent developments and future prospects. *Journal of Nanobiotechnology, 16*(1), 71.

104. Perrault, S. D., Walkey, C., Jennings, T., Fischer, H. C., & Chan, W. C. (2009). Mediating tumor targeting efficiency of nanoparticles through design. *Nano Letters, 9*(5), 1909–1915.

105. Ragelle, H., Danhier, F., Préat, V., Langer, R., & Anderson, D. G. (2017). Nanoparticle-based drug delivery systems: A commercial and regulatory outlook as the field matures. *Expert Opinion on Drug Delivery, 14*(7), 851–864.

106. Raja, H. N., Ud Din, F., Shabbir, K., Khan, S., Alamri, A. H., Al Awadh, A. A., Lahiq, A. A., & Alasiri, A. (2023). Sodium alginate-based smart gastro-retentive drug delivery system of revaprazan loaded SLNs: Formulation and characterization. *International Journal of Biological Macromolecules, 253*, 127402.

107. Ramezani, F., & Faris, R. (2024). Odii Peter Egwuatu, Merit Oluchi Ori, Humphrey Sam Samuel, Francis-Dominic Makong Ekpan. *Eurasian Journal of Science and Technology, 4*(3).

108. Reamer, A., Icerman, L., Youtie, J. L., & United States Economic Development Administration. (2003). *Technology Transfer and Commercialization: Their Role in Economic Development.* United States Economic Development Administration.

109. Riley, R. S., & Day, E. S. (2017). Gold nanoparticle-mediated photothermal therapy: Applications and opportunities for multimodal cancer treatment. *Wiley Interdisciplinary Reviews: Nanomedicine and Nanobiotechnology, 9*(4), e1449.

110. Roy, R., Parashar, V., Chauhan, L., Shanker, R., Das, M., Tripathi, A., & Dwivedi, P. D. (2014). Mechanism of uptake of ZnO nanoparticles and inflammatory responses in macrophages require PI3K mediated MAPKs signaling. *Toxicology in Vitro, 28*(3), 457–467.

111. Rudramurthy, G. R., Swamy, M. K., Sinniah, U. R., & Ghasemzadeh, A. (2016). Nanoparticles: Alternatives against drug-resistant pathogenic microbes. *Molecules, 21*(7), 836.

112. Sahin, U., Muik, A., Derhovanessian, E., Vogler, I., Kranz, L. M., Vormehr, M., Baum, A., Pascal, K., Quandt, J., Maurus, D., Brachtendorf, S., Lörks, V., Sikorski, J., Hilker, R., Becker, D., Eller, A. K., Grützner, J., Boesler, C., Rosenbaum, C., Kühnle, M. C., Luxemburger, U., Kemmer-Brück, A., Langer, D., Bexon, M., Bolte, S., Karikó, K., Palanche, T., Fischer, B., Schultz, A., Shi, P. Y., Fontes-Garfias, C., Perez, J. L., Swanson, K. A., Loschko, J., Scully, I. L., Cutler, M., Kalina, W., Kyratsous, C. A., Cooper, D., Dormitzer, P. R., Jansen, K. U., & Türeci, Ö. (2020). COVID-19 vaccine BNT162b1 elicits human antibody and T(H)1 T cell responses. *Nature, 586*(7830), 594–599.

113. Sainz, V., Conniot, J., Matos, A. I., Peres, C., Zupancic, E., Moura, L., Silva, L. C., Florindo, H. F., & Gaspar, R. S. (2015). Regulatory aspects on nanomedicines. *Biochemical and Biophysical Research Communications, 468*(3), 504–510.

114. Salamanca-Buentello, F., & Daar, A. S. (2021). Nanotechnology, equity, and global health. *Nature Nanotechnology, 16*(4), 358–361.

115. Saraf, S. (2009). Process optimization for the production of nanoparticles for drug delivery applications. *Expert Opinion on Drug Delivery, 6*(2), 187–196.

116. Saraiva, C., Praça, C., Ferreira, R., Santos, T., Ferreira, L., & Bernardino, L. (2016). Nanoparticle-mediated brain drug delivery: Overcoming blood-brain barrier to treat neurodegenerative diseases. *Journal of Controlled Release, 235*, 34–47.

117. Sarwal, A., Singh, G., Singh, K., & Garg, S. (2018). Recent interventions for nanotechnology-based drug products: Insights into the regulatory aspects. *Current Pharmaceutical Design, 24*(43), 5219–5228.

118. Satterfield, T., Kandlikar, M., Beaudrie, C. E. H., Conti, J., & Harthorn, B. H. (2009). Anticipating the perceived risk of nanotechnologies. *Nature Nanotechnology, 4*(11), 752–758.

119. Siddiqi, N. J., Abdelhalim, M. A. K., El-Ansary, A. K., Alhomida, A. S., & Ong, W. (2012). Identification of potential biomarkers of gold nanoparticle toxicity in rat brains. *Journal of Neuroinflammation, 9*, 1–7.

120. Siegel, R. A., Kirtane, A. R., & Panyam, J. (2016). Assessing the benefits of drug delivery by nanocarriers: A partico/pharmacokinetic framework. *IEEE Transactions on Biomedical Engineering, 64*(9), 2176–2185.

121. Silva, M. M., Calado, R., Marto, J., Bettencourt, A., Almeida, A. J., & Gonçalves, L. M. D. (2017). Chitosan nanoparticles as a mucoadhesive drug delivery system for ocular administration. *Marine Drugs, 15*(12), 370.

122. Slingsby, B. T., & Kurokawa, K. (2013). The Global Health Innovative Technology (GHIT) Fund: Financing medical innovations for neglected populations. *The Lancet Global Health, 1*(4), e184–e185.

123. Soares, S., Sousa, J., Pais, A., & Vitorino, C. (2018). Nanomedicine: Principles, properties, and regulatory issues. *Frontiers in Chemistry, 6*, 356901.

124. Sohail, S., Shah, F. A., Zaman, S. uz, Almari, A. H., Malik, I., Khan, S. A., Alamro, A. A., Zeb, A., & ud Din, F. (2023). Melatonin delivered in solid lipid nanoparticles ameliorated its neuroprotective effects in cerebral ischemia. *Helion, 9*(9).

125. Song, J., Chappell, J. C., Qi, M., VanGieson, E. J., Kaul, S., & Price, R. J. (2002). Influence of injection site, microvascular pressure, and ultrasound variables on microbubble-mediated delivery of microspheres to muscle. *Journal of the American College of Cardiology, 39*(4), 726–731.

126. Swamy, M. K., & Sinniah, U. R. (2016). Patchouli (Pogostemon cablin Benth.): Botany, agrotechnology, and biotechnological aspects. *Industrial Crops and Products, 87*, 161–176.

127. Tang, B., Peng, Y., Yue, Q., Pu, Y., Li, R., Zhao, Y., Hai, L., Guo, L., & Wu, Y. (2020). Design, preparation, and evaluation of different branched biotin modified liposomes for targeting breast cancer. *European Journal of Medicinal Chemistry, 193*, 112204.

128. Tang, Y., Wang, X., Li, J., Nie, Y., Liao, G., Yu, Y., & Li, C. (2019). Overcoming the reticuloendothelial system barrier to drug delivery with a "don't-eat-us" strategy. *ACS Nano, 13*(11), 13015–13026.

129. Tavano, R., Gabrielli, L., Lubian, E., Fedeli, C., Visentin, S., Polverino De Laureto, P., Arrigoni, G., Geffner-Smith, A., Chen, F., & Simberg, D. (2018). C1q-mediated complement activation and C3 opsonization trigger recognition of stealth poly(2-methyl-2-oxazoline)-coated silica nanoparticles by human phagocytes. *ACS Nano, 12*(6), 5834–5847.

130. Thapa, R. K., & Kim, J. O. (2023). Nanomedicine-based commercial formulations: Current developments and future prospects. *Journal of Pharmaceutical Investigations, 53*(1), 19–33.

131. Vauthier, C., Labarre, D., & Ponchel, G. (2007). Design aspects of poly(alkylcyanoacrylate) nanoparticles for drug delivery. *Journal of Drug Targeting, 15*(10), 641–663.

132. Wang, L., Zhao, W., & Tan, W. (2008). Bio conjugated silica nanoparticles: Development and applications. *Nano Research, 1*(2), 99–115.

133. Wang, M., Zuris, J. A., Meng, F., Rees, H., Sun, S., Deng, P., Han, Y., Gao, X., Pouli, D., Wu, Q., Georgakoudi, I., Liu, D. R., & Xu, Q. (2016). Efficient delivery of genome-editing proteins using bio reducible lipid nanoparticles. *Proceedings of the National Academy of Sciences U.S.A., 113*(11), 2868–2873.

134. Wang, Q., Alshaker, H., Böhler, T., Srivats, S., Chao, Y., Cooper, C., & Pchejetski, D. (2017). Core shell lipid-polymer hybrid nanoparticles with combined docetaxel and molecular targeted therapy for the treatment of metastatic prostate cancer. *Scientific Reports, 7*(1), 5901.

135. Wang, W., Pang, J., Su, J., Li, F., Li, Q., Wang, J., Ibarlucea, B., Liu, X., Li, Y., Zhou, W., Wang, K., Han, Q., Liu, L., Zang, R., Rümmeli, M. H., Li, Y., Liu, H., Hu, H., & Cuniberti, G. (2022). Applications of nanogenerators for biomedical engineering and healthcare systems. *InfoMat, 4*(2), e12262.

136. Wang, Y., Yang, P., Zhao, X., Gao, D., Sun, N., Tian, Z., Ma, T., & Yang, Z. (2018). Multifunctional cargo-free nanomedicine for cancer therapy. *International Journal of Molecular Sciences, 19*(10), 2963.

137. Wickline, S. A., & Lanza, G. M. (2003). Nanotechnology for molecular imaging and targeted therapy. *Circulation, 107*(8), 1092–1095.

138. Wojnicki, M., Luty-Błocho, M., Hessel, V., Csapó, E., Ungor, D., & Fitzner, K. (2018). Micro droplet formation towards continuous nanoparticle synthesis. *Micromachines (Basel), 9*(5).

139. Wong, C., Stylianopoulos, T., Cui, J., Martin, J., Chauhan, V. P., Jiang, W., Popović, Z., Jain, R. K., Bawendi, M. G., & Fukumura, D. (2011). Multistage nanoparticle delivery system for deep penetration into tumor tissue. *Proceedings of the National Academy of Sciences, 108*(6), 2426–2431.

140. Woodward, R. (2009). *The Organization for Economic Co-Operation and Development (OECD)*. Routledge.

141. World Health Organization. (2019). *Global Observatory on Health Research and Development.*

142. Xu, C., Lei, C., & Yu, C. (2019). Mesoporous silica nanoparticles for protein protection and delivery. *Frontiers in Chemistry, 7*, 290.

143. Yamaguchi, Y., & Igarashi, R. (2006). Nanotechnology for therapy of type 2 diabetes. *Nihon Rinsho. Japanese Journal of Clinical Medicine, 64*(2), 295–300.

144. Yang, Q., Jones, S. W., Parker, C. L., Zamboni, W. C., Bear, J. E., & Lai, S. K. (2014). Evading immune cell uptake and clearance requires PEG grafting at densities substantially exceeding the minimum for brush conformation. *Molecular Pharmaceutics, 11*(4), 1250–1258.

145. Yin, H., Kanasty, R. L., Eltoukhy, A. A., Vegas, A. J., Dorkin, J. R., & Anderson, D. G. (2014). Non-viral vectors for gene-based therapy. *Nature Reviews Genetics, 15*(8), 541–555.

146. Zhang, S., Wang, Y., Zhang, S., Huang, C., Ding, Q., Xia, J., Wu, D., & Gao, W. (2023). Emerging anesthetic nanomedicines: Current state and challenges. *International Journal of Nanomedicine, 18*, 3913–3935.

147. Zhang, Y., Zhang, Y., Han, Y., & Gong, X. (2022). Micro/nanorobots for medical diagnosis and disease treatment. *Micromachines, 13*(5), 648.

INDEX

O

P

U

V

W

Z